# NON-ULCER DYSPEPSIA : PATHOPHYSIOLOGICAL AND THERAPEUTIC APPROACHES

*Editors*

J.-P. GALMICHE
R. JIAN
M. MIGNON
Ph. RUSZNIEWSKI

**Editions John Libbey Eurotext**
6, rue Blanche, 92120 Montrouge, France
Tél. : (1) 47 35 85 52

**John Libbey and Company Ltd**
13 Smiths Yard, Summerley Street, London SW18 4HR, England
Tel. : (1) 947 27 77

**John Libbey CIC**
Via Spallanzani 11, 00161, Rome, Italy

© 1991, John Libbey Eurotext, Paris

Il est interdit de reproduire intégralement ou partiellement le présent ouvrage — loi du 11 mars 1957 — sans autorisation de l'éditeur ou du Centre Français du Copyright, 6 bis, rue Gabriel-Laumain, 75010 Paris, France.

# NON-ULCER DYSPEPSIA : PATHOPHYSIOLOGICAL AND THERAPEUTIC APPROACHES

**International Symposium**
**Cannes**
**September, 20-21, 1991**

*Presidents*
**J.-P. Etienne**
**H. Michel**

*Scientific organization*
**J.-P. Galmiche**
**R. Jian**
**M. Mignon**

*Scientific secretaries*
**Ph. Ruszniewski**
**M. Pappo**

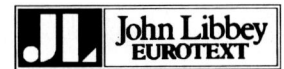

**British Library Cataloguing in Publication Data**

Non-ulcer dyspepsia : pathophysiological
and therapeutic approaches.
I. Galmiche J.-P.
616.33207

ISBN 0-86196-3288
ISSN 0768-3154

# Contents

List of contributors .................................................................................. VII

Foreword ................................................................................................. XI

## SESSION I. Introduction, epidemiology and fundamental mechanisms.

1. Non-ulcer dyspepsia: from the iceberg to the tower of Babel. R. Jian (Paris) ........................................................................... 3
2. The epidemiology of non-ulcer dyspepsia. O. Nyrén (Uppsala) ............. 7
3. Gastric motor response to food. A. Dubois (Bethesda) .......................... 15
4. Sensory visceral innervation. C. Rozé (Paris) ....................................... 33
5. Control of gastric tone. F. Azpiroz (Barcelona) .................................... 47
6. Stress and upper gut motility disorders: mechanisms involved. L. Buéno (Toulouse) ................................................................... 59
7. Control of appetite and satiety. D. Rigaud (Paris) ................................ 67

## SESSION II. Pathophysiology.

8. Motor disturbances: 1. Manometry. V. Stanghellini, M. Ricci Maccarini, C. Ghidini, R. Corinaldesi, L. Barbara (Bologna) ........................ 79
9. Motor disturbances: 2. Abnormalities of gastric myoelectrical activity. A. Smout, H. Jebbink, P. Bruijs, D. Fone (Utrecht) ..................... 89

10. Disturbances of gastric emptying. *S. Bruley des Varannes (Nantes)* ...... 105

11. Role of acid and pepsin. *H. Petersen (Trondheim)* .................................. 121

12. Duodenogastric reflux. *S. Müller-Lissner (München)* ............................... 129

## SESSION III. Pathophysiology (continued).

13. Gastric mucosal barrier and non-steroidal anti-inflammatory drugs. *F. Halter (Bern)* ........................................................................................ 139

14. Weakness of gastric mucosal barrier: myth or reality? *Ch. Florent, B. Flourié, B. Desaint, C. Legendre (Paris)* .................................................. 147

15. *Helicobacter pylori*, gastritis and non-ulcer dyspepsia. *P. Mainguet, J.-C. Debongnie (Brussels)* ...................................................................... 155

16. Food allergy and the immune intestinal barrier: facts, doubts and fancy. *J.-F. Colombel, B. Mesnard, P. Desreumaux (Lille)* .......................... 165

17. Abnormal perception of visceral pain. *M. Lémann, J.-P. Dederding, B. Flourié, J.-C. Rambaud, R. Jian (Paris)* .................................................. 175

18. Psychosomatic heterogeneity in essential dyspepsia supports syndromatic clinical presentation. *S. Bonfils (Paris)* .................................. 183

## SESSION IV. Management of non-ulcer dyspepsia.

19. An introduction to the management of non-ulcer dyspepsia. Is a rational approach currently available? *M. Mignon, Ph. Ruszniewski (Paris)* ......................................................................................................... 197

20. Pharmacological bases of therapeutics. *C. Scarpignato (Parma)* ............. 201

21. Randomized clinical trials in patients with dyspepsia. *T. Poynard, B. Mory, D. Levoir, J.-P. Pignon, S. Naveau, J.-C. Chaput (Clamart)* ..... 227

22. Diagnostic strategy. *G. Vantrappen (Louvain)* ........................................... 239

23. Therapeutic strategy. *J.-P. Galmiche, T. Vallot (Nantes and Paris)* ........ 247

24. Prospects and priorities for research in non-ulcer dyspepsia. *R.C. Heading (Edinburgh)* ........................................................................... 265

# List of contributors

**Aspiroz F.,** Digestive System Research Unit, Hospital General Vall d'Hebron, 08035 Barcelona, Spain
**Barbara L.,** Istituto di Clinica Medica e Gastroenterologia, Policlinico S. Orsola, via Massarenti, 9, 40128 Bologna, Italia
**Bernades P.,** Service de Gastroentérologie, Hôpital Beaujon, 100, bd du Général-Leclerc, 92118 Clichy Cedex, France
**Bigard M.-A.,** Service des Maladies de l'Appareil digestif, CHU de Brabois, Route de Neufchâteau, 54500 Vandœuvre-les-Nancy, France
**Bommelaer G.,** Service d'Hépato-gastroentérologie, Hôtel-Dieu, av. Vercingétorix, 63003 Clermont-Ferrand Cedex, France
**Bonfils S.,** INSERM U. 10, Hôpital Bichat, 170, bd Ney, 75877 Paris Cedex 18, France
**Bretagne J.-F.,** Service de Gastroentérologie, Hôpital de Pontchaillou, rue Henri Le Guilloux, 35033 Rennes, France
**Bruijs P.,** Department of Gastroenterology, University Hospital, 3508 GA Utrecht, The Netherlands
**Bruley des Varannes S.,** Service de Gastroentérologie, Hôpital G. et R. Laennec, 44035 Nantes Cedex, France
**Buéno L.,** Laboratoire de Pharmacologie, INRA, 180, chemin des Tournefeuilles, 31300 Toulouse, France
**Cerf M.,** Service de Gastroentérologie, Hôpital Louis-Mourier, 178, rue des Renouillers, 92700 Colombes, France
**Chaput J.-C.,** Service de Gastroentérologie, Hôpital Antoine-Béclère, 157, rue de la Porte-de-Trivaux, 92141 Clamart, France
**Chaussade S.,** Service d'Hépatogastroentérologie, Hôpital Cochin, 27, rue du Fg St-Jacques, 75674 Paris Cedex 14, France
**Colombel J.-F.,** Service des Maladies digestives, Hôpital Claude Huriez, 59037 Lille Cedex, France
**Corinaldesi R.,** Istituto di Clinica Medica e Gastroenterologia, Policlinico S. Orsola, via Massarenti, 9, 40128 Bologna, Italia
**Dapoigny M.,** Service d'Hépato-gastroentérologie, Hôpital de l'Hôtel-Dieu, av. Vercingétorix, 63003 Clermont-Ferrand Cedex, France
**Debongnie J.-C.,** Cliniques Universitaires St-Luc, Université Catholique de Louvain, Service de Gastroentérologie, 10, avenue Hippocrate, 1200 Bruxelles, Belgique
**Dederding J.-P.,** Service de Gastroentérologie, Hôpital Saint-Louis, 1, avenue Claude-Vellefaux, 75475 Paris Cedex 10, France

*List of contributors*

**Delchier J.-C.,** Service de Gastroentérologie, Hôpital Henri-Mondor, 51, avenue De-Lattre-de-Tassigny, 94000 Créteil, France

**Desaint B.,** Service de Gastroentérologie, Hôpital Saint-Antoine, 184, rue du Fg St-Antoine, 75012 Paris, France

**Desreumaux P.,** INSERM U. 167 — CNRS 624, Institut Pasteur de Lille, 59000 Lille, France

**Dubois A.,** Department of Medicine, Uniformed Services of the Health Sciences, F. Edward Hébert School of Medicine, 4301 Jones Bridge Road, Bethesda, MD 20814-4799, Maryland, USA

**Ducrotté Ph.,** Service de Gastroentérologie, Hôpital Charles-Nicolle, 1, rue de Germont, 76031 Rouen Cedex, France

**Etienne J.-P.,** Service de Gastroentérologie, CHU de Bicêtre, 78, rue du Général-Leclerc, 94275 Le Kremlin-Bicêtre Cedex, France

**Florent Ch.,** Service de Gastroentérologie, Hôpital Saint-Antoine, 184, rue du Fg St-Antoine, 75012 Paris, France

**Flourié B.,** INSERM U. 290, Hôpital Saint-Lazare, 107 bis, rue du Fg St-Denis, 75010 Paris Cedex, France

**Fone D.,** Department of Gastroenterology, University Hospital, 3508 GA Utrecht, The Netherlands

**Fournet J.,** Service de Gastroentérologie, CHRU — Hôpital Michalon, 38043 Grenoble Cedex, France

**Frexinos J.,** Service de Nutrition et Gastroentérologie, Hôpital de Rangueil, Chemin du Vallon, 31054 Toulouse, France

**Galmiche J.-P.,** Service de Gastroentérologie, CHU Nord G. et R. Laennec, BP 1005, 44035 Nantes Cedex, France

**Ghidini C.,** Istituto di Clinica Medica e Gastroenterologia, Policlinico S. Orsola, via Massarenti, 9, 40128 Bologna, Italia

**Halter F.,** Inselspital, Gastroenterologische Abteilung, CH — 3030 Bern, Switzerland

**Heading R.,** Department of Medicine, Royal Infirmary, University of Edinburgh, Scotland, UK

**Hostein J.,** Service de Gastroentérologie, CHRU — Hôpital Michalon, 38043 Grenoble Cedex, France

**Janssens J.,** Universitaire Ziekenhuizen, Gasthuisberg, Herestraat 49, 3000 Louvain, Belgique

**Jebbink H.,** Department of Gastroenterology, University Hospital, 3508 GA Utrecht, The Netherlands

**Jian R.,** Service de Gastroentérologie, Hôpital Saint-Louis, 1, avenue Claude-Vellefaux, 75475 Paris Cedex 10, France

**Legendre C.,** Service d'Anatomie Pathologique, Hôpital Saint-Antoine, 184, rue du Fg St-Antoine, 75012 Paris, France

**Lémann M.,** Service de Gastroentérologie, Hôpital Saint-Louis, 1, avenue Claude-Vellefaux, 75475 Paris Cedex 10, France

**Levoir D.,** Service de Gastroentérologie, Hôpital Antoine-Béclère, 157, rue de la Porte-de-Trivaux, 92141 Clamart, France

**Mainguet P.,** Cliniques Universitaires St-Luc, Université Catholique de Louvain, Service de Gastroentérologie, 10, avenue Hippocrate, 1200 Bruxelles, Belgique

*List of contributors*

**Mesnard B.,** Service des Maladies digestives, Hôpital Claude Huriez, 59037 Lille Cedex, France

**Michel H.,** Service des Maladies de l'Appareil digestif, Hôpital Saint-Eloi, 4, avenue Bertin-Sans, 34059 Montpellier Cedex, France

**Mignon M.,** Service de Gastroentérologie, Hôpital Bichat, 46, rue Henri-Huchard, 75877 Paris Cedex 18, France

**Mory B.,** Service de Gastroentérologie, Hôpital Antoine-Béclère, 157, rue de la Porte-de-Trivaux, 92141 Clamart, France

**Müller-Lissner S.,** Gastroenterologische Abteilung, Klinik Innenstadt, Ziemssenstrasse 1, D-8000 München, Germany

**Naveau S.,** Service de Gastroentérologie, Hôpital Antoine-Béclère, 157, rue de la Porte-de-Trivaux, 92141 Clamart, France

**Nyrén O.,** University Hospital, Department of Surgery, S. 75185 Uppsala, Sweden

**Pappo M.,** Département Médical, Laboratoires Glaxo, 43, rue Vineuse, 75016 Paris, France

**Petersen H.,** Section of Gastroenterology, Department of Medicine, University Hospital, Trondheim, Norway

**Pignon J.-P.,** Service de Gastroentérologie, Hôpital Antoine-Béclère, 157, rue de la Porte-de-Trivaux, 92141 Clamart, France

**Poynard T.,** Service de Gastroentérologie, Hôpital Antoine-Béclère, 157, rue de la Porte-de-Trivaux, 92141 Clamart, France

**Rambaud J.-C.,** Service de Gastroentérologie, Hôpital Saint-Lazare, 107, rue du Fg St-Denis, 75010 Paris, France

**Ricci Maccarini M.,** Istituto di Clinica Medica e Gastroenterologia, Policlinico S. Orsola, via Massarenti, 9, 40128 Bologna, Italia

**Rigaud D.,** Service de Nutrition, Hôpital Bichat, 46, rue Henri-Huchard, 75877 Paris Cedex 18, France

**Rozé C.,** Laboratoire de Biologie et Physiologie des Cellules digestives, INSERM U. 239, Hôpital Bichat, 16, rue Henri-Huchard, 75877 Paris Cedex 18, France

**Ruszniewski Ph.,** Service de Gastroentérologie, Hôpital Bichat, 46, rue Henri-Huchard, 75877 Paris Cedex 18, France

**Scarpignato C.,** Université de Parme, Istituto di Farmacologia, Ospedale Maggiore, 43100 Parma, Italia

**Smout A.,** Department of Gastroenterology, University Hospital, 3508 GA Utrecht, The Netherlands

**Stanghellini V.,** Istituto di Clinica Medica e Gastroenterologia, Policlinico S. Orsola, via Massarenti, 9, 40128 Bologna, Italia

**Vallot T.,** Service de Gastroentérologie, Hôpital Bichat, 46, rue Henri-Huchard, 75877 Paris Cedex 18, France

**Vantrappen G.,** Universitaire Ziekenhuizen, Gasthuisberg, Herestraat 49, 3000 Louvain, Belgique

**Zeitoun P.,** Service de Gastroentérologie, Hôpital Robert Debré, rue Alexis Carrel, 51092 Reims Cedex, France

# Foreword

The term dyspepsia comes from the Greek words δυσ and πεπτειν which mean bad or difficult digestion. The expression "non-ulcer dyspepsia" (NUD), although widely used in the literature, does not cover a precise and homogeneous area; on the contrary, it artificially regroups a heterogeneous set of symptoms and upper digestive complaints, more or less well-defined, but whose common denominator is the absence of organic lesions. From a practical point of view, however, NUD corresponds to a situation that is very frequently met by the clinician, be he a general practitioner or a gastroenterologist. No doubt this explains the success and generalized use of this term... and the large number of meetings and working parties that it has provoked.

What therefore is the justification for a new symposium on this subject in 1991? Firstly, the term NUD certainly does not have the same meaning in all countries. One of our aims was therefore to bring together French teaching hospital gastroenterologists and their Anglo-Saxon or Scandinavian colleagues in order to confront and discuss their experience and opinions in this domain. However, our objectives were not limited simply to the search for a consensus on the diagnostic and therapeutic methods that should be used when dealing with a dyspeptic patient. Without denying the importance of a pragmatic approach, we felt that a large part of this symposium should be devoted to pathophysiology. Progress, in the domain of both nosology and therapeutics, can only result from an improvement in the knowledge of basic physiology, and that of exploratory techniques suitable for use in humans. Certain parts of the NUD spectrum, for example gastro-oesophageal reflux disease without oesophagitis, have already benefited from this pathophysiological approach during the last decade. A progressive dismantling of NUD into better defined and more homogeneous entities is therefore the only rational and satisfactory approach for the future.

While waiting until we get to this pathophysiological — if not aetiological — objective, we must still take care of the present by treating our patients in the most efficient way possible, but also by keeping in mind the importance of economizing the means employed. In parallel, the development of new molecules by the pharmaceutical industry leads us to conduct therapeutic trials the success of which in detecting favourable effects largely depends on the pertinence of the questions raised and the methodology used to answer them. For all these reasons, it appears to us that a considerable time for discussion in small workshops should complement the more theoretical lectures. These workshops have been prepared through a questionnaire sent to all the French teaching hospital gastroenterologists.

Our initial intention was to produce a single publication of all the lecture transcripts and the results of the workshop discussions. By forcing us to postpone the symposium, initially planned for January 1991, the Gulf War decided otherwise! The punctuality of the orators sending us their manuscripts in good time has enabled us to publish them during the Cannes symposium (September, 20-21, 1991). We would like to extend our grateful thanks to the authors of the various chapters of the publication

*Foreword*

for their excellent contribution and we hope that the reader will find elements which will be useful for both his scientific culture and his practical experience. We will later publish the results of the survey carried out on French teaching hospital gastroenterologists and the minutes of the workshop discussions. We are indebted to our publisher, John Libbey Eurotext, for having adapted to circumstances by allowing for the subsequent insertion of these further documents in the cover of the publication. Finally, we would like to thank Glaxo France Laboratories for their support and active participation in this very fruitful and stimulating symposium.

J.-P. GALMICHE, R. JIAN,
M. MIGNON and Ph. RUSZNIEWSKI

# SESSION I

# Introduction, epidemiology and fundamental mechanisms

Chairman: J.-C. RAMBAUD

# 1

# Non-ulcer dyspepsia: from the iceberg to the tower of Babel

R. JIAN

*Service de Gastroentérologie, Hôpital Saint-Louis, 75010 Paris, France*

Non-ulcer dyspepsia (NUD) is a common but loosely defined entity that usually covers all symptoms referable to the upper digestive tract, but not related to any focal lesion or systemic disease. NUD is thus easily distinguished from organic diseases. Separation of NUD from other functional disorders like gastro-oesophageal reflux (GOR) without oesophagitis and irritable bowel syndrome is more difficult, mainly because these syndromes frequently occur together in the same patients.

In order to improve physiological and therapeutic approaches to NUD, several attempts [1-3] have been made to subdivide or to focus this entity into more specific categories (Table I). Dysmotility-like dyspepsia probably forms the largest and most well-defined subgroup of NUD. It is characterized by the presence of symptoms related to meal ingestion, including early satiety, more or less painful feeling of epigastric distension or heaviness, bloating, nausea and vomiting, and sensation of abnormally prolonged digestion. GOR-like dyspepsia is a group comprising those patients who have typical symptoms of reflux, but without endoscopically proven oesophagitis. The only, but highly questionable, reason to include such typical GOR symptoms in NUD is the big overlap that exists between these two entities. Ulcer-like dyspepsia and aerophagia are probably small subgroups of NUD. The idiopathic subgroup isolated by the working party includes all NUD patients who do not fit into the previous groups; the term "unclassified" should be preferred to "idiopathic", which falsely suggests that the absence of causative factor is limited to this subgroup of NUD. More generally, it must be emphasized that the predictive value of these classifications for the presence of specific objective anomalies and for specific therapeutic responses remains undefined and is probably very poor.

The pathophysiology of NUD is also a matter of debate. NUD may be either considered as a psychofunctional disorder or as a somatic disorder. In the psychofunctional concept [4], subjects suffering from dyspeptic symptoms seek

**Table I.** Classification of non-ulcer dyspepsia.

| Working party 1 (1) | Working party 2 (2) | Personal (3) |
|---|---|---|
| Dysmotility-like | Flatulent dyspepsia | Chronic idiopathic dyspepsia |
| GOR-like | ? | GOR without oesophagitis |
| Ulcer-like | Non-ulcer dyspepsia | Unexplained epigastric pain |
|  | Biliary dyspepsia | (burning, ulcer- or biliary-like) |
| Aerophagia | ? | Belching, merycism |
| Idiopathic | ? | Unclassified |

**Table II.** Causative factors evidenced or suspected in non-ulcer dyspepsia.

Gastro-oesophageal reflux
Gastro-duodenal motor disturbances (gastric stasis)
Duodeno-gastric reflux
Biliary dyskinesia
Gastric secretory anomalies
Gastric mucosal defects, gastritis, *Helicobacter* infection
Decreased gastric transmural potential difference
Sensory anomalies (to distension of proximal stomach)
Psychological disorders, abnormal responses to stress

medical advice for reasons more related to psychological characteristics than to the nature or the intensity of their symptoms; thus patients seek care because of a feeling of general discomfort more or less expressed, and no real visceral anomalies distinguish them from the mass of healthy subjects. This iceberg concept has been weakened in recent years by several findings: (1) a psychological or psychiatric therapeutic approach to NUD is usually inefficient; (2) several objective digestive anomalies have been found in NUD; (3) the pathophysiology of the dyspepsia occurring in people who do not seek care cannot be explained by psychological anomalies which seem no more frequent than those observed in asymptomatic subjects. In the somatic concept, dyspeptic symptoms are related to anomalies emerging within the digestive tract; psychological factors may be involved, but only as a trigger of local digestive disturbances. Indeed, objective GOR and gastric stasis have each been evidenced in more than 50% of NUD patients [5, 6]. Further progress has been made in elucidating their mechanism and treatment. However the objective approach to NUD has been complicated by the evidence of many other more or less well proven anomalies (Table II) which often occur simultaneously in the same patient and are neither constant nor specific. Moreover, no clear correlation can usually be shown between the intensity of these anomalies and that of the symptoms. Thus, the somatic theory has led to a degree of incoherence and unintelligibility resembling the tower of Babel.

The failure of these two approaches may be due to the fact that NUD cannot be explained by a simple causality, but results from a process of interacting sociopsychological and biological factors that set up vicious circles [7]. Despite these difficulties, we cannot ignore the fact that NUD is a real health problem that affects more than 30% of the population and costs $50 to 70 per person per year, at least in the Swedish evaluation [8]. Further improvement in the clinical and therapeutic approach to NUD by the gastroenterologist therefore continues to be necessary and must be supported by a better knowledge of its pathophysiology, provided that we always keep in mind the practical clinical implications of our research.

# References

1. Colin-Jones DG, Bloom B, Bodemar G, Crean GP, Freston J, Gugler R, Malagelada JR, Nyrén O, Petersen H, Piper D. Management of dyspepsia: report of a working party. Lancet 1988;1:576-9.
2. Barbara L, Camilleri M, Corinaldesi R, Crean GP, Heading RC, Johnson AG, Malagelada JR, Stanghellini V, Wienbeck M. Definition and investigation of dyspepsia. Consensus of an international *ad hoc* working party. Dig Dis Sci 1989;34:1272-6.
3. Jian R. Approche objective de la psychologie des troubles fonctionnels intestinaux. Rev Fr Gastroenterol 1986;22:63-5.
4. Devroede G. Syndrome de l'intestin irritable: maladie de l'intestin, maladie de la personnalité? Gastroenterol Clin Biol 1990;14:3C-4C.
5. Jian R, Ducrot F, Ruskoné A, Chaussade S, Rambaud JC, Modigliani R, Rain JD, Bernier JJ. Symptomatic, radionuclide and therapeutic assessment of chronic idiopathic dyspepsia. A double-blind placebo-controlled evaluation of cisapride. Dig Dis Sci 1989;34:657-64
6. Schwizer W, Hinder RA, DeMeester TR. Does delayed gastric emptying contribute to gastroesophageal reflux disease? Am J Surg 1989;157:74-81
7. Sjodin I, Svedlund J. Psychological aspects of non-ulcer dyspepsia: a psychosomatic view focusing on a comparison between the irritable bowel syndrome and peptic ulcer disease. Scand J Gastroenterol 1985;20 (suppl 109):51-8.
8. Nyrén O, Adami HO Gustavsson S, Loof L, Nyberg A. Social and economic effects of non-ulcer dyspepsia. Scand J Gastroenterol 1985;20 (suppl 109):41-7.

# 2

# The epidemiology of non-ulcer dyspepsia

O. NYRÉN

*Department of Surgery, University Hospital, Uppsala, Sweden*

When the causes of a disease are unknown, the science of epidemiology may add significant contributions to the understanding of the aetiology of that disease. The descriptive epidemiology, i.e. the incidence and prevalence rates in various populations, sex differences, geographical distribution, and secular trends, may provide important clues as to the causal mechanisms. Moreover, analytical epidemiological investigations (cohort of case-control studies) may further increase the knowledge about risk factors and possible aetiologies. It therefore seems appropriate to utilize epidemiological methods in the exploration of non-ulcer dyspepsia, a disorder of virtually unknown aetiology. In this paper, some problems associated with the application of such methods in this particular area will be discussed, and the published reports on the descriptive epidemiology of non-ulcer dyspepsia will be reviewed. Furthermore, examples of data derived from a population-based analytical epidemiological study will be given.

## The epidemiology of non-ulcer dyspepsia — potential problems

Establishing prevalence and incidence rates of non-ulcer dyspepsia in the community is a formidable task. The most important stumbling block is the lack of generally accepted, uniform definitions of the disease. Although the term *dyspepsia* has been said to defy definition [1], it is widely used in clinical practice [2]. The original meaning of the Greek term dyspepsia was "bad digestion". This implies that the symptoms should be referable to the gastrointestinal tract, and more specifically to that part of the gastrointestinal tract which is thought to be involved in the digestion of nutrients, rather than the process of defaecation. Consequently, most physicians make a distinction between dyspepsia, which has become synonymous with symptoms believed to originate in the *upper* gastrointestinal tract, and symptoms thought to emanate from the bowel. This conception is shared in several newly proposed definitions for the term dyspepsia: episodic or persistent symptoms thought by the physician to be referable to the proximal gastrointestinal tract [3-7]. Although this definition may be a realistic reflection of current usage of the term, it is far from ideal as a basis for systematic investigation. It combines a somewhat arbitrary collection of symptoms with an interpretation put upon them. Knowing that the symptomatic overlap with the bowel-related "irritable bowel syndrome" is considerable [8-10], it is very much a matter of opinion whether a patient will be labelled as having dyspepsia or the irritable bowel syndrome. Moreover, even if the borderline between dyspepsia and irritable bowel were strictly defined, dyspepsia is still not a single disease entity. It is merely a symptomatic common denominator of several organic and non-organic disorders, which may not even be confined to the gastrointestinal tract. Clearly, this limits both the reproducibility and the validity of epidemiological and clinical studies in this condition.

Even if there were a general consensus on definitions of dyspepsia and dyspepsia subgroups among doctors, laymen would still have a slightly different view on abdominal symptomatology [2]. The term dyspepsia is not in common parlance; patients prefer the term indigestion, which covers a number of different symptoms as far as laymen are concerned: to some it means heartburn, to others epigastric pain or discomfort, and to still others it means symptoms consistent with a diagnosis of the irritable bowel syndrome [2]. Consequently, it is inappropriate in an epidemiological study to ask specifically about the presence of "dyspepsia" or "indigestion". In order to reach some degree of validity, questions need to be asked about each single symptom separately. Even so, semantic problems will be encountered [3]. Since most individuals may experience casual symptoms or sensations from the gastrointestinal tract at some point, it is a matter of personal interpretation (or of how the threshold is set) whether those sensations will be reported as complaints or not. Therefore, it is crucial how the questions in an epidemiological questionnaire are phrased. As dyspepsia often appears in bouts with long symptom-free periods in between, the length of the period which is covered by the survey would also seem to be crucial. Moreover, since dyspeptic symptoms are poor indicators of organic diseases, the prevalence of the latter cannot be established with certainty unless each individual is thoroughly investigated. Thus, population-based epidemiological studies do not generally produce data on the frequency of non-ulcer dyspepsia, but rather on the frequency of dyspepsia. In the latter category, non-organic dyspepsia dominates, but a certain proportion of the subjects will have organic dyspepsia. Another problem related to the utilization of epidemiological methods in dyspepsia is the very high prevalence of the disorder in the population. If the risk of having the disease is close to, or even greater than, the risk of not having it, those who are unaffected constitute a minority which may differ from those who have the disease in more respects than those directly related to the aetiology of the disease. Morever, standard statistical methods involve an assumption that the risk of falling ill in the disease studied is small or moderate among non-exposed individuals.

## Prevalence and incidence rates in various communities

Given all these hurdles, the concordance between published epidemiological studies is surprisingly high (Table I). Doll *et al.* [11] found that 31% of 6,000 Londoners had

**Table I.** The prevalence of dyspepsia in the community.

| Authors [ref. number] | Country | Prevalence of dyspepsia % | (period) |
|---|---|---|---|
| Doll et al. (1951) [11] | England | 31 | (5 years) |
| Tibblin (1966) [12] | Sweden | 37 | (ever) |
| Weir and Backett (1968) [13] | Scotland | 26 | (5 years) |
| Banke (1975) [14] | Denmark | 26 | (ever) |
| Thompson and Heaton (1980) [15] | England | 21* | (1 year) |
| Hollnagel et al. (1982) [16] | Denmark | 25 | (1 year) |
| Drossman et al. (1982) [17] | USA | 25 | (1 year) |
| Shirlow and Mathers (1985) [18] | Australia | 34 | (ever) |
| Tibblin (1985) [19] | Sweden | 19 | (3 months) |
| Johnsen et al. (1988) [20] | Norway | 23/18 | (Males/females) |
| Jones and Lydeard (1989) [21] | England | 38 | (6 months) |
| Jones (1989) [22] | England/Scotland | 41 | (6 months) |
| Talley et al. (1990) [23] | USA | 9.5 | (1 year) |
| Agréus et al. (1991) [24] | Sweden | 54 | (3 months) |
| *Heartburn* | | | |
| Nebel et al. (1976) [25] | USA | 36 | (ever) |
| Kjellén and Tibbling (1981) [26] | Sweden | 16 | |
| Thompson and Heaton (1982) [27] | England | 34 | (1 year) |

\* strictly defined dyspepsia: 7%

experienced dyspepsia — mostly minor complaints — during the preceding 5 years. The prevalence of peptic ulcers was estimated at approximately 6% and 1.5% in men and women, respectively. The 3-month, 5-year and life-time period prevalences of dyspepsia in Scottish men were reported by Weir and Backett [13] to be 23%, 26% and 29% respectively. Interestingly, the majority were classified as having ulcer-like dyspepsia, and one third had a peptic ulcer diagnosed. By repeating the survey 3 years later, the investigators were able to estimate the annual incidence rate at 1.6%; 1.7% recovered annually from their dyspepsia. Somewhat higher figures were reported by Jones and Lydeard [21]: the 6-month prevalence rate was found to be 38%, and the life-time incidence was 63%. In a second study performed in various areas of England and Scotland, the same author found a 6-month prevalence rate of 41% [22]. Shirlow and Mathers [18] reported from Australia that 34% of the studied population had experienced dyspepsia at some time. Tibblin [12] found similar rates among middle-aged Swedish men: 37% had undergone a barium meal at some time due to dyspepsia. Agréus et al. [24] reported the highest figures published so far: the 3-month prevalence rate in a semi-rural Swedish population was 54.3%. In contrast, the lowest figures stem from the United States [23]: abdominal pain localized to the upper abdomen more than six times a year was reported by 9.5% of the population. In Norway, the prevalence rates were found to be 23% and 18% for men and women, respectively [20]. Banke [14] estimated the life-time incidence of dyspepsia in Denmark at 26%. Another Danish study addressed the question of the relationship between dyspepsia and the irritable bowel syndrome: in people 40 years of age the life-time incidence and one-year prevalence of epigastric pain was estimated at 31% and 25%, respectively [16]. No less that 62% of those who reported symptoms had complaints which were compatible with the irritable bowel diagnosis. Drossman *et al.* [17] found that approximately one in four Americans experience abdominal pain more than six times yearly and that 17% have disturbed defaecation. A similar study from England, focusing on the prevalence of irritable bowel syndrome, showed that 30% of the studied population reported some kind of abdominal or gastrointestinal symptom during the past year: 21% had recurrent abdominal pain — 14% with symptoms typical of irritable bowel syndrome, and 7% with dyspepsia but without features of irritable bowel syndrome; 10% had disturbed defaecation without other symptom. Only one in five symptomatic individuals consulted a physician [15]. The same research group also studied the prevalence of heartburn [27]: 34% had experienced heartburn at least once in one year, 10% at least once every week, and 4% every day. These figures are well in accordance with data from the United States [25], but are higher than the prevalence rates found in Sweden [26].

## Age and gender

The prevalence of dyspepsia decreases quite consistently with age [13, 14, 19, 21, 24], whereas the prevalence of heartburn remains stable [24] or increases [25]. The proportion of individuals with dyspepsia who seek help from the health care system increases with age [22]. The findings with regard to sex differences are conflicting: whereas some studies have failed to show any consistent differences, Agréus *et al.* [24] showed higher prevalence rates among women, particularly for symptoms of the irritable bowel syndrome and "dysmotility-like dyspepsia". Banke [14] reported that the prevalence rates did not decrease with age in women as opposed to men, where there was a marked decline.

## Consultations for dyspepsia

Clearly, those who decide to consult a doctor with dyspepsia do not constitute a representative sample of all those in the community with that symptomatology. There are several factors that are associated with the mere act of seeking medical advice — probably irrelevant as far as the aetiology is concerned — which make consulters differ from non-consulters [28]: for instance, consulters are more worried about the possible seriousness of their symptoms, and they are more likely to have experienced disruptive or threatening life events than those dyspeptic individuals — with equally severe complaints — who do not consult [28]. However, even though the incidence and prevalence in the population may reflect aetiological factors better than do consultation patterns, the delineation of the consulting population is still of utmost interest. The obvious advantage of studying consulting populations rather than non-consulters is that in the former a larger proportion has been investigated. Thus, the admixture of organic cases is minimized.

Most physicians are all too familiar with the large number of patients presenting with epigastric pain or discomfort without any apparent anatomical or physiological correlates. In a Swedish survey investigation in a sample of 135,597 outpatient consultations in general practice as well as at hospital outpatient departments, the clinical diagnosis of "gastritis" — which in Sweden is equivalent to non-ulcer dyspepsia — accounted for 1.9% of all outpatient consultations, or an estimated number of 47 annual consultations per 1,000 inhabitants [29]. That figure was more than five times as much as the corresponding figure for duodenal ulcer and gastric ulcer diseases combined. As opposed to duodenal ulcer disease, in which there was a predominance of men, the male/female ratio in "gastritis" was 1:1 [29]. The findings in Sweden are well in accordance with international figures: approximately 2% of all general practice consultations are reserved for dyspepsia, which thus accounts for about one third of all gastroenterological consultations in this country [29-32]. The annual incidence of consultations due to dyspepsia (the proportion of the general population seeing a doctor for dyspepsia *for the first time*) has been estimated at 1% [33]. Owing to the vast proportions of this patient category, the economic consequences of dyspepsia for society are clearly considerable [34].

## Case-control analysis of risk factors

In a population-based case-control study, 178 well-characterized patients with non-ulcer dyspepsia and an equal number of age- and sex-matched community controls completed a comprehensive questionnaire covering background factors such as marital status, educational level, housing standard, job characteristics, medical history, personality, and smoking, coffee, alcohol and drug consumption habits [35]. In a multivariate logistic regression analysis, multiple somatic non-abdominal symptoms showed the strongest association with non-ulcer dyspepsia — the odds ratio (OR) was 2.8, 95% confidence limits (95%CL) 2.0-3.9 for each additional symptom. Economic worries (OR=3.1, 95%CL 1.5-6.5), a history of psychiatric consultations (OR=3.9, 95%CL 1.6-9.7), and residential mobility (OR for >3 dwellings during the past 10 years was 2.3, 95%CL 1.2-4.4) also remained as independent significant risk factors in the multivariate analysis (Table II). Factors traditionally considered to be risk factors, such as coffee drinking, smoking, alcohol consumption, and ingestion of aspirin and non-steroidal anti-inflammatory drugs were not significantly associated with an increased risk of developing non-ulcer dyspepsia. In fact, coffee drinking was

**Table II.** Factors associated with an increased risk of developing non-ulcer dyspepsia. When controlled in a multivariate stepwise logistic regression model for the confounding effects of 20 factors which were significantly associated with non-ulcer dyspepsia in a preliminary univariate analysis, the factors shown in the table remained independent, significant risk factors [35].

| Factor | Odds ratio | 95% confidence limits |
|---|---|---|
| Multiple somatic non-abdominal symptoms | 2.8 | 2.0-3.9 |
| Economic worries | 3.1 | 1.5-6.5 |
| Psychiatric consultations | 3.9 | 1.6-9.7 |
| Residential mobility | 2.3 | 1.2-4.4 |

negatively associated with the condition. With epidemiological methodology it was shown that psychosocial factors appear to be important in the aetiology of non-ulcer dyspepsia.

## References

1. Thompson WG. Non-ulcer dyspepsia. Can Med Assoc J 1984;130:565-9.
2. Kingham JG, Fairclough PD, Dawson AM. What is indigestion? J R Soc Med 1983;76:183-6.
3. Knill-Jones RP. A formal approach to symptoms in dyspepsia. Clin Gastroenterol 1985;14:517-29.
4. Dobrilla G. Functional dyspepsia: problems of classification, pathophysiology, diagnosis and therapy. In: Cheli R, Molinary F, eds. *Pirenzepine — Knowledge and New Trends.* Verona: Cortina International, 1986:43-8.
5. Heatley RV, Rathbone BJ. Dyspepsia: a dilemma for doctors? Lancet 1987;2:779-82.
6. Colin-Jones DG, Bloom B, Bodemar G, Crean GP, Freston J, Gugler R, Malagelada JR, Nyrén O, Petersen H, Piper D. Management of dyspepsia: report of a working party. Lancet 1988;1:576-9.
7. Barbara L, Camilleri M, Corinaldesi R, Crean GP, Heading RC, Johnson AG, Malagelada JR, Stanghellini V, Wienbeck M. Definition and investigation of dyspepsia. Consensus of an international *ad hoc* working party. Dig Dis Sci 1989;34:1272-6.
8. Dotevall G, Svedlund J, Sjödin I. Symptoms in irritable bowel syndrome. Scand J Gastroenterol 1982;17(suppl 79): 16-9.
9. Talley NJ, Piper DW. The association between non-ulcer dyspepsia and other gastrointestinal disorders. Scand J Gastroenterol 1985;20:896-900.
10. Sielaff F. Coincidence between chronic dyspepsia and irritable bowel syndrome. Eur J Gastroenterol Hepatol 1990;2(suppl 1): S105-6.
11. Doll R, Avery Jones F, Buckatzsch MM. Occupational factors in the aetiology of gastric and duodenal ulcers, with an estimate of their incidence in the general population. Medical Research Council Special Reports, Series 276. London: HMSO, 1951:7-96.
12. Tibblin G. Ulcers. 3. The frequency of ulcers among 50-year-old men. Lakartidningen 1966;63:4825-6.
13. Weir RD, Backett EM. Studies of the epidemiology of peptic ulcer in a rural community: prevalence and natural history of dyspepsia and peptic ulcer. Gut 1968;9:75-83.
14. Banke L. Ulcussygdommens epidemiologi. Copenhagen: F.A.D.L., 1975.
15. Thompson WG, Heaton KW. Functional bowel disorders in apparently healthy people. Gastroenterology 1980;79:283-8.
16. Hollnagel H, Norrelund N, Larsen S. Gastrointestinal symptoms among 40-year olds in Glostrup. An epidemiological study. Ugeskr Laeger 1982;144:267-73.
17. Drossman DA, Sandler RS, McKee DC, Lovitz AJ. Bowel patterns among subjects not seeking health care. Use of a questionnaire to identify a population with bowel dysfunction. Gastroenterology 1982;83:529-34.
18. Shirlow MJ, Mathers CD. A study of caffeine consumption and symptoms: indigestion, palpitations, tremor, headache and insomnia. Int J Epidemiol 1985;14:239-48.
19. Tibblin G. Introduction to the epidemiology of dyspepsia. Scand J Gastroenterol 1985;20(suppl 109):29-33.
20. Johnsen R, Straume B, Forde OH. Peptic ulcer and non-ulcer dyspepsia — a disease and a disorder. Scand J Prim Health Care 1988;6:239-43.
21. Jones R, Lydeard S. Prevalence of symptoms of dyspepsia in the community. Br Med J 1989;298:30-2.
22. Jones R. Dyspeptic symptoms in the community. Gut 1989;30:893-8.

*Epidemiology*

23. Talley NJ, Phillips SF, Zinsmeister AR, Melton LJ. Dyspepsia subgroups in a community: a random population-based study. Am J Gastroenterol 1990;85:1241.
24. Agréus L, Svärdsudd K, Tibblin G, Nyrén O. The epidemiology of dyspepsia: symptom clusters and demographic characteristics. Gastroenterology 1991:A1(abstr).
25. Nebel OT, Fornes MF, Castell DO. Symptomatic gastroesophageal reflux: incidence and precipitating factors. Am J Dig Dis 1976;21:953-6.
26. Kjellén G, Tibbling L. Manometric oesophageal function, acid perfusion test and symptomatology in a 55-year-old general population. Clin Physiol 1981;1:405-15.
27. Thompson WG, Heaton KW. Heartburn and globus in apparently healthy people. Can Med Assoc J 1982;126:46-8.
28. Lydeard S. Jones R. Factors affecting the decision to consult with dyspepsia: comparison of consulters and non-consulters. JR Coll Gen Pract 1989;39:495-8.
29. Loof L, Adami HO, Agenäs I, Gustavsson S, Nyberg A, Nyrén O. The diagnosis and therapy survey October 1978 — March 1983, health care consumption and current drug therapy in Sweden with respect to the clinical diagnosis of gastritis. Scand J Gastroenterol 1985;20(suppl 109):35-9.
30. Davies SWY. A year in general practice. J R Coll Gen Pract 1958;1:315-29.
31. Morrell DC, Gage HG, Robinson NA. Symptoms in general practice. J R Coll Gen Pract 1971;21:32-43.
32. Kristensen P, Sandbakken P, Johannessen T, Loge I, Hafstad PE, Petersen H, Fjosne U, Kleveland PM. Gastrointestinal diseases in general practice. A general practice register. Tidsskr Nor Laegeforen 1985;105:728-31.
33. Gear MW, Barnes RJ.Endoscopic studies of dyspepsia in a general practice. Br Med J 1980;280:1136-7.
34. Nyrén O, Adami HO, Gustavsson S, Lööf L, Nyberg A. Social and economic effects of non-ulcer dyspepsia. Scand J Gastroenterol 1985;20(suppl 109):41-7.
35. Nyrén O. Non-ulcer dyspepsia. Studies on epidemiology, pathophysiology, and therapy. [Thesis]. Uppsala: Acta Universitatis Upsaliensis Faculty of Medicine, 1985, Abstr 527.

Non-ulcer dyspepsia: pathophysiological and therapeutic approaches. Eds J.-P. Galmiche, R. Jian, M. Mignon, Ph. Ruszniewski, John Libbey Eurotext, Paris © 1991, pp. 15-31.

# 3

# Gastric motor response to food

A. DUBOIS

*Laboratory of Gastrointestinal and Liver Studies, Digestive Diseases Division, Department of Medicine, Uniformed Services University of the Health Sciences, Bethesda, MD 20814-4799, USA*

## Introduction

The stomach has three main functions in relation to feeding: it acts as a reservoir, allowing short term storage of food; it initiates peptic digestion; and it insures a timely delivery of liquified and partly digested nutrients to the small intestine. In addition, the sphincteric regions of the cardia and pylorus prevent reflux of material that may be noxious to the oesophageal and gastric mucosae, while allowing smooth aboral progression of gastrointestinal contents. Before discussing the normal and abnormal gastric responses to food, it is necessary to review gastric anatomy as well as the methods available to evaluate the functions of the stomach.

## Anatomy

### Regional organization

The stomach comprises a proximal and a distal region (Fig. 1). The proximal stomach may be divided in a fundus and a corpus. However, in contrast to what is observed in certain species, there is no clearcut separation between these two regions in man. The proximal stomach relaxes during feeding, allowing accommodation of the cavity to food and secretions with only a very small increase in intraluminal pressure (receptive relaxation). In addition, peristaltic waves that travel across the corpus and the distal stomach are initiated in a pacemaker located in the proximal stomach. Because its mucosa contains acid-secreting parietal cells, it has also been named the oxyntic gland area (from the Greek οξυνειν : to make acid).

The distal stomach or antrum has stronger muscles than the proximal stomach with which it cooperates to propel gastric contents in an aboral direction. The antrum also belongs to the functional antropyloroduodenal pump, which promotes grinding and sieving of solid food, and normally prevents excessive duodenogastric reflux.

In addition, the stomach is separated from the rest of the gastrointestinal tract by two sphincteric areas: the lower oesophageal sphincter, also called distal oesophageal sphincter, or cardia, and the pyloric sphincter. Relaxation of these sphincters allows passage of food, while their contractions prevent gastro-oesophageal and duodenogastric reflux.

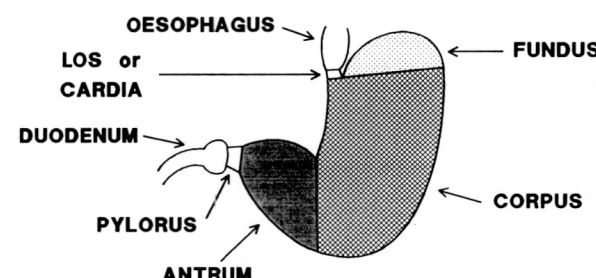

**Figure 1.** Schematic representation of the anatomy of the stomach.

## Smooth muscles

As in the rest of the digestive tract, the stomach smooth muscles consist of two main layers. The outer, longitudinal muscle is in continuity with the oesophagus and duodenum, curling towards the submucosa at the level of the pylorus to form this sphincteric area. The inner, circular muscle is interrupted at this level. In addition, the proximal stomach contains a third, inner layer of muscle which is found immediately between the circular muscle and the submucosa [1]. This oblique muscle appears to be in continuity with the muscles of the lower oesophageal sphincter. The arrangement of these muscles explains how the different portions of the stomach can produce the coordinated propulsion and retropulsion of the intragastric contents, as well as the functional organization of the two gastric sphincters.

## Innervation

The stomach is innervated by extrinsic nerves and by an intramural myenteric plexus.

### *Extrinsic nerves (vagus nerves and splanchnic nerves)*

*Vagus nerves.* The right and level vagi originate from numerous rootlets from the lateral sides of the medulla oblongata. Below the diaphragm, they lie anteriorly and posteriorly to the oesophagus and stomach. At the level of the lower oesophageal sphincter, both trunks give rise to branches innervating the anterior and posterior walls of the stomach. The anterior trunk gives off pyloric branches travelling within the lesser omentum (nerve of Latarjet), while the posterior aspect of the distal antrum and the pylorus are innervated by the coeliac branch.

The vagus nerves contain 80% afferent fibres and 20% motor neurones. Afferent fibres conduct potentials from gastric mechano- and chemoreceptors to the central nervous system, while the motor fibres are either preganglionic cholinergic, postganglionic noradrenergic, or non-adrenergic non-cholinergic. Preganglionic parasympathetic nerves synapse with the myenteric (Auerbach) and submucosal (Meissner) plexuses. Their stimulation increases gastric contractility and peristalsis, relaxes the pylorus, and may enhance gastric emptying of both solids and liquids. Postganglionic noradrenergic nerves also innervate the myenteric and submucosal plexuses; in addition, a number of noradrenergic nerve endings are present in the circular muscles and near the mucosal cells. Stimulation of noradrenergic nerves produces relaxation of the stomach, inhibition of gastric motility and contraction of the pyloric sphincter, thus resulting in an inhibition of gastric emptying of both solids and liquids. The stimulation of non-adrenergic, non-cholinergic nerves produces relaxation of the stomach and allows accommodation of food. These nerves contain several neurotransmitters that vary according to the species, but the neurotransmitter that is responsible for their effect has not yet been defined. Vasoactive intestinal polypeptide (VIP), ATP (purinergic), or serotonin may be involved, but none of these substances has satisfied all the criteria that are required for them to be recognized physiological neurotransmitters in the stomach.

*Splanchnic nerves.* They contain mostly postganglionic noradrenergic nerves originating in the thoracic chains and the coeliac and mesenteric ganglia. Their branches follow the blood vessels to the gastric wall. Cholinergic nerves are probably also present since electrical stimulation of the peripheral end of the cut splanchnic nerves produces atropine-sensitive contraction of the stomach. Sensory nerves also travel along these tracts to convey impulses from the stomach to the central nervous system.

*Myenteric plexus*

The organization of the myenteric plexus is extremely complex, and it closely resembles that of the central nervous system. In the stomach, as in other parts of the gut, the intramural nerves contain and release one or several neurotransmitters (acetylcholine, one or several peptides, etc.), and they are innervated by cholinergic preganglionic axons. Postganglionic noradrenergic nerves entering the myenteric plexus innervate the smooth muscle both indirectly by synapsing with myenteric ganglia, and directly by entering the inner circular muscle. However, they do not appear to innervate the longitudinal outer layer.

## Methods available for studying gastric motility

### Electrical activity

Gastric electrical activity requires continuous undisturbed contact of electrodes with the wall of the stomach. In animals this may be achieved by suturing the electrodes to the tissues, which is rarely an option in humans. Silver/silver chloride monopolar or bipolar electrodes have been inserted into suction cups placed at the tip of flexible tubes [2]. This type of tube may be introduced into the stomach through nasogastric intubation. Once the tube is in the stomach and its position has been verified by cineradiography, suction is applied in order to maintain the electrode in place. Alternatively, magnetic attraction has been exerted across the abdominal wall to ensure close apposition of the electrodes with the gastric wall [3]. In both cases however, there is concern that the procedure may create artifactual stimulation of gastric activity.

**Mechanical activity**

Most early studies of gastric activity were performed by visual observation of the movements of the stomach. This could be done in laparotomized animals or through the abdominal wall in cachectic patients. Another approach was possible in patients with gastrostomies [4]. Finally, radiographic pictures and cineradiography have allowed very important observations [5]. However, all these techniques usually fail to provide quantitative data and are commonly used only as an aid to the interpretation of results obtained using the methods described below.

*Extraluminal measurements*

These techniques provide important quantitative data regarding gastric contractility. They use either force transducers or displacement transducers sutured onto the serosa of the stomach [6, 7]. The problem with both transducers, however, is that they tend to malfunction because of breakage of foil strain gauges or growth of fibrous tissue into the moving parts of displacement transducers. Moreover, they have to be implanted surgically, which limits their use to animal experimental studies.

*Intraluminal measurements*

In contrast to the situation in the tube-shaped oesophagus or intestine, intraluminal measurements are difficult in the relatively large gastric cavity. Postprandially, the stomach is filled with variable and large volumes of fluids, solids, and air. Based on the Pascal principle one can predict that intraluminal manometry will not provide reliable recording of the contractile activity of the proximal stomach [8]. Continuously perfused catheters or intraluminal transducers are probably not reliable in the body of the stomach or in the proximal antrum, although they can be used in the immediate vicinity of the sphincters [9]. Small or large balloons, distended with air, usually provide better recordings, but they may trigger local motor reflexes and the tracings obtained with this technique may not represent true physiological events.

**The electrogastrogram (EGG)**

Early investigators reported that electrodes placed on the abdomen permit recording of gastrointestinal electrical potentials at 3 per minute [10, 11]. More recently, it was shown that these potentials originate in the stomach [12] and that they reflect accurately both the electrical and mechanical gastric activity [13]. Therefore, the EGG represents an attractive alternative to serosal or mucosal gastric electromyography, while possibly allowing an indirect evaluation of gastric emptying [14]. However, more work is needed to better define the exact characteristics of gastric activity that is reflected in the EGG.

## Gastric emptying

The methods available to evaluate gastric emptying can be separated into six major classes. The first three methods require nasogastric intubation. In contrast, the other three techniques are non-invasive, although two of them require exposure to ionizing radiations.

### Aspiration of gastric contents

Two types of tests have been developed. The first one is called the Ewald test meal [15]. It consists of administering a mixed solid and liquid meal at time 0. Thirty to sixty minutes later, a nasogastric tube is passed and the stomach contents are completely aspirated. The saline load test [16] is similar in its principle, but differs because it explores only the emptying of liquids, i.e., a 750 ml saline load. Both techniques suffer severe limitations. First, the volume present in the stomach may not be totally reaspirated. In the case of the Ewald solid test meal, in addition, the solid particles usually clog the tube. Furthermore, the volume of fluids secreted into the stomach, which can represent a large fraction of the gastric volume, cannot be determined. Thus, these tests will give similar results whether a large residual volume is due to slow emptying associated with normal gastric secretion or to hypersecretion associated with normal emptying.

The saline load test may be improved if the technique is modified to include a non-absorbable marker in the liquid meal. This is the so-called serial test meal technique, originally developed by Salamanca in Spain [17], and by Hunt in England [18]. The problem with this technique, as well as with the saline load tests, is that it does not allow repeated measurements of gastric emptying over the entire course of the emptying of a meal, unless one accepts the physiological impact of the complete aspiration and immediate reinjection of the total volume of the gastric contents.

### Gastric dye dilution technique

This method and its subsequent improvements permit repeated determination of the volume of the gastric contents, without the need for complete emptying of the stomach [19-22]. In addition, it permits concurrent calculations of gastric secretion and gastric emptying rates [19, 22] and allows measurement of emptying during fasting [22]. This technique is simple to perform, as it requires only gastric intubation, spectrophotometric measurements of the marker, and determination of concentration of acid and other components of gastric juice in the samples aspirated from the stomach. Calculations are easily performed using programmable calculators or mini-computers [23]. However, it suffers certain limitations in that it requires homogeneous mixing of the gastric contents at the time of the samplings and is therefore not applicable to studies of emptying of solids.

### Intraduodenal dye dilution technique

This method also allows concurrent determination of gastric secretion and gastric emptying, although it does not allow measurement of emptying during fasting. This technique has been developed almost simultaneously in the United States [24, 25], in France [26], and in Sweden [27]. The method is based on dilution techniques previously developed to measure propulsion of fluids in the jejunum [28, 29], and has been extensively described by Malagelada *et al.* [30]. The calculations are based on a number of assumptions and approximations, and it is possible that some of the errors are magnified as each equation uses values calculated in the previous one [31]. In addition, there is no published experimental evidence showing that perfusion of the duodenum with physiological saline at 2 to 10 ml/min does not affect gastric emptying and secretion. Nonetheless, this method is useful as it allows the determination of the rates of gastric emptying for liquids as well as solids. Finally, it has provided valuable information regarding the pathophysiology of gastric emptying and of gastric secretion.

*Radiological methods*

These methods have been used to study gastric emptying since radiology was developed [5]. Radiological techniques are usually limited to an estimation of the time needed to completely empty barium from the stomach. If this time is longer than three hours, gastric retention may be suspected. As barium is not physiological, it has been mixed with ground steak, a preparation called the steak and barium meal [32] or, more commonly, the "barium burger" [33]. Normally, all the barium should be emptied from the stomach in five hours. However, one should remember that barium is probably rapidly separated from the steak, which means that this test is of questionable physiological significance, and it evaluates only the effect of a steak on the emptying of barium from the stomach.

A similar technique uses radio-opaque pellets of barium-impregnated polyethylene [34]. These 3-mm diameter pellets are mixed with a standard mixed meal and appear to be evacuated at a rate comparable to that calculated using radioisotopic techniques [35]. The problem with this method, however, is that it evaluates the emptying of non-digestible solids, and its physiological meaning remains to be established.

*Radionuclide imaging*

This method is based on the detection of gamma photons by a gamma camera, which consists of a large number of photomultiplier tubes placed next to each other. A collimator placed in front of the gamma camera allows only the passage of photons that are perpendicular to the detector, an effect similar to that of the lens of an optical camera. The amplified signal is then transmitted to a cathode ray tube which can be used to visualize the image. Quantitative analysis of this image can be performed at a later time as the signal is concurrently acquired on a computer interfaced with the camera. This technique allows calculation of gastric emptying rates [36, 37] and permits the concurrent determination of the emptying of two different isotopes [38]. Therefore, if one of these isotopes is bound to solid particles and the other stays in the liquid phase, one can measure simultaneously the emptying of both components of a meal. The solid phase can be firmly tagged if $^{99m}$Technetium sulphur colloid is injected intravenously into a live chicken, because the Kupfer cells of its liver bind the colloid [39]. The chicken is then killed and its liver is incorporated into a meal which can be fed to a patient. $^{111}$Indium or $^{113}$Indium chelated to a non-absorbable marker (such as diethylene pentacetic acid, DTPA) is added to water or milk in order to tag the liquid phase. However, the amount of radioactivity measured will vary with the depth of tissue and with the amount of radioisotope separating the region of the stomach containing the isotope and the gamma camera [40]. This geometry problem is particularly critical in the stomach, as its proximal portion is more posterior than the distal portion. To obviate this problem, it is presently recommended that one should record an image from two opposed detectors, i.e., one from the front and one from the back of the subject or to use another correction factor for depth penetration. Radionuclide imaging can also be used to measure duodenogastric reflux. $^{99m}$Tc-HIDA is injected intravenously, taken up by the liver and excreted into the duodenum. $^{99m}$Tc is observed in the area of the stomach if reflux does occur.

## Ultrasonic methods

Recently, several groups have attempted to measure gastric emptying using sonographic techniques. As ultrasounds are reflected by interfaces, they can be used to measure the volume of an organ. However, these reports are still preliminary, and the methods have several limitations especially in the presence of air in the stomach.

# Normal response of the stomach to food

## Fasting activity

### Gastric electrical and motor activity

The subject of *in vitro* and *in vivo* recording of gastric motility has been reviewed extensively [41, 42]. Gastric electrical activity is characterized by the presence of slow waves, also called electrical control activity (ECA), or basic electric rhythm (BER) or pacesetter potential (PSP). These membrane potentials may be recorded both intra- and extracellularly at 5/min in dogs and at 3/min in primates, and in the presence as well as in the absence of contractions. In the absence of mechanical contraction, extracellular electrical activity appears as a succession of triphasic waves, with a large negative potential preceded and followed by a smaller positive deflection. During stomach contractions, this triphasic event is followed by a "second potential" (or plateau potential) which is typically a 4-8 sec positive or negative deflection in most of the stomach. In the terminal antrum, fast action potentials (spikes or electrical response activities, ERA) are superimposed onto the second potential. Both ECA and ERA propagate along the greater curvature at a speed that progressively increases from 0.1 cm/sec in the corpus to 4 cm/sec in the distal antrum. Acetylcholine and adrenergic agonists respectively stimulate and inhibit the ERA but not the ECA.

Contractile activity of the stomach is characterized by tonic contractions in the proximal stomach and by phasic contractions in the antrum. The tone of the fundus and corpus may be recorded using large balloons inflated in the proximal stomach, demonstrating that swallowing is immediately followed by receptive relaxation. This reflex allows accommodation of food in the stomach without an increase in intragastric pressure. No electrical activity is recorded from the proximal stomach during gastric relaxation, but this could be due to technical defects. In the corpus, phasic contractions may be superimposed on tonic contractions, but these waves may be caused by the pressure applied by the balloon onto the gastric mucosa.

In the distal stomach, fasting mechanical activity is characterized by cyclic fluctuations of the migrating motor complexes [43]. Irregular non-propagated contractions during phase I progressively evolve into phase II contractions and culminate with the phase III peristaltic waves that propagate towards the pylorus at a speed that increases distally (Fig. 2, left side of the tracing) [44].

*Gastric emptying*

Although gastric emptying is usually studied only after meals, it is a continuous process which goes on even during fasting. Fasting gastric emptying has two functions. First, it permits the continuous transfer of gastric secretions and swallowed saliva to the duodenum. Secondly, it allows the emptying of undigestible solids smaller than

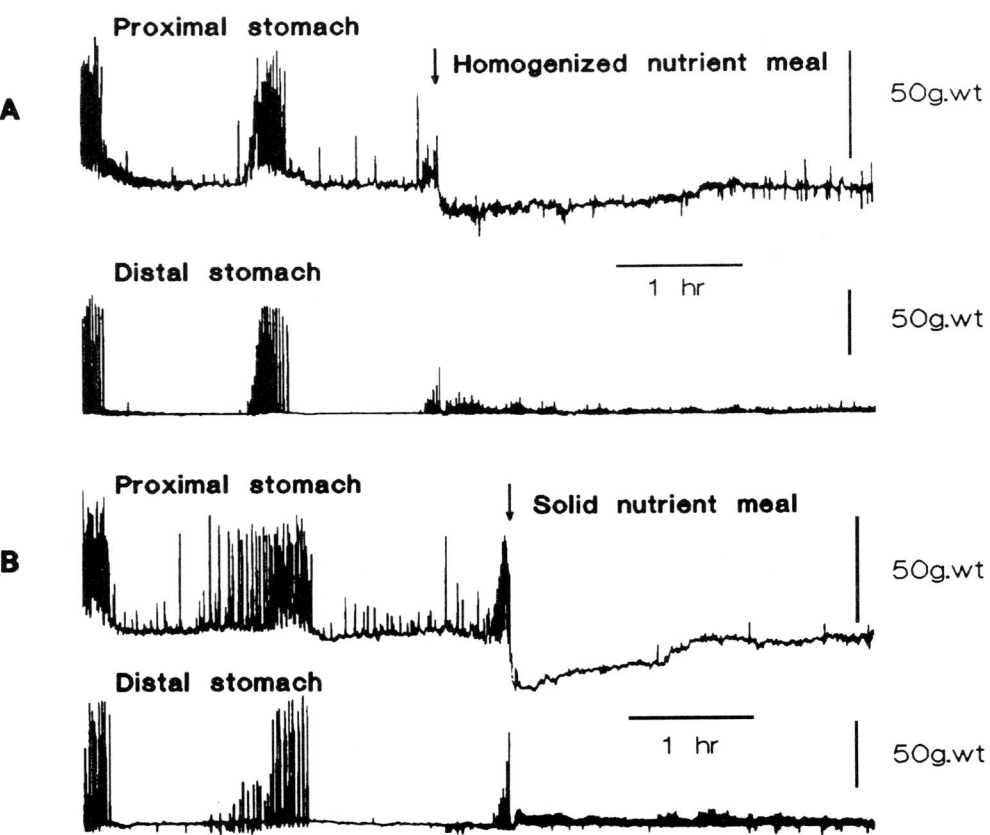

**Figure 2.** Effect of oral administration of two types of meals on gastric activity as recorded in dogs using extraluminal force transducers. Note that the cyclical MMC pattern observed during fasting (on the left of the figure) is replaced by continuous irregular activity of smaller amplitude after the meal. In addition, relaxation of the proximal stomach is relatively greater after the solid nutrient meal (bottom tracing) than after the homogenized meal (top tracing). (From Gill *et al.* [44], with permission).

approximately 25 mm or one inch in diameter, which occurs at the end of the postprandial period, concurrently with bursts of spikes and powerful phase III contractions.

**Response to meals**

*Gastric filling*

During swallowing of food or drinks, the stomach relaxes and can accommodate large volumes with very little increase in intragastric pressure. This relaxation occurs mostly in the proximal stomach, and is greater after solid meals than after homogenized meals (Fig. 2) [44]. This relaxation is also observed, although to a lesser extent, after non-nutrient meals (Fig. 3), but not after intraduodenal administration of meals (Fig. 4 and 5) [44]. Recording of electrical potentials during gastric relaxation failed to demonstrate a typical event reflecting this activity. Section of the vagus nerve abolishes gastric relaxation, but the neurotransmitter responsible for this response has not been identified. It is neither noradrenergic nor cholinergic, and is therefore called non-adrenergic non-cholinergic. This subject is reviewed in greater detail by Dr. Aspiroz in the chapter "Control of gastric tone".

*Mixing and grinding of food*

In dogs prepared with serosal strain gauges, oral or intraduodenal administration of solid-liquid nutrient meals abolished the cyclic pattern of gastric MMC, which is replaced by weaker but continuous contractions (Fig. 2 and 4) [44]. In contrast, oral or intraduodenal administration of non-nutrient meals did not interrupt the cyclical pattern of the MMC (Fig. 3 and 5) [44]. In man, postprandial contractions have been recorded only in the distal antrum after liquid-solid meals when using intraluminal strain gauges but they were not observed after homogenized meals [45]. In another study also in man, large gastric contractions have been observed after liquid meals when using intraluminal low compliance perfused catheters (Fig. 6) [46]. In addition, the amplitude of the EGG also increases following meals, and this increase is related to gastric emptying (see below) [14].

Non-occlusive gastric waves progress toward the pylorus, pushing the gastric contents that are lining the walls into the duodenum. Larger particles tend to accumulate away from the gastric walls, in a zone where the flow is reversed [47]. As a result, the larger particles are pressed between the ring of contraction to flow back and to be dispersed into the proximal stomach. There, the slow tonic contractions of the corpus again propel the particles toward the antrum where they are caught by the next peristaltic wave. This to-and-fro motion produces trituration of food and explains both the sieving and the grinding of particles which are known to occur after consumption of solid food. It is worth noticing that grinding may occur through the effect of rapid flow of particles through a small opening, even in the absence of a totally occlusive contraction waves.

*Emptying*

Gastric emptying occurs concurrently with mixing and grinding during the postprandial period. Liquids are emptied exponentially, that is at a rate that is proportional to the

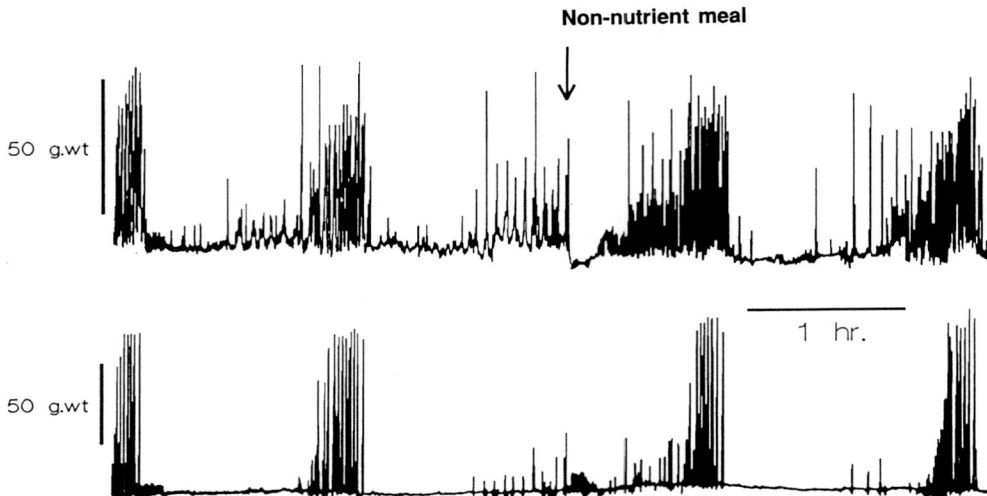

**Figure 3.** Effect of oral administration of a non-nutrient meal on gastric activity as recorded in dogs using extraluminal force transducers. Note that the cyclical MMC pattern observed during fasting (on the left of the figure) is not interrupted by this type of meal, although a small relaxation of the proximal stomach is observed. (From Gill et al. [44], with permission).

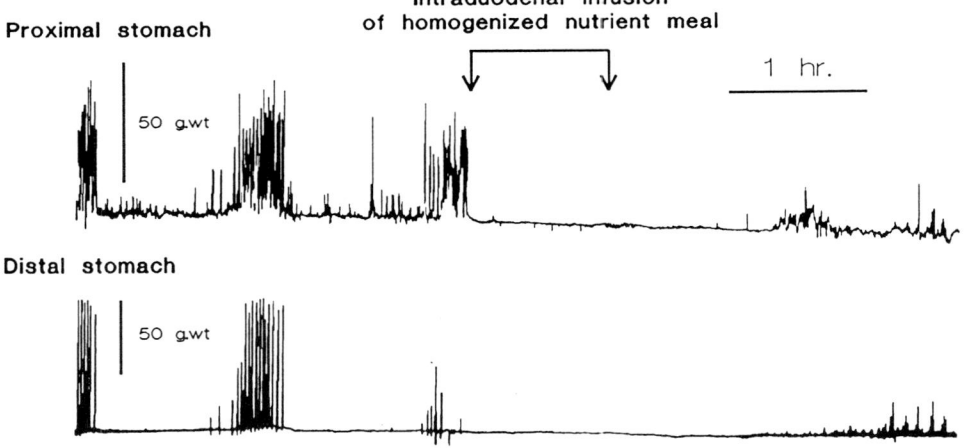

**Figure 4.** Effect of intraduodenal infusion of a homogenized nutrient meal on gastric activity as recorded in dogs using extraluminal force transducers. Note that the cyclical MMC pattern observed during fasting (on the left of the figure) is abolished after the meal and that irregular activity of smaller amplitude reappears only 2 hours later. In addition, no relaxation of the proximal stomach is observed when food bypasses the stomach. (From Gill et al. [44], with permission).

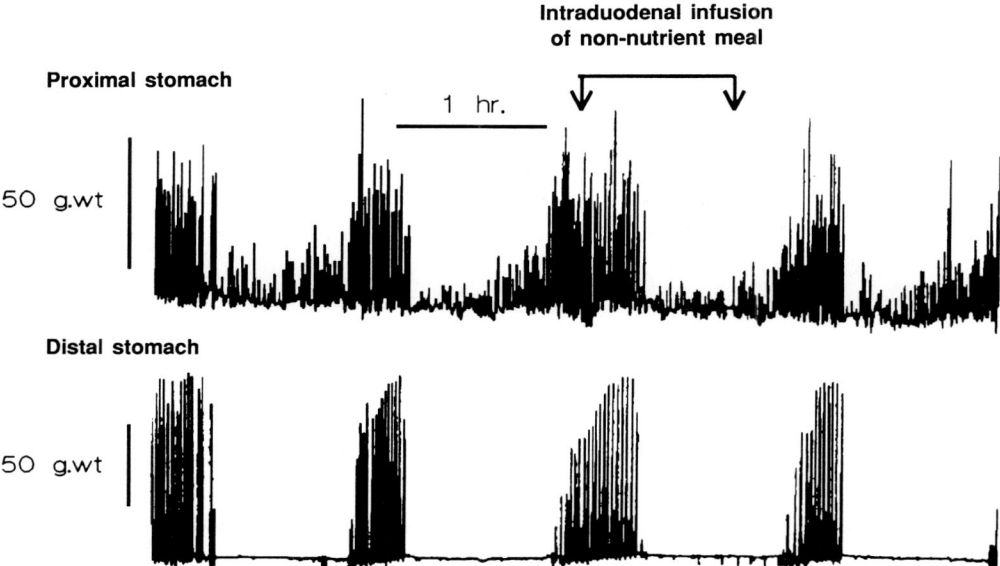

**Figure 5.** Effect of intraduodenal infusion of a homogenized non-nutrient meal on gastric activity as recorded in dogs using extraluminal force transducers. Note that the cyclical MMC pattern observed during fasting (on the left of the figure) is not interrupted by this type of meal, and that no relaxation is observed in the proximal stomach. (From Gill et al. [44], with permission).

intragastric volume [48]. To express emptying of liquids independently from the stimulatory effect of gastric distension, one should use the fractional rate of emptying, which is equal to the rate of emptying divided by the intragastric volume [22]. Since 99% of the solids are emptied only after having been ground to particles less than 2 mm, solids are emptied more slowly than liquids and at a rate inversely proportional to the diameter of the particles present in the stomach [49]. Thus, the delay between emptying of liquids and that of solids probably results from the fact that solids need to be processed by the stomach before being emptied. Large (greater than 5 mm diameter), indigestible solids are retained by the stomach during the entire digestive period and are emptied by MMCs after all digestible food has left the stomach. The maximum diameter of the particles that can be emptied from the stomach is 25 mm or less because the pylorus has limited distensibility. In addition, the chemical composition and the energy content of meals modify emptying [50].

The electrical and mechanical activity of the stomach during the grinding and emptying phases of gastric digestion is complex and appears less organized than fasting cycling of MMCs. Because a better knowledge of gastric activity during the immediate postprandial period would be required to enhance our understanding of gastric functional diseases, more studies should concentrate on this question.

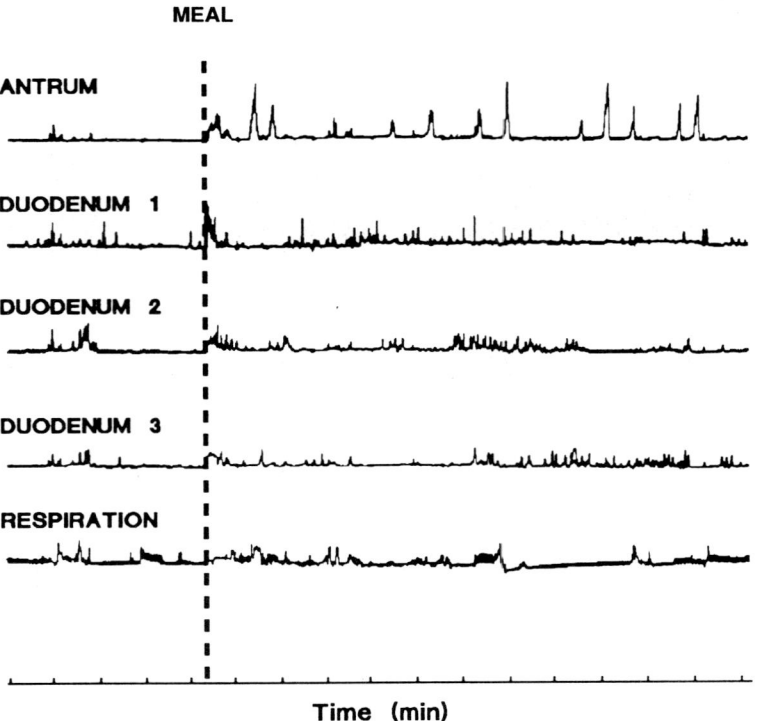

**Figure 6.** Effect of a 789 kJ (199 kcal) liquid-solid meal on gastroduodenal activity in man as recorded using a low compliance perfusion system. The meal contained 20.5 g carbohydrate, 11 g protein, and 8.1 g fat, administered in a 240 ml volume. Note the increase in amplitude and duration of the gastric contractions following the meal. (From Thompson et al. [46], with permission).

*Duodenogastric reflux*

The rate and direction of flow through the pylorus depends on the difference between intragastric and intraduodenal pressures, although this has not yet been proven experimentally. Whatever the cause of movements of gastroduodenal contents, some of the duodenal fluids may enter the stomach under physiological conditions, both postprandially and during fasting. Postprandial reflux is probably not damaging, since food and gastric secretion dilute and neutralize duodenal fluids. During fasting however, reflux of duodenal, pancreatic and biliary enzymes may cause significant damage to the gastric mucosa.

**Regulation of gastric motility**

The functioning of the stomach is controlled by impulses that can be triggered by external (visual, olfactory, auditory, motion) or internal (e.g., pneumonia, peritoneal irritation) stimuli perceived by the central nervous system and conveyed to the stomach through nervous or humoral mechanisms. In addition, gastric emptying is delayed when the acidity and energy concentration of the gastroduodenal contents increase, an effect mediated by neurohumoral vectors released following stimulation of chemoreceptors located in the wall of the stomach and duodenum [51]. Similarly, gastroduodenal mechanoreceptors mediate the stimulation of gastric motility induced by distension of the stomach, as well as the inhibition produced by overdistension. It is worth noticing that hormones and neurotransmitters which affect gastric motility may stimulate the gastric antrum while inhibiting the corpus. In addition, their effect on the movements of the gastric contents within and out of the stomach results from the complex integration of each of these actions. Therefore, only *in vivo* studies of gastric emptying allow the definition of the pathophysiological effect of various transmitters. In addition, *in vivo* and *in vitro* studies of mechanical and electrical activity of the stomach permit the analysis and the interpretation of these effects.

*Nervous factors*

In general, cholinergic nerves stimulate, while noradrenergic nerves inhibit, gastric contractions. In addition, many peptides have been observed within the neurones of the intramural plexus, and these peptides play an important role in the regulation of gastric motility [52]. However, these effects on contractions may result in increased or decreased gastric emptying. The nervous control of the stomach relies on extrinsic nerves, which connect the central nervous system to the stomach, and on intramural myenteric plexuses.

*Hormonal factors*

Many hormones have been found to modify gastric motor activity, but their physiological role or their involvement in gastric pathology is often difficult to establish.

*Secretin.* This hormone, which was the first to be described, is known to delay gastric emptying of liquids [53, 54]. Since secretin is released by infusion of physiological amounts of acid into the duodenum, it could play a role in the normal regulation of gastric emptying. Generally, secretin relaxes fundal and antral smooth muscle and contracts the pylorus, which may occur because secretin decreases the responsiveness of gastric smooth muscle to other neural and hormonal stimuli.

*Cholecystokinin (CCK).* Like secretin, CCK delays gastric emptying at very low doses and could also play a physiological role in the regulation of gastric emptying and secretion [53, 55]. Both hormones also suppress gastric secretion which could further decrease intragastric digestion, thereby delaying grinding and emptying of solid food. CCK may suppress emptying by inhibiting the spontaneous contraction of gastric muscle, or by increasing the contractility of antral circular muscles.

We recently evaluated the role of cholecystokinin (CCK) in the regulation of gastric emptying following four mixed solid-liquid meals in monkeys [56]. We administered 80 ml meals tagged with $^{99m}$Tc sulphur-colloid and $^{111}$In-DTPA to six rhesus monkeys and measured gastric emptying using scintigraphy. We determined plasma CCK before, 30, 60 and 90 min after the meals using a specific radioimmunoassay. After a 2 kcal/kg meal, emptying of solids was linear and emptying of liquids was faster and exponential, EGG amplitude increased only during the first 30 min after the meal ($P < 0.05$) and plasma CCK did not increase significantly. A carbohydrate-rich, isosmotic, 5 kcal/kg meal slowed emptying of solids and liquids and increased plasma CCK ($P<0.05$). A lipid-enriched, isosmotic, 5 kcal/kg meal also inhibited emptying and increased plasma CCK, but the effect was less than after the carbohydrate meal. A hyperosmotic, balanced, 5 kcal/kg meal slowed emptying similarly, but caused no significant change in plasma CCK. To determine the role of CCK in these postprandial responses, we administered the specific antagonist L-364,718 (i.v., 40 min before the meals) at 1 mg/kg, a dose that had abolished the inhibition of gastric emptying induced by a 70 min infusion of 4 ng.kg$^{-1}$.min$^{-1}$ of CCK-8. After isosmotic 5 kcal/kg meals, L-364,718 increased emptying and further increased plasma CCK after the 2 kcal/kg meal or after the hyperosmotic 5 kcal/kg meal. Thus, CCK appears to play a role in the effect of isosmotic, but not hyperosmotic, caloric meals on gastric emptying. In addition, L-364,718 enhances emptying of food energy into the duodenum, which could be responsible for the potentiation of postprandial plasma CCK release.

*Gastrin.* The gastrins and their analogue pentagastrin delay gastric emptying through relaxation of the fundus and contraction of the antrum [57, 58]. However, these actions occur only when high doses are administered, suggesting that gastrin may not play a physiological role in the regulation of gastric motility.

*Motilin* is the only gastrointestinal peptide that has been found to stimulate gastric emptying [59]. This action appears to result from a direct effect on the smooth muscles of both the proximal and the distal stomach. Plasma motilin concentrations are higher at the time of the initiation of the gastric migrating myoelectric complexes (MMC), but it is still unclear whether motilin initiates these MMCs or if the MMCs release motilin.

*Other hormones.* Vasoactive intestinal polypeptide, gastric inhibitory polypeptide, pancreatic polypeptide, and glucagon have been found to alter gastric smooth muscle activity but their physiological role in the regulation of gastric emptying is unknown. More studies will be needed before such a role can be established.

**Paracrine mechanisms**

Little is known about the effect of the release of local agents on gastric emptying. Prostaglandins of the E, F and I class(es) have been found in significant amounts in the stomach wall and in the gastric juice. Since prostaglandins have a major effect on gastric emptying, they could play a role in the physiological and pathological regulation of gastric motility [60].

# References

1. Rayl JE, Balison JR, Thomas HF, Woodward ER. Combined radiographic, manometric and histological localization of the canine lower esophageal sphincter. J Surg Res 1972;13:307-14.
2. Couturier D, Rozé C, Couturier-Turpin MH, Debray C. Electromyography of the colon *in situ*. An experimental study in man and in the rabbit. Gastroenterology 1969;56:317-22.
3. Abell TL, Malagelada JR. Glucagon-evoked gastric dysrhythmias in humans shown by an improved electrogastrographic technique. Gastroenterology 1985;88:1932-40.
4. Dubois A, Johnson LF. William Beaumont: frontier physician and founding father of gastric physiology. J Clin Gastroenterol 1985;7:472-4.
5. Cannon WB. The mechanical factors of digestion. In: Hill L, Bulloch W, eds. *International Medical Monographs*. New York: Longmans, Green & Co, 1911.
6. Bass P, Wiley JN. Contractile force transducer for recording muscle activity in unanesthetized animals. J Appl Physiol 1972;32:567-70.
7. Mendel C, Pousse A, Lambert A, Sava P, Grenier JF. Recording of canine intestinal chronic longitudinal movements. In: Christensen J, ed. *Proceedings of the 7th International Symposium on Gastrointestinal Motility*. New York: Raven Press, 1979:323-30.
8. You CH, Chey WY. Study of electromechanical activity of the stomach in humans and in dogs with particular attention to tachygastria. Gastroenterology 1984;86:1460-8.
9. Camilleri M, Malagelada JR, Brown ML, Becker G, Zinsmeister AR. Relation between antral motility and gastric emptying of solids and liquids in humans. Am J Physiol 1985;249:G580-5.
10. Alvarez WC. The electrogastrogram and what it shows. JAMA 1922;78;1116-9.
11. Martin A, Thillier JL. L'électro-gastroentérographie (E.GE.G). Press Med 1971;79:1235-7.
12. Brown BH, Smallwood RH, Duthie HL, Stoddard CJ. Intestinal smooth muscle electrical potentials recorded from surface electrodes. Med Biol Eng 1975;13:97-103.
13. Smout AJ, Van der Schee EJ, Grashuis JL. What is measured in electrogastrography? Dig Dis Sci 1980;25:179-87.
14. Bruley des Varannes S, Mizrahi M, Dubois A. Relation between postprandial gastric emptying and cutaneous electrogastrogram in primates. Am J Physiol (Gastrointest Liver Physiol) 1991;261 (in press).
15. Ewald CA, Boas J. Beitrage zur Physiologie und Pathologie der Verdauung. Virchows Arch Pathol Anat Physiol 1885;101:325-75.
16. Goldstein H, Boyle JD. The saline load test — a beside evaluation of gastric retention. Gastroenterology 1965;49:375-80.
17. Salamanca FE de, Jr. Las técnicas de exploración functional gàstrica aplicadas al estudio de la fisiología del perro. Medicina (Madr) 1950;18:308-61.
18. Hunt JN, Spurrell WR. The pattern of emptying of the human stomach. J Physiol (Lond) 1951;113:157-68.
19. Hildes JA, Dunlop DL. A method for estimating the rates of gastric secretion and emptying. Can J Med Sci 1951;29:83-9.
20. George JD. New clinical method for measuring the rate of gastric emptying: the double sampling test meal. Gut 1968;9:237-42.
21. Hunt JN. A modification to the method of George for studying gastric emptying. Gut 1974;15:812-3.
22. Dubois A, Van Erdewegh P, Gardner JD. Gastric emptying and secretion in Zollinger-Ellison syndrome. J Clin Invest 1977;59:255-63.
23. Dubois A, Dorval ED. Do we need to measure gastric output and how? Gastroenterology 1984;86:1631-2.
24. Go VL, Hofman AF, Summerskill WH. Simultaneous measurements of total pancreatic, biliary, and gastric outputs in man using a perfusion technique. Gastroenterology 1970;58:321-8.

25. MacGregor IL, Gueller R, Watts HD, Meyer JH. The effect of acute hyperglycemia on gastric emptying in man. Gastroenterology 1976;70:190-6.
26. Bernier JJ, Lebert A. Vitesse de l'évacuation de l'estomac et du duodénum au cours de l'hyperglycémie provoquée *per os*. Biol Gastroenterol (Paris) 1971;4:351-2.
27. Johansson C. Studies of gastrointestinal interactions. Scand J Gastroenterol 1974;9 (suppl 28):1-60.
28. Dillard RL, Eastman H, Fordtran JS. Volume-flow relationship during the transport of fluid through the human small intestine. Gastroenterology 1965;49:58-66.
29. Barreiro MA, McKenna RD, Beck IT. Determination of transit time in the human jejunum by the single injection indicator-dilution technic. Am J Dig Dis 1968;13:222-33.
30. Malagelada JR, Longstreth GF, Summerskill WH, Go VL. Measurement of gastric functions during digestion of ordinary solid meals in man. Gastroenterology 1976;70:203-10.
31. Dubois A. Methods for studying propulsion and retropulsion of the alimentary tract contents. In: Tichen DA, ed. *Techniques in the Life Sciences*. Amsterdam: Elsevier 1982;P202/1-18.
32. Stordy SN, Greig JH, Bogoch A. The steak and barium meal: a method for evaluating gastric emptying after partial gastrectomy. Am J Dig Dis 1969;14:463-9.
33. Raskin HF. Barium-burger roentgen study for unrecognized, clinically significant, gastric retention. South Med J 1971;64:1227-35.
34. Hinton JM, Lennard-Jones JE, Young AC. A new method for studying gut transit times using radioopaque markers. Gut 1969;10:842-7.
35. Bertrand J, Metman EH, Dorval ED, Rouleau P, D'Hueppe A, Itti R, Philippe L. Etude du temps d'évaluation gastrique de repas normaux au moyen de granules radio-opaques. Applications cliniques et validation. Gastroenterol Clin Biol 1980;4:770-6.
36. Griffith GH, Owen GM, Campbell H, Shields R. Gastric emptying in health and gastroduodenal disease. Gastroenterology 1968;54:1-7.
37. Chaudhuri TK. Use of $^{99m}$Tc-DTPA for measuring gastric emptying time. J Nucl Med 1974;15:391-5.
38. Heading RC, Tothill P, McLoughlin GP, Shearman DJ. Gastric emptying rate measurement in man. A double isotope scanning technique for simultaneous study of liquid and solid components of a meal. Gastroenterology 1976;71:45-50.
39. Meyer JH, MacGregor IL, Gueller R, Martin P, Cavalieri R. $^{99m}$Tc-tagged chicken liver as a marker of solid food in the human stomach. Am J Dig Dis 1976;21:296-304.
40. Tothill P, McLoughlin GP, Heading RC. Techniques and errors in scintigraphic measurements of gastric emptying. J Nucl Med 1978;19:256-61.
41. Szurszewski JH. Electrical basis for gastrointestinal motility. In: Johnson LR, ed. *Physiology of the Gastrointestinal Tract*, New York: Raven Press, 1987:383-422.
42. Sarna SK. *In vivo* myoelectric activity: methods, analysis and interpretation. In: Wood JD ed. *Handbook of Physiology, Gastrointestinal Motility and Circulation*. Bethesda: Am Physiol Soc, 1988.
43. Code CF, Marlett JA. The interdigestive myoelectric complex of the stomach and small bowel of dogs. J Physiol (Lond) 1975;246:289-309.
44. Gill RC, Pilot MA, Thomas PA, Wingate DL. Effect of feeding on motor activity of canine stomach. Dig Dis Sci 1989;34:865-72.
45. Rees WD, Go VL, Malagelada JR. Antroduodenal motor response to solid-liquid and homogenized meals. Gastroenterology 1979;76:1438-42.
46. Thompson DG, Richelson E, Malagelada JR. Perturbation of gastric emptying and duodenal motility through the central nervous system. Gastroenterology 1982;83:1200-6.
47. Dubois A. The Stomach. In: Wingate DL, Christensen J, eds. *A guide to Gastrointestinal Motility*. London: John Wright and Sons Ltd, 1983:101-27.
48. Hunt JN, Spurrell WR. The pattern of emptying of the human stomach. J Physiol (Lond) 1951;113:157-68.

49. Hinder RA, Kelly KA. Canine gastric emptying of solids and liquids. Am J Physiol 1977;233:E335-40.
50. Hunt JN, Stubbs DF. The volume and energy content of meals as determinants of gastric emptying. J Physiol (Lond) 1975;245:209-25.
51. Hunt JN. Regulation of gastric emptying by neurohumoral factors and by gastric and duodenal receptors. In: Dubois A, Castell DO, eds. *Esophageal and Gastric Emptying.* Boca Raton: CRC Press, 1984:65-71.
52. Davison JS. Innervation of the gastrointestinal tract. In: Wingate DL, Christensen J, eds. *A guide to Gastrointestinal Motility.* London: John Wright and Sons Ltd, 1983:1-47.
53. Chey WY, Hitanant S, Hendricks J, Lorber SH. Effect of secretin and cholecystokinin on gastric emptying and gastric secretion in man. Gastroenterology 1970;58:820-7.
54. Kleibeuker JH, Beekhuis H, Piers DA, Schaffalitzky de Muckadell OB. Retardation of gastric emptying of solid food by secretin. Gastroenterology 1988;94;122-6.
55. Debas HT, Farooq O, Grossman MI. Inhibition of gastric emptying is a physiological action of cholecystokinin. Gastroenterology 1975;68:1211-7.
56. Dubois A, Bruley S, Mizrahi M, Fiala N, Solomon T, Turkelson C. Role of cholecystokinin in the regulation of gastric function after caloric meals. Gastroenterology 1991;100: A439(abstr).
57. Hunt JN, Ramsbottom N. Effect of gastrin II on gastric emptying and secretion during a test meal. Br Med J 1967;4:386-7.
58. Cooke AR, Chvasta TE, Weisbrodt NW. Effect of pentagastrin on emptying and electrical motor activity of the dog stomach. Am J Physiol 1972;223:934-8.
59. Debas HT, Yamagishi Y, Dryburgh JR. Motilin enhances gastric emptying of liquids in dogs. Gastroenterology 1977;73:777-80.
60. Dubois A. E prostaglandins and the stomach. Pathophysiological mediators or therapeutic agents? In: Samuelsson B, Ramwell PW, Paoletti R, eds. *Advances in Prostaglandin and Thromboxane Research.* Volume 8. New York: Raven Press, 1980:1581-6.

# 4

# Sensory visceral innervation

C. ROZÉ

*INSERM U. 239, 16 rue Henri Huchard, 75018 Paris, France*

During the last decades, it has progressively been realized that sensory nerves connecting the gastrointestinal system to the central nervous system (CNS) were much more numerous than had previously been thought. This new view arose mainly from morphological studies combining degeneration experiments with electron microscopy of transverse sections of peripheral nerves such as the vagus. It then appeared that the number of small-diameter, unmyelinated fibres had been grossly underestimated, and that at least 80% of fibres in the abdominal vagus were afferent fibres [1, 2]. This, together with similar observations on sympathetic nerves (although the proportion of afferent fibres is smaller), led to a new concept of the organization of the gut-brain relationships, in which a large number of afferent fibres, originating in the gut, convey messages towards several hierarchically arranged integrative centres: prevertebral ganglia, spinal cord, medulla oblongata and brain. The many afferent signals are processed in these different centres, and the appropriate commands are conveyed back to the gut through the classical sympathetic and parasympathetic motor pathways, by a comparatively small number of motor and/or secretory fibres.

We shall summarize in this chapter some methods allowing the study of sensory neurones, and the main receptors and sensory pathways that are involved in the normal gut function, focusing primarily upon sensory innervation of stomach and small intestine.

## Methods for the study of sensory neurones

### Morphology

Electron microscopy allows the precise determination of the true number of small diameter unmyelinated fibres in peripheral nerves such as the vagus. The fibres can be classified in terms of diameter and conduction velocity as myelinated A α (20-12 μ), A β and A γ (12-5 μ), A δ (5-2 μ), myelinated B (<3 μ) and unmyelinated C (<1.2 μ). Since most sensory fibres from the gut are unmyelinated, and tightly wrapped up into Schwann cells, only electron microscopy, combined with degeneration experiments after appropriate sections, allows their correct counting and classification as sensory or motor.

The study of receptor morphology has yielded less information, since most sensory terminals in the gut appear to be free nerve endings. The membrane of sensory endings is expected to possess certain specific receptors, channels or enzymes supporting their sensory function, but these are so far unknown and still undetectable by present methods.

Immunocytochemistry, combined with degeneration experiments, has enabled us to identify the main peptide transmitters or modulators present in afferent neurones and to trace their pathways. Among these, the most abundantly represented are substance P (SP), other tachykinins (neurokinin A, neuropeptide K), and calcitonin-gene-related peptide (CGRP) [3, 4]. Several peptides are usually associated within the same neurone, and the relationship between the immunocytochemical fingerprint of each sensory neurone with its physiological function is generally not known.

Anterograde and retrograde axonal transport [5] has been extensively used to trace the pathways and projections of sensory neurones. Horseradish peroxidase, which is transported in neurones by fast axonal flow, has been shown to be very useful in this prospect, either alone or associated with a lectin such as wheat germ agglutinin, which adheres to membrane glycoproteins of nerve terminals and is taken up in large amounts by endocytosis. Diagrams such as those illustrated in Figure 1 can be obtained with such methods.

**Physiology**

Most data concerning intestinal receptors and their function have been obtained by recording neural activity with electrodes placed on afferent fibres or in the close vicinity of nerve cell bodies of the large T-shaped primary sensory neurones in sensory ganglia. Dissection and recording from single fibres in the peripheral end of a visceral nerve after section was first undertaken by Adrian [6], and then by many others [7-11]. Recording in sensory ganglia such as the nodose ganglia with extracellular microelectrodes [12] is especially suitable for recording the activity of unmyelinated neurones. Intracellular recording with microelectrodes has been used to record from neurones in the myenteric, prevertebral and spinal ganglia [13, 14]. The main drawback of these methods is that they necessitate anaesthesia of the animals, so they can be used in acute conditions only. The method of crossed nerve suture has been proposed to allow chronic studies in awake animals. Its principle lies in the reinnervation of a motor nerve destined to a striated muscle by the central ends of sensory neurones (or alternatively by the peripheral end of motor neurones). However, on sensory neurones few data have been published using this method [15].

Destruction and stimulation of peripheral or central parts of the central nervous system have also produced interesting results. Selective destruction or stimulation of sensory fibres is generally difficult. However, the use of capsaicin, a neurotoxin extracted from the hot red pepper, has recently shed some light on the function of some sensory neurones in the digestive tract. Capsaicin seems remarkably specific for a subpopulation of primary sensory neurones and can induce stimulation or destruction of these neurones according to the dose.

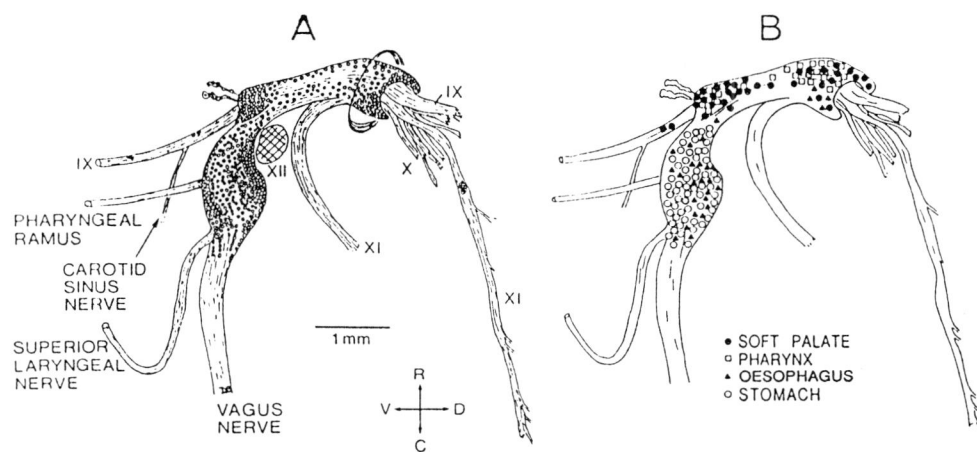

**Figure 1.** Tracing of cell bodies of sensory neurones innervating the pharynx and upper gut in the nodose ganglion of the rat. **A.** Anatomical arrangement of the right sensory ganglionic mass of the IXth and Xth cranial nerves. The position of the XIIth nerve is indicated in cross-section. Distribution of sensory perikarya (cell bodies) in the ganglia is indicated by open circles (methylene blue staining). A continuous series of perikarya bridges the inferior ganglion (nodose) of the Xth nerve with the superior and inferior ganglia of the IXth and with the superior ganglion of the Xth nerve. The opening of the jugular foramen is indicated schematically near the proximal end of the ganglion cell mass. **B.** After injection of wheat germ agglutinin - horseradish peroxidase (WGA-HRP) in various parts of the upper digestive tract, labelled perikarya occur following the retrograde transport of WGA-HRP. Sensory neurones innervating the stomach are confined to the nodose ganglion, whereas those innervating the oesophagus are found in both the nodose ganglion and the postero-medial glossopharyngeal vagal cuff. (Orientation arrows: R: rostral, C: caudal, V: ventral, D: dorsal). (From ref. [50], with permission).

## Receptor types and functions

Sensory endings able to detect a great variety of physical and chemical parameters have been described functionally in the gut. Morphologically they consist in ramified free and thin nerve endings issuing out of the Schwann cell sheath. They can for clarity be divided in mechanoreceptors sensitive to pressure, tension, pinch, etc., chemoreceptors, detecting the presence and concentration of a variety of chemicals, and other receptors such as thermoreceptors and polymodal receptors sensitive to various chemical and physical stimuli including osmolality (Table I).

**Table I.** Receptors in the digestive tract: location and fibre pathway. Extensive references concerning each receptor type will be found in [16].

| Receptors | Location | Fibre pathway |
|---|---|---|
| **Mechanoreceptors** | | |
| Muscular | Oesophagus, GI tract, colon, gallbladder | Vagus |
| | Colon, rectum | Pelvic |
| | GI tract | Splanchnic |
| Mucosal | Oesophagus, GI tract | Vagus |
| | Colon, rectum | Pelvic |
| Serosal | Mesentery (LES, pylorus) | Vagus |
| | Mesentery (intestine, gallbladder) | Splanchnic |
| Pacinian corpuscles | Mesentery | Splanchnic |
| **Chemoreceptors** | | |
| Alkali and acid | GI mucosa | Vagus |
| Glucoreceptors (glucose and other carbohydrates) | Gastric and intestinal mucosa | Vagus |
| | Intestinal mucosa | Splanchnic |
| Amino acid receptors | Intestinal mucosa | Vagus |
| Fatty acid receptors | Intestinal mucosa | Vagus |
| **Thermoreceptors** | | |
| Cold | Oesophageal and GI mucosa | Vagus |
| Warmth | Oesophageal and GI mucosa | Vagus |
| Cold, warmth | Oesophageal and GI mucosa | Vagus |
| **Polymodal receptors** (mechanical, thermal, chemical, osmotic stimulation) | GI mucosa | Vagus |

## Mechanoreceptors

They are usually separated in two major groups: slowly adapting, and rapidly adapting mechanoreceptors [16].

*Slowly adapting mechanoreceptors.* These can be activated by various events such as distension, contraction or stretch, that occur during normal gut function, and produce pressure or volume changes. This kind of nerve unit discharges regularly as long as the mechanical stimulation is maintained. Slowly adapting mechanoreceptors have a low triggering threshold, so that many of them are spontaneously active in normal conditions. Most of them are located in the gut muscle and they have been previously referred to as "in series" tension receptors, but this terminology is probably inadequate. Some slowly adapting mechanoreceptors are also found in the gut serosa.

***Rapidly adapting mechanoreceptors.*** These usually have a high stimulation threshold, so that they are not spontaneously active in normal conditions. They are mainly found in mucosa and serosa, and stop firing shortly after the beginning of the stimulation. Some of them show an "off" response. Pacinian corpuscles of the mesentery belong to this category, and are connected centrally by $A\beta$ myelinated fibres, the largest diameter visceral fibres.

## Chemoreceptors

Several types of digestive chemoreceptors are now known. They are located in the mucosa, immediately beneath the epithelial cells, and correspond to one of several classes: acid- and alkaline-sensitive in the stomach and intestine [17, 18], glucoreceptors with various sensitivities to glucose and other sugars [19-21], receptors for amino acids [22], and fatty acids [23]. Most of these are specific in the sense that they pulse in response to a single substance, or a single group of substances; their response usually increases with the concentration, indicating a dose-response behaviour. Some others (part of the pH- and amino acid-sensitive units) are less specific since they are responsive to several classes of substances. Finally some of them are polymodal (see below).

## Other receptors

***Thermoreceptors.*** Receptors to cold, warm, and mixed receptors, have been demonstrated in the oesophagus, stomach and small intestine [24, 25]. These receptors respond to temperature changes, which are especially likely to occur in the stomach (where temperatures of 20° C and 44° C have been measured after ice-cold or hot drinks [26]).

***Osmoreceptors*** had been postulated from the work of Hunt's group on gastric emptying [27]. Some mucosal receptors in the stomach and small intestine [28, 29] have been shown to respond to several hypo- and hypertonic solutions, and to plain water, and were at first described as osmoreceptors. However, other factors such as the chemical nature and the molecular weight of the solutes also intervene [30]. This suggests that these receptors are not true "osmoreceptors", but rather polymodal receptors, i.e. a class of receptors able to discharge in response to various chemical as well as physical (mechanical and thermal) stimuli.

***Are there nociceptors?*** Before the detailed description of diverse chemo- and mechanoreceptors in the gastrointestinal tract, the idea prevailed that free sensory nerve endings without morphological specialization might be equivalent to somatic nociceptors. These free endings would not be activated by the normal events in the gut, but, due to their high threshold, they would be activated during unusually high mechanical or chemical stimulation, then inducing discomfort and pain. In that sense, mucosal and serosal receptors that adapt rapidly and have high thresholds resemble nociceptors, as well as high threshold polymodal receptors. On the other hand, the presence of specialized nociceptors is not absolutely necessary to explain the facts. In nocuous circumstances, intense and abnormal stimulation of a series of receptors that are normally activated by stimuli of lower intensity may produce an overall activity that differs significantly from that found in normal circumstances. Thus, the amount of stimulation and the diffusion of stimulation to neighbouring structures (for example in the spinal cord) may both induce diffuse noxious sensations and the somatic projections that are well-known in visceral pain.

## Afferent neural pathways

The main pathways and projections of sensory neurones of the gut are summarized in Figure 2.

### Local (intrinsic) projections

Local sensory neurones within the enteric nervous system are less well-defined than extrinsic (for example vagal) sensory neurones. The presence of sensory neurones in the enteric nervous system is attested by the peristaltic reflex that functions in an isolated segment of intestine. Thus, local stimulation of sensory endings can evoke both anal relaxation and oral contraction of the gut. The reflexes that are initiated by stimuli applied to the mucosa and those initiated by radial stretch have similar characteristics. Thus, it seems straightforward to postulate two sensory inputs to each of two common motor neurones: the enteric excitatory motor neurone and the enteric inhibitory motor neurone [3]. Cell bodies of the sensory neurones are located in the myenteric plexus (at least in the guinea-pig intestine). It is not known, however, whether the same or different sensory neurones activate the excitatory and inhibitory motor neurones, nor whether they synapse directly or through one or several interneurones.

Electrophysiological studies with extracellular microelectrodes made it possible to record mechanosensitive units in the myenteric ganglia, which display slowly adapting, rapidly adapting, and tonic discharge characteristics [13]. The mechanosensitive activity that can be recorded at the myenteric ganglia does not originate from mechanoreceptors located within the mucosa. It seems that the most probable location of the generator region of these deep tension receptors is within the periganglionic connective tissue [13]. Some of the units recorded may correspond to sensory neurones and others to interneurones.

### Vagal sensory neurones

Primary sensory neurones innervating the gastrointestinal area and travelling via the vagus nerve are T-shaped cells, the cell bodies of which are located within the nodose ganglia. The long peripheral process (bringing messages from the gut) and the shorter central process (projecting upon the nucleus tractus solitarius (NTS) in the medulla oblongata) are both now considered as axons [31].

Most fibres (>80%) in the abdominal vagus are sensory, small diameter unmyelinated C axons. They travel mixed with the motor fibres, but some separation

## Sensory visceral innervation

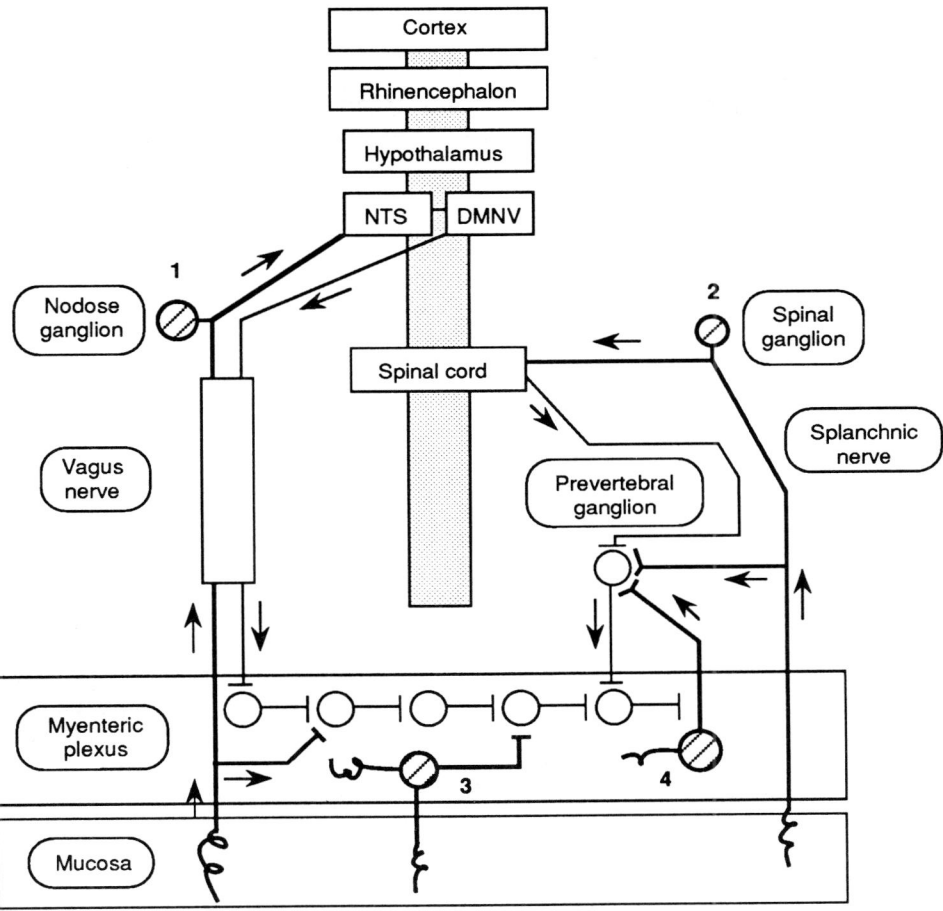

**Figure 2.** Main neural pathways connecting the digestive tract and the central nervous system. NTS= nucleus tractus solitarius; DMNV=dorsal motor nucleus of the vagus. The cell bodies of sensory neurones are symbolized by hatched circles. **1.** Vagal sensory neurone. A branching pattern is schematized at the sensory terminal of this neurone. This may be the anatomical basis for "axon reflexes": depolarization induced by activation of the sensory ending may depolarize another branch of the neurone, inducing transmitter release near to a neurone (illustrated) or another structure (i.e. vessel, secretory cell). This type of branching may occur for every kind of gut sensory neurone. **2.** "Sympathetic" sensory neurone **3.** Intrinsic sensory neurone responsible for organization of the peristaltic reflex. The effector neurones (excitatory and inhibitory) innervating gut muscle are not represented. **4.** Intrinsic neurone conveying sensory information to the prevertebral sympathetic ganglia.

between motor and sensory fibres exists within the nodose ganglia, at least in species such as the pig, sheep, and cat, in which motor fibres form distinct ventral bundles [32, 33].

The central process usually has a smaller diameter than the peripheral process; in the nodose ganglion, the incoming influx depolarizes first the peripheral process, then the stem process and the cell body, and probably simultaneously the central process. It seems that some modulation of the incoming influxes can occur at the level of the cell body and the stem process within the ganglion, by several mechanisms. These include: electrotonic influence by field potential of other active neighbouring cell bodies, inhibition by synaptic influences from fibres impinging upon the cell body or the stem process, chemical modulation by locally released substances (5HT, substance P, etc.).

Within the nodose ganglia, ganglion cells form clusters surrounded by a fibre network. Some grouping of ganglion cells occurs according to their site of origin: pulmonary, cardiovascular and gastrointestinal areas have been described within the nodose ganglia [34].

**Sensory neurones travelling in sympathetic nerves**

No clear distinction can be drawn between the functions of sensory neurones with axons travelling in the parasympathetic vagal and pelvic nerves, or in splanchnic nerves. However, it is generally agreed that sympathetic neurons are mostly responsible for the painful sensations originating in the viscera. Primary neurons travelling in the splanchnic nerves have their cell body located in the dorsal root ganglion. Apart from a few exceptions, afferent fibres enter the spinal cord by the dorsal root, so there is an anatomical separation of sensory and motor fibres at this level. Section of dorsal roots will therefore destroy only the sensory components of sympathetic nerves. A large segmental dispersion occurs, since at least the T6 to T12 roots participate in the formation of splanchnic nerves, depending upon the species.

This pathway contains primary sensory neurones analogous to the previously described vagal neurones, conducting information from several sorts of free endings (muscular and serosal mechanoreceptors, mucosal glucoreceptors, serosal thermoreceptors) and from Pacinian corpuscles localized in the mesentery.

Apart from these neurones directly connecting the gut and mesentery to the spinal cord, immunohistochemical techniques combined with degeneration studies have shown several kinds of neurochemically defined fibres projecting from the gut to the prevertebral ganglia. Neurotransmitters detected in these fibres in the guinea-pig small intestine include CCK, dynorphin, enkephalins, GRP and VIP. Since systematic double staining studies have shown that these five substances are colocalized in a single group of neurones of the myenteric plexus [3], it is likely that these neurones represent either sensory neurones or interneurones that convey information to prevertebral ganglia. Physiological experiments have shown that prevertebral ganglia represent an important integrative centre participating in the control of the final tone of noradrenergic motor neurones destined for the gut [35], and it is thus essential that afferent information from the gut receptors is transmitted to the prevertebral ganglia.

**Central projections**

The input point of vagal afferent gastrointestinal information into the brain is the NTS. Primary neurones of spinal ganglia first connect with secondary neurones in the dorsal horn of the medulla, which are in fact somato-sensory neurones, receiving inputs from both visceral and somatic (mainly nociceptive and polymodal) primary afferents. These secondary neurones run to the brain through the spinothalamic or spinoreticular bundles. Ascending projections, involving a number of interneurones, involve the hypothalamus, rhinencephalon and cortex. In addition, a direct connection of the NTS to the dorsal motor nucleus of the vagus has also been demonstrated, allowing direct control of efferent vagal fibres by afferent ones. These diverse projections allow the afferent information to be processed and elaborated in terms of secretory, motor and behavioural effector functions. Multiple descending pathways have been found that can modulate efferent function: for example, there are cortical projections to the NTS, and to the midbrain areas involved in the regulation of descending pain modulating systems such as the periaqueductal grey, which themselves can modulate the activity of the secondary afferent spinal neurones.

Gastrointestinal information is not only relevant to gastrointestinal motility and secretion. Some divergence occurs between digestive and non-digestive regulation. Gastric distension, for instance, produces an increase in blood pressure [36, 37]. It has also been shown that physiological information coming from different visceral receptors (i.e. gastric mechanoreceptors and hepatic glucoreceptors) may converge onto the same neurone in the dorsal motor nucleus of the vagus [38]. Thus both convergence and divergence in the CNS are essential mechanisms contributing to the final elaboration of complex reflexes and behaviours.

**Local transmitter release by sensory neurones**

Sensory endings in the gut were seen at first as a receptive and afferent system whose function was limited to the elaboration of centripetal influxes. This concept was questioned, however, when it was found (more than a century ago) that antidromic stimulation of the peripheral stump of transected dorsal roots or sensory nerves induced vasodilatation and other signs of inflammation in the skin [4]. In the last twenty years, evidence has accumulated that sensory neurones may not only serve a sensory role, but also take part in local effector systems in regulating blood flow, vascular permeability, trophic and immunological processes, and smooth muscle contractility. This probably occurs through the common innervation of several peripheral structures by branches of the same sensory neurone. This particular branching pattern allows the local release of regulatory transmitters such as substance P and other neuropeptides by one branch of the neurone following activation of the sensory ending of another branch ("axon reflex"). Transmitters may probably even be released by the sensory branch itself following its activation. It should also be realized that the sensory endings possess neurotransmitter receptors and can be excited by substances issued from neighbouring cells. Various mediators and neurotransmitters (acetylcholine, bradykinin, substance P, serotonin, etc.) have been shown to activate some types of gut sensory fibres.

**Information derived from capsaicin experiments**

Few methods are available to selectively excite or destroy gut sensory fibres in conscious animals. Capsaicin (8-methyl-N-vanillyl-6-nonenamide), a pungent ingredient found in a variety of red peppers of the genus *Capsicum*, acts as a selective neurotoxin for some afferent neurones. Most experiments with this drug have been carried out in small rodents (rats, mice, guinea pigs). At low doses (in the µg/kg range), capsaicin exerts a powerful excitatory effect on peripheral sensory endings, this effect being apparently confined to unmyelinated afferent C fibres. Although the precise mechanism of capsaicin excitation has not yet been determined, some evidence suggests that an increase in conductance to calcium ions may be involved. Excitation is soon followed by desensitization to the drug and by a block of nerve conduction which is also seen after local application of capsaicin to peripheral axons. Systemic administration of high doses (in the mg/kg range) has a definitely neurotoxic effect on a population of sensory neurones, the extent of damage depending on the dosage, route of administration, animal species and age of the animals. The most extensive and consistent lesions are produced by the systemic treatment of newborn rats: a single dose of 50 mg/kg capsaicin results in a permanent loss, by degeneration, of 50-90% of all unmyelinated afferent fibres. The value of capsaicin as a pharmacological tool is critically dependent upon the specificity of its action on sensory neurones. There is thus far no clear-cut evidence that capsaicin has direct excitatory or neurotoxic actions on non-sensory neurones, in the dosage conditions described above. Capsaicin sensitive sensory neurones represent only one part of sensory neurones, and cannot yet be equated with any group of afferents classified by morphological or functional criteria. Neurochemically, capsaicin induces a depletion of substance P and of a number of other transmitters: GRP (gastrin releasing peptide), CGRP, CCK (cholecystokinin), galanin, neurokinin A, neuropeptide K, somatostatin, VIP (vasoactive intestinal peptide). Even with increasing capsaicin doses, not all substance P afferents are destroyed, indicating that only a subpopulation of sensory fibres is capsaicin sensitive.

There is evidence that capsaicin-sensitive neurones innervate the gastrointestinal tract [39], whereas, fortunately, capsaicin appears to lack any action on enteric neurones. Afferent nerve endings seem to have vascular and motility effects on the alimentary canal, by axon reflexes or through the more complex intervention of the enteric nervous system. In the stomach and intestine, the vascular effects of activation of afferents or administration of substance P include vasodilatation, but not increase in vascular permeability inducing protein extravasation [40].

Intragastric application of capsaicin enhances blood flow in the mucosa of the rat stomach [41-43] and this effect is probably involved in the apparent participation of capsaicin-sensitive sensory neurones to gastric mucosal defence mechanisms. Indeed, ablation of capsaicin sensitive neurones aggravates gastric lesions in a variety of experimental ulcer models [44], whereas activation of capsaicin-sensitive nerve endings in the rat gastric mucosa by low dose capsaicin affords protection against ulcerogenic factors [43]. This sensory-nerve-mediated protection of gastric mucosa might be primarily due to the release of protective factors from afferent nerve endings in the stomach. An increase in mucosal blood flow would be an effective mechanism for this protection. Among the possible candidates, tachykinins, CGRP, somatostatin and CRF have been shown to increase mucosal blood flow. Somatostatin and CGRP have in fact been shown to protect the rat stomach from lesion formation [45, 46].

Apart from their intervention in the regulation of gastric mucosal blood flow, capsaicin-sensitive neurones have been shown to participate in certain effects of CCK. CCK8 decreases food intake in the rat and this effect was attenuated after capsaicin pretreatment [47]. CCK8 also decreases gastric motility in the gastric corpus and delays gastric emptying by acting upon capsaicin sensitive vagal afferent fibres [48]. However, vagal sensory fibres are not all capsaicin sensitive: it is possible, in rats, to record with microelectrodes the activity of neurones in the dorsal motor nucleus of the vagus which pulse in response to gastric distension or after nearby intra-arterial injection of bombesin in the stomach wall. These responses are capsaicin insensitive [49], suggesting that peripheral afferents which are activated by CCK8 and bombesin are different, although both peptides are able to suppress food intake.

## Summary and conclusion

The digestive tract is abundantly innervated by afferent neurones which convey information from a series of receptors to integrative neural centres. The receptors include mechanoreceptors, chemoreceptors, thermoreceptors and polymodal receptors. Whether true nociceptors exist in the gut is a debated question. However, high threshold polymodal receptors that are unlikely to fire under physiological conditions might be candidates for this function.

Sensory neurones are intrinsic and extrinsic. Intrinsic neurones regulate peristaltic reflexes, and some of them project to prevertebral ganglia. The cell bodies of extrinsic sensory neurones are located in cervical and spinal ganglia, and their axons travel in the vagus, pelvic and splanchnic nerves. Information is processed at several levels: prevertebral ganglia, spinal cord, medulla oblongata, hypothalamus, rhinencephalon, cortex. Convergence and divergence of information at these levels explain why digestive afferences participate in elaboration of complex digestive, vascular and behavioural responses.

## References

1. Agostoni E, Chinnock JE, Daly de Burgh M, Murray JG. Functional and histological studies on the vagus nerve and its branches to the heart, lungs and abdominal viscera in the cat. J Physiol (Lond) 1957;135:182-205.
2. Mei N, Condamin M, Boyer A. The composition of the vagus nerve of the cat. Cell Tissue Res 1980; 209:423-31.
3. Furness JB, Costa M. *The Enteric Nervous System*. Edinburgh: Churchill Livingstone, 1987.
4. Holzer P. Local effector functions of capsaicin-sensitive sensory nerve endings: involvement of tachykinins, calcitonin gene-related peptide and other neuropeptides. Neuroscience 1988;24:739-68.
5. Hammerschlag R, Brady ST. Axonal transport and the neuronal cytoskeleton. In: Siegel GJ, ed. *Basic Neurochemistry: Molecular, Cellular, and Medical Aspects*. 4th ed. New York: Raven Press, 1989:457-78.
6. Adrian ED. Afferent impulses in the vagus nerve endings. J Physiol (Lond) 1933;61:49-72.
7. Niijima A. Afferent impulse discharges from glucoreceptors in the liver of the guinea pig. Ann N Y Acad Sci 1969;157:690-700.
8. Paintal AS. Vagal sensory receptors and their reflex effects. Physiol Rev 1973;53:159-227.
9. Iggo A. Gastrointestinal tension receptors with unmyelinated afferent fibres in the vagus. Q J Exp Physiol 1957;42:130-41.
10. Andrews PL, Grundy D, Scratcherd T. Vagal afferent discharge from mechanoreceptors in different regions of the ferret stomach. J Physiol (Lond) 1980;298:513-24.
11. Sharkey KA, Cervero F. An *in vitro* method for recording single unit afferent activity from mesenteric nerves innervating isolated segments of rat ileum. J Neurosci Methods 1986;16:149-56.

12. Mei N. Enregistrement de l'activité unitaire des afférences vagales. Réception par microélectrodes au niveau du ganglion plexiforme. Ann Biol Anim Biochim Biophys 1962;2:361-4.
13. Wood JD. Physiology of the enteric nervous system. In: Johnson LR, ed. *Physiology of the Gastrointestinal Tract*. Volume 1. 2nd ed. New York: Raven Press, 1987:67-110.
14. Julé Y, Krier J, Szurszewski JH. Patterns of innervation of neurones of the inferior mesenteric ganglion of the cat. J Physiol (Lond) 1983;344:293-304.
15. Falempin M, Mei N, Rousseau JP. Vagal mechanoreceptors of the inferior thoracic oesophagus, the lower oesophageal sphincter and the stomach in the sheep. Pflugers Arch 1978;373:25-30.
16. Mei N. Sensory structures in the viscera. In: Ottoson D, ed. *Progress in Sensory Physiology*. Volume 4, Berlin: Springer Verlag, 1983:1-42.
17. Iggo A. Gastric mucosal receptors with vagal afferent fibres in the cat. Q J Exp Physiol 1957;42:398-409.
18. Andrews CJ, Andrews WH. Receptors, activated by acid, in the duodenal wall of rabbits. Q J Exp Physiol Cogn Med Sci 1971;56:221-30.
19. Sharma KN, Nasset ES. Electrical activity in mesenteric nerves after perfusion of gut lumen. Am J Physiol 1962;202:725-30.
20. Hardcastle J, Hardcastle PT, Sanford PA. Effect of actively transported hexoses on afferent nerve discharge from rat small intestine. J Physiol (Lond) 1978;285:71-84.
21. Mei N. Vagal glucoreceptors in the small intestine of the cat. J Physiol (Lond) 1978;282:485-506.
22. Jeanningros R. Vagal unitary responses to intestinal amino acid infusion in the anesthetized cat: a putative signal for protein-induced satiety. Physiol Behav 1962;28:9-21.
23. Melone J. Vagal receptors sensitive to lipids in the small intestine of the cat. J Auton Nev Syst 1986;17:231-41.
24. Gupta BN, Nier K, Hensel H. Cold sensitive afferents from the abdomen. Pflugers Arch 1979;380:203-4.
25. El Ouazzani T, Mei N. Electrophysiological properties and role of the vagal thermoreceptors of lower esophagus and stomach of cat. Gastroenterology 1982;83:995-1001.
26. Mei N. Propriétés et rôle des fibres sensitives et des intérocepteurs digestifs. In: Encyclopédie Médico-Chirurgicale, Nutrition: Digestion et absorption. Paris: Masson 1984;10351 A10:1-6.
27. Hunt JN, Knox MT. Regulation of gastric emptying. In: *Handbook of Physiology, Alimentary Canal*. Volume 4. Washington: Am Physiol Soc, 1968:1917-35.
28. Leek BF. Abdominal and pelvic visceral receptors. Br Med Bull 1977;33:163-8.
29. Clarke GD, Davison JS. Mucosal receptors in the gastric antrum and small intestine of the rat with afferent fibres in the cervical vagus. J Physiol (Lond) 1978;284:55-67.
30. Garnier L, Mei N. Do true osmoreceptors exist at intestinal level? J Physiol (Lond) 1982;327:97P-98P.
31. Mei N. La sensibilité viscérale. J Physiol (Paris) 1981;77:597-612.
32. Darcy B, Falempin M, Laplace JP, Rousseau JP. Importance de la voie vagale sensitive: recherche d'une technique de déafférentation sélective chez le porc et le mouton. Ann Biol Anim Biochim Biophys 1979;19:881-8.
33. Mei N. Existence d'une séparation anatomique des fibres vagales efférentes et afférentes au niveau du ganglion plexiforme du chat. J Physiol (Paris) 1966;58:253-4.
34. Mei N. Mécanorécepteurs vagaux cardio-vasculaires et respiratoires chez le chat. Exp Brain Res 1970;11:480-501.
35. Szurszewski JH, Weems WA. A study of peripheral input to and its control by postganglionic neurones of the inferior mesenteric ganglion. J Physiol (Lond) 1976;256:541-56.
36. Pozo F, Fueyo A, Esteban MM, Rojo-Ortega JM, Marin B. Blood pressure changes after gastric mechanical and electrical stimulation in rats. Am J Physiol 1985;249:G739-44.

37. Pittam BS, Ewart WR, Appia F, Wingate DL. Physiological enteric stimulation elicits cardiovascular reflexes in the rat. Am J Physiol 1988;255:G319-28.
38. Appia F, Ewart WR, Pittam BS, Wingate DL. Convergence of sensory information from abdominal viscera in the rat brain stem. Am J Physiol 1986;251:G169-75.
39. Holzer P, Schluet W, Lippe IT, Sametz W. Involvement of capsaicin-sensitive sensory neurons in gastrointestinal function. Acta Physiol Hung 1987;69:403-11.
40. Lundberg JM, Brodin E, Hua X, Saria A. Vascular permeability changes and smooth muscle contraction in relation to capsaicin-sensitive substance P afferents in the guinea pig. Acta Physiol Scand 1984;120:217-27.
41. Limlomwongse L, Chaitauchawong C, Tongyai S. Effect of capsaicin on gastric acid secretion and mucosal blood flow in the rat. J Nutr 1979;109:773-7.
42. Lippe IT, Pabst MA, Holzer P. Intragastric capsaicin enhances rat gastric acid elimination and mucosal blood flow by afferent nerve stimulation. Br J Pharmacol 1989;96:91-100.
43. Holzer P, Pabst MA, Lippe IT, Peskar BM, Peskar BA, Livingston EH, Guth PH. Afferent nerve-mediated protection against deep mucosal damage in the rat stomach.Gastroenterology 1990;98:838-48.
44. Holzer P, Sametz W. Gastric mucosal protection against ulcerogenic factors in the rat mediated by capsaicin-sensitive afferent neurons. Gastroenterology 1986;91:975-81.
45. Maggi CA, Evangelista S, Giuliani S, Meli A. Anti-ulcer activity of calcitonin gene-related peptide in rats. Gen Pharmacol 1987;18:33-4.
46. Moreau JP, De Feudis FV. Pharmacological studies of somatostatin and somatostatin analogues: therapeutic advances and perspectives. Life Sci 1987;40:419-37.
47. Ritter RC, Ladenheim EE. Capsaicin pretreatment attenuates suppression of food intake by cholecystokinin. Am J Physiol 1985;248:R501-4.
48. Raybould HE, Taché Y. Cholecystokinin inhibits gastric motility and emptying via a capsaicin-sensitive vagal pathway in rats. Am J Physiol 1988;225:G242-6.
49. Ewart WR, Jones MV, Primi MP. Bombesin changes excitability or rat brain stem neurones sensitive to gastric distension. Am J Physiol 1990;258:G841-7.
50. Altschuler SM, Bao XM, Bieger D, Hopkins DA, Miselis RR. Viscerotopic representation of the upper alimentary tract in the rat: sensory ganglia and nuclei of the solitary and spinal trigeminal tracts. J Comp Neurol 1989;248-68.

# 5

# Control of gastric tone

F. AZPIROZ

*Hospital General Vall d'Hebron, Autonomous University of Barcelona, Spain*

The stomach accomplishes a reservoir function comprising meal reception, temporal storage and progressive intestinal delivery [1]. During ingestion the stomach relaxes to accommodate the meal. Subsequently, a progressive gastric contraction during the postprandial period gently forces gastric content caudally and produces gastric emptying. This reservoir function of the stomach is accomplished by the tonic (sustained) muscular activity of the gastric walls, which is named gastric tone.

**Physiological role of gastric tone**

Electrophysiological studies have shown that the wall of the proximal stomach has the particular ability to generate a tonic contraction, because its membrane potential is above the threshold for contraction [2]. This tonic contraction is neurally modulated. Cholinergic stimuli induce a partial depolarization, enhancing tonic contraction, whereas non-adrenergic, non-cholinergic stimuli induce repolarization, and consequently decrease tonic contraction. In contrast, the membrane potential in antral muscle is far below the threshold for contraction and it rapidly depolarizes in response to neural cholinergic stimuli, causing phasic contractions [2]. Muscle strips from the proximal stomach exposed to a fixed tension undergo a larger elongation (fraction stretch) than muscle strips from the distal stomach tested under similar conditions [3]. Given the greater distensibility of the proximal stomach, gastric contents largely accommodate in this area [3, 4]. Furthermore, mechanoreceptors located in the proximal stomach signal the degree of distension, whereas antral mechanoreceptors signal information concerning the amplitude, rate and duration of antral contractions [3]. Hence, intragastric content accumulates largely in the proximal stomach, which behaves as a reservoir of regulable capacity. Gastric tone, i.e. the wall tension (and hence intragastric pressure) resulting from a given intragastric volume, determines the capacity of the stomach. At low gastric tone the capacity of the stomach enlarges, accommodating large volumes of ingested material. Conversely, a progressive tonic contraction during the postcibal period gradually reduces gastric capacity and produces gastric emptying.

The concept of the tonic motor activity of the proximal stomach acting as the driving force for gastric emptying [5] is supported by three main lines of evidence. First, studies in dogs showed accelerated liquid emptying after partial resection of the proximal stomach (fundectomy) [6]. Similar effects were observed after proximal gastric vagotomy [7, 8] and were explained on the basis of gastric wall rigidity or dystonia subsequent to denervation [9]. Second, there is direct relationship between intragastric pressure (maintained constant at predetermined levels by means of a hydrostatic barostat) and the rate of emptying of liquids [10]. However, these data only suggest a relationship between gastric capacity and emptying, but they do not directly prove that the motor activity of the proximal stomach determines emptying of liquids. The third line of evidence includes the results of hormonal studies, which may be summarized as follows. Gastrin causes relaxation of the proximal stomach [11-13], stimulates antral phasic contractility [14], and delays gastric emptying of liquids [15, 16]. In particular the observation that gastrin delays gastric emptying of an alkaline solution after distal gastrectomy suggests a correlation between muscular activity of the proximal stomach and gastric emptying [15]. Cholecystokinin similarly decreases the pressure in the distended stomach [17] and delays gastric emptying [18, 19], even after pyloroplasty or antropyloric resection [19]. Conversely, motilin increases intragastric pressure [17] and accelerates gastric emptying of liquids after distal gastrectomy [20].

In a series of experiments we have demonstrated the correlation between gastric tone and gastric emptying. In healthy volunteers we measured simultaneously gastric emptying of a solid-liquid meal by radioscintigraphy and gastric tone by a gastric barostat [21]. The gastric barostat maintains a constant pressure level within an air-filled intragastric bag by means of an electronic feedback regulation of air volume (Fig. 1). Hence the barostat measures gastric tone as isobaric volume variations; a small intragastric volume reflects a high gastric tone (gastric contraction) and an isobaric expansion reflects a gastric relaxation (low gastric tone) [22, 23]. During fasting the stomach exhibits a tonic contraction and adapts a small volume of air in the bag of the barostat. Ingestion of a meal produced an additional isobaric air expansion of the stomach of similar magnitude, reflecting a pronounced accommodative relaxation. Subsequently, the stomach gradually contracted and regained tone as gastric emptying progressed. When gastric emptying was accomplished, gastric tone had returned to the preprandial level [21].

Studies by other investigators suggest that the tonic contraction of the proximal stomach plays a role in the process of intragastric redistribution of contents that takes place during the postprandial period [24, 25]. Stimuli that induce a marked gastric relaxation (i.e., duodenal fat infusion) decrease the emptying force [26] and thereby the antral content returns to the more distensible proximal stomach and gastric emptying stops [27]. Similarly, postprandial administration of atropine to dogs stops gastric emptying, even though both the antrum and the pylorus are relaxed by the drug [28]. Therefore it seems that gastric tone provides the emptying force and feeds the antropyloric pump, which exerts a regulated resistance to liquid outflow and accomplishes the sieving and grinding process of solid particles [1, 5].

## Control of gastric tone

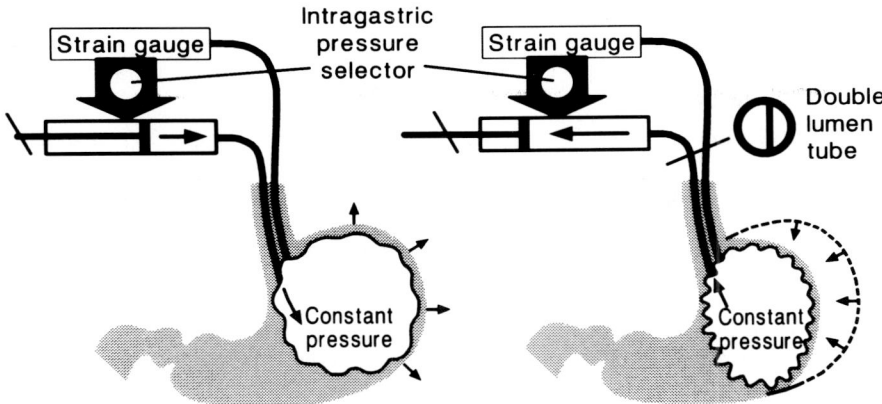

**Figure 1.** Barostat maintains a constant pressure (previously selected) within intragastric bag. When stomach relaxes, system injects air (left); when stomach contracts, air is aspirated (right). (From Azpiroz and Malagelada, ref. [23]).

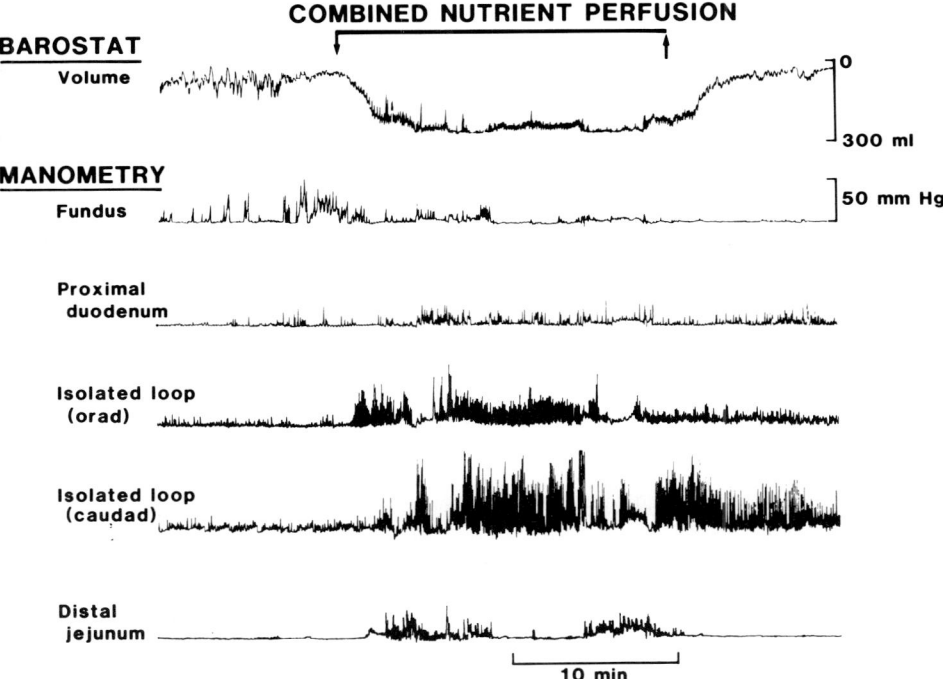

**Figure 2.** Canine gastric tone, monitored by barostat, and gut pressure activity, monitored by manometry, during perfusion of combined nutrients into an isolated loop of jejunum. Note gastric relaxation (barostat volume increase) and increased motor activity in isolated loop. (From Azpiroz and Malagelada, ref. [26]).

## Regulatory mechanisms of gastric tone

### Role of nutrients

The profiles of gastric tone during the postcibal period is finely regulated to accomplish its physiological function. Intestinal nutrients trigger feedback regulatory mechanisms which modify gastric tone and hence the nutrient load delivered into the small intestine. In a series of studies in a canine model with isolated loops of either proximal or distal intestine, we demonstrated that a mixture of absorbable nutrients (fat, carbohydrate and protein) elicited a strong gastric relaxatory response whether it was infused into the distal or into the proximal small bowel (Fig. 2) [26]. Alternatively, individual nutrient-induced responses were site-specific, particularly with perfusion of carbohydrate (no effect proximally and a strong relaxatory effect distally) and fat (the opposite effects of carbohydrate) [26]. Hence, chyme composition along the small intestine regulates gastric tone.

Nutrient-mediated intestinal effects on gastric tone share some characteristics with enterogastric reflexes that affect secretion and emptying [29, 30]; for instance, the diversity of responses depending on the nutrient and the intestinal region perfused. It also appears that enteral effects on gastric tone are different from those on gastric secretion and emptying, suggesting that a different class of mechanisms is involved. It has recently been shown that ileal lipids in humans inhibit gastric emptying by a pyloric mechanism [27]. Conceivably ileal lipids may also exert a regulation on gastric tone in humans, in contrast to dogs. Conversely, the potent gastric relaxation induced by carbohydrate in the distal intestine may also operate in humans, because treatment with an amylase inhibitor that causes carbohydrate malabsorption inhibits gastric emptying [31].

### The vagus

The fact that gastric tone can be substantially reduced (gastric relaxation) by food ingestion or intestinal nutrient perfusion suggests that the stomach maintains a tonic contraction during fasting. *In vivo* studies that record the spontaneous activity of vagal efferent fibres during basal conditions in the dog (conscious, fasting and resting animals) suggest the existence of a tonic excitatory input to the stomach [32, 33]. However, in conflict with this postulate, vagotomy has been consistently reported to increase gastric tone [34-41], refuting the classic concept that the vagus exerts a cholinergic stimulatory action on the stomach [41]. A careful review of the published work reveals that the studies were performed under conditions other than basal (that is gastric distension, acute experimental conditions, chronic vagotomy) and this may account for the incongruent results. Indeed, gastric distension, or surgical manoeuvres and anaesthesia in acute experiments, may induce changes in gastric tone [37, 40, 42-44]. Chronic vagotomy may be followed by adaptive changes secondary either to the lack of trophic effect consecutive to denervation, or to the release of mechanisms due to the suppression of feedback control [45, 46].

In our laboratory we have studied the basal vagal input on gastric tone under physiological conditions. The vagus is a mixed nerve, incorporating cholinergic, adrenergic and non-adrenergic, non-cholinergic fibres [33]. Efferent fibres join the nerve trunk at different levels, for instance, adrenergic fibres join the nerve mainly at a thoracic level [47], and some fibres, for instance fibres innervating the lower oesophageal sphincter, leave the nerve to join the intramural plexus at the mediastinal oesophagus [46, 48]. We therefore examined the effect of reversible vagal blockade by cooling [49, 50] at either the cervical or the supradiaphragmatic level in conscious dogs. The dogs were prepared with a chronic model, either isolating both cervical vagal trunks in a cutaneous tunnel or including the supradiaphragmatic vagi within an implanted cooling jacket [51]. Vagal blockade at either level produced gastric relaxation, which indicates a vagal excitatory input on gastric tone (Fig. 3). Cholinergic blockade (atropine) mimicked the effect of vagal blockade and a cholinergic agonist (bethanechol) increased gastric tone regardless of vagal blockade. Therefore the excitatory vagal input is probably mediated by a cholinergic (muscarinic) mechanism. This conclusion is supported by *in vitro* investigations that show a gradual depolarization and consequent tonic contraction of fundic muscle fibres in response to neural cholinergic stimulation [2]. Consequently, it seems that basal gastric tone in the fasted state is maintained by an extrinsic cholinergic input, which is vagally mediated at both the cervical and the supradiaphragmatic levels.

**The adrenergic system**

Adrenergic blocking agents (phentolamine plus propanolol) had no effect on basal gastric tone, which indicates the absence of basal adrenergic input on gastric tone during fasting. Adrenergic stimulation (adrenaline) induced gastric relaxation. Gastric relaxation has also been demonstrated in response to electrical stimulation of the greater splanchnic nerve [34]. This adrenergically mediated relaxation may involve a dual effect: inhibition of acetylcholine release from intramural cholinergic neurones ($\alpha$-receptors) and direct inhibition of the smooth muscle ($\beta$-receptors) [33]. Hence, although there is no basal adrenergic input on gastric tone, adrenergic stimulation, as it occurs during stress [52], may produce gastric relaxation.

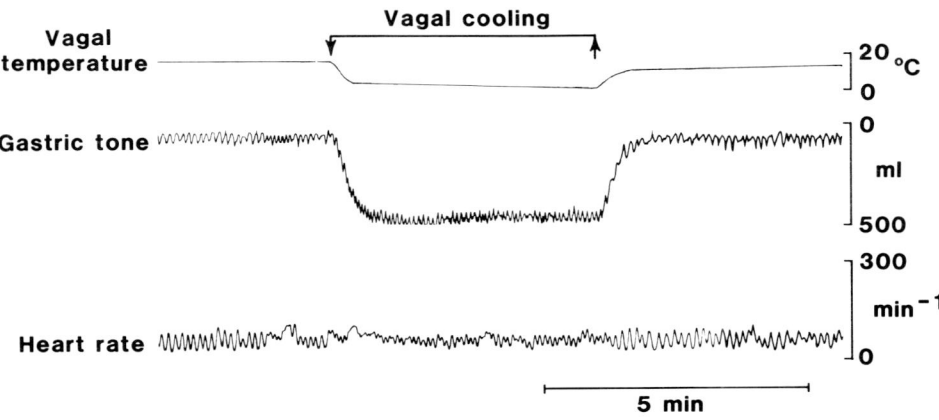

**Figure 3.** Supradiaphragmatic vagal cooling in a canine model. Note pronounced gastric relaxation without change in heart rate. (From Azpiroz and Malagelada, ref. [51]).

## Non-adrenergic, non-cholinergic regulation

However, the reflex gastric relaxation in response to nutrients is produced by a different type of mechanism [53]. In a similar canine model we observed that the gastric relaxatory response to intestinal nutrient perfusion was not abolished by a dose of bethanechol that completely neutralizes the effect of vagal cooling (Fig. 4) [53]. Hence a mechanism other than inhibition of the cholinergic excitatory input participates in this relaxatory response. On the other hand, the effect of intestinal nutrients is not suppressed by pharmacological adrenergic blockade. Therefore intestinal nutrients elicit a gastric relaxatory mechanism that is not cholinergic or adrenergic. Indeed, during intestinal nutrient perfusion and simultaneous administration of bethanechol (either alone or combined with adrenergic blockers), gastric tone was low (gastric relaxation). However, gastric tone markedly increased during the time vagal cooling was applied. Thus vagal cooling interrupts the relaxatory effect of intestinal nutrients and, in the absence of this relaxatory input, gastric tone increases, driven by the cholinergic background (provided by intravenous bethanechol). After vagal warming, vagal conductivity is re-established and the relaxatory stimulus returns gastric tone to the previous relaxed state [53]. Hence, it seems that gastric relaxation induced by intestinal nutrients is mediated, at least in part, by a non-adrenergic, non-cholinergic mechanism that is activated by fibres contained in the vagus at both cervical and supradiaphragmatic levels. It cannot be excluded that additional mechanisms participate in this relaxatory reflex, for instance a concomitant decrease in the excitatory basal input. Indeed, *in vivo* studies suggest that during reflex gastric relaxation efferent vagal discharge into the proximal stomach is increased in inhibitory fibres, but also decreased in excitatory fibres [32, 54].

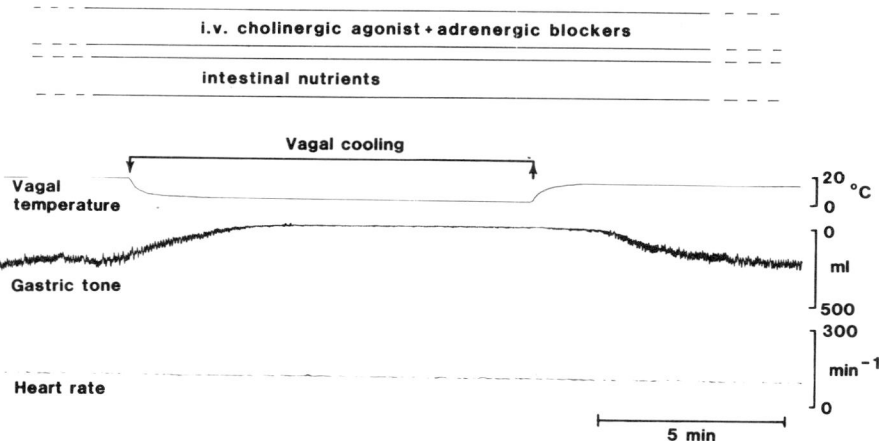

**Figure 4.** Supradiaphragmatic vagal cooling during continuous intravenous infusion of bethanechol plus adrenergic blockers and simultaneous intestinal nutrient perfusion in a canine model. Note low base-line gastric tone (relaxation induced by nutrients); during vagal cooling (relaxatory effect blocked) gastric tone increased (by pharmacological cholinergic effect). (From Azpiroz and Malagelada, ref. [53]).

Non-adrenergic, non-cholinergic gastric relaxation has been described in response to electrical vagal stimulation [37, 38, 40, 55]. However, the specific neurotransmitter or neurotransmitters involved have not been elucidated. Dopamine has been suggested as a potential gastric relaxatory neurotransmitter [56]. However, domperidone, a selective dopamine receptor blocker, does not affect gastric relaxation produced by electrical stimulation of the vagus [55]. Furthermore, in our laboratory, we have observed that domperidone does not change gastric tone during intestinal nutrient perfusion. Other studies point to either purinergic or peptidergic neurotransmitters [39, 55, 57]. Also, a serotoninergic intermediate neurone synapsing with vagal inhibitory preganglionic fibres has been postulated [58]. However, the non-adrenergic, non-cholinergic pathway of gastric relaxation may not represent a single, but rather multiple mechanisms.

## Pathophysiology of gastric tone in relation to dyspeptic symptoms

The physiological regulation of gastric tone accomplishes a normal gastric reservoir function, so that meal-distension of the stomach during gastric accommodation and the gastric emptying process are unperceived. A distortion of this regulation may result in symptomatic perception, because gastric tone indirectly determines the sensitivity of the stomach to distension. Distension of the stomach with an air-filled bag in healthy subjects produces symptoms that resemble those reported by dyspeptic patients after meal ingestion [59]. At the same intragastric volumes the intragastric pressures (wall tension) and the intensity of perception are lower when the stomach is relaxed (for instance by intravenous glucagon) than when the stomach is contracted (basal conditions) [59]. Interestingly, an apparently antagonistic effect is observed when gastric distension is produced at standardized levels of intragastric pressure with the barostat. At the same distending pressures (isobaric distensions) the intragastric volumes (wall elongation) and the intensity of perception are greater when the stomach is relaxed than when the stomach is contracted [59]. Hence, the prevailing gastric tone determines the symptomatic response to distension; symptoms may be elicited by either excessive tension on a contracted stomach or by excessive elongation of a relaxed organ.

A dysregulation of gastric tone may affect the gastric function and/or produce symptoms by meal accommodation. For instance, severe gastric tone impairment results in gastric stasis. Patients with the postsurgical gastroparesis syndrome are a good model to study this effect, since they lack other gastric mechanisms involved in the regulation of gastric emptying, such as the antroduodenal area [1, 5, 19]. In a group of such patients with normal intestinal manometry and delayed gastric emptying of both solids and liquids, we demonstrated a gastric tone impairment in the residual gastric pouch [23]. However, a dysregulation of gastric tone may produce symptoms without affecting gastric emptying. Since during basal conditions gastric tone is normally high, most regulatory mechanisms operating during the postprandial period are inhibitory; these relaxatory mechanisms prevent volume-dependent wall tension increments after meal ingestion [21]. In a group of healthy subjects we simulated a defective gastric accommodation by annulling the role of gastric tone using a gastric barostat [60]. A low intragastric pressure produced a slight acceleration of gastric emptying and was largely unperceived. High intragastric pressure produced significant symptomatic perception, but, interestingly, without a further modification of gastric emptying [60]. It seems that normally gastric tone provides the emptying force by gently pushing intragastric content distally, whereas other mechanisms (i.e., antroduodenal resistance to flow) modulate the final gastric outflow [1, 61]. Therefore, a dysregulation of gastric tone may induce symptoms, while compensatory mechanisms prevent major derangements in gastric emptying.

Stimuli that are not operational in physiological conditions may also induce changes in gastric tone. For instance, duodenal distension elicits a reflex gastric relaxation, characterized by a short latency, quick recovery after withdrawal of the stimulus and lack of fatigue and carry-over effects [62]. Combining the vagal cooling technique with pharmacological experiments in a chronic canine model, we demonstrated that this reflex is, at least in part, mediated by a non-adrenergic, non-cholinergic vagal mechanism [62].

While stimuli involved in the digestive process are largely unperceived, mechanical stimuli in the gut may induce symptomatic perception as well as visceral reflexes [63, 64]. Human experiments in our laboratory indicate that the sensorial and reflex visceral responses are independently elicited by specific mechanisms [65]. Distension of the first duodenal portion elicits perception and gastric relaxation (Fig. 5). Interestingly, unperceived (low level) distensions at this site induce significant relaxation, and, therefore, gastric relaxation is not secondary to perception (subcortical reflex). Conversely, distension of the proximal jejunum elicits a similar symptomatic response to equivalent (isobaric) duodenal distension, but does not induce gastric relaxation [65]. Thus perception is not dependent on the reflex gastric relaxation. However, we cannot ascertain whether this dissociation between perception and reflex gastric

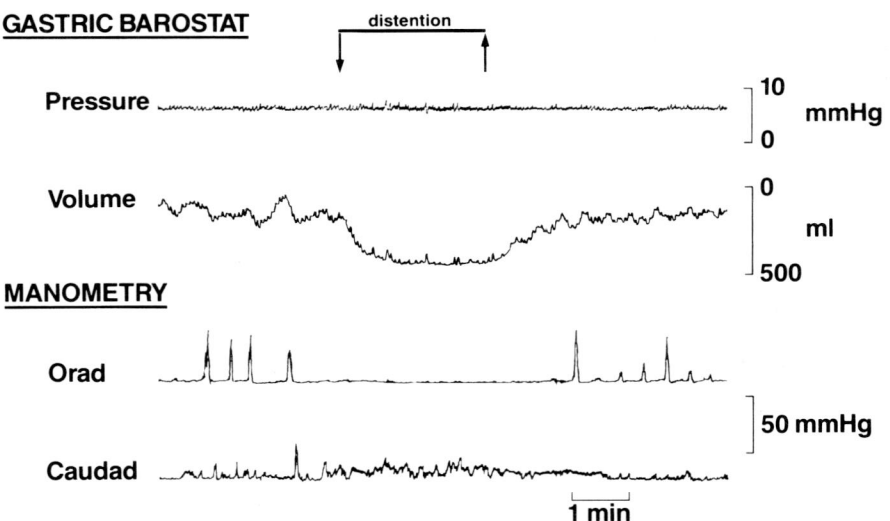

**Figure 5.** Balloon-distension of the first duodenum in a healthy volunteer. Note marked gastric relaxation (volume increase) recorded by gastric barostat; balloon location monitored by orad (antral) and caudad (duodenal) manometric ports. (From Azpiroz and Malagelada, ref. [64]).

relaxation in response to intestinal distension prevails at higher levels of distension. Conceivably, at higher levels, nociception could induce gastric relaxatory reflexes, and conversely, a profound gastric relaxatory response could contribute to epigastric discomfort.

Under physiological conditions enterogastric distension-triggered reflexes may not play a major regulatory role, since inert (saline) intestinal perfusion, mimicking the postprandial flow rate, does not induce changes in canine tone, whereas specific nutrients do [26, 53]. However, since the sensorial and gastric tone responses are elicited by specific mechanisms [65], both responses may be independently altered in pathological conditions. For instance, we have recently demonstrated in our laboratory that dyspeptic patients may have a gastric hyporeactivity to duodenal distending stimuli, whereas duodenal sensitivity to distension is normal [66].

It has been shown that somatic stimuli relay at a central level to produce gastrointestinal motor effects [67]. This type of somatovisceral reflex also participates in the regulation of gastric tone. For instance, pain perception by hand immersion in cold water induces a gastric relaxatory response [68]. Interestingly, we have found that this somatovisceral reflex is normal in dyspeptic patients [68], in contrast to the abnormal duodenogastric reflex previously alluded to [66]. These data indicate that dyspeptic patients may display a selective alteration of a specific mechanism regulating gastric tone.

Even if meal-related symptoms may be the result of a dysregulation of gastric tone, it is important to stress that the sensorial response to gastric distension (gastric sensitivity) may be selectively altered in certain conditions. Experimentally we can modify the sensorial responses to visceral stimuli without affecting the corresponding reflex viscerovisceral responses. For instance, a somatic stimulus, such as transcutaneous electrical nerve stimulation applied on the hand at a level that produces discomfort but no visceral effects, increases the tolerance to gut distension (either gastric or duodenal) without interfering with the reflex visceral responses (i.e., the gastric relaxatory response to duodenal distension) [69]. In clinical conditions this selective sensorial alteration can also be observed in patients with functional dyspepsia, who display gastric hypersensitivity to distension but normal duodenal sensitivity [66, 68, 70].

Since dyspeptic patients may exhibit a normal basal gastric tone [68] and gastric emptying [71] their symptoms may originate in more subtle forms of gastric dysfunction, such as an abnormal reflex reactivity or a visceral hypersensitivity, that still remain to be characterized.

**Acknowledgments.** The author thanks Mrs. Montserrat Domenech for secretarial assistance.

# References

1. Malagelada JR, Azpiroz F. Determinants of gastric emptying and transit in the small intestine. In: *Handbook of Physiology. Gastrointestinal System. Motility and Circulation.* Bethesda: Am Physiol Soc 1989:909-37.

2. Morgan KG, Muir TC, Szurszewski JH. The electrical basis for contraction and relaxation in canine fundal smooth muscle. J Physiol (Lond) 1981;311:475-88.
3. Andrews PL, Grundy D, Scratcherd T. Vagal afferent discharge from mechanoreceptors in different regions of the ferret stomach. J Physiol (Lond) 1980;298:513-24.
4. Schulze-Delrieu K. Volume accommodation by distension of gastric fundus (rabbit) and gastric corpus (cat). Dig Dis Sci 1985;28:625-32.
5. Kelly KA. Gastric emptying of liquids and solids: roles of proximal and distal stomach. Am J Physiol 1980;239:G71-6.
6. Wilbur BG, Kelly KA, Code CF. Effect of gastric fundectomy on canine gastric electrical and motor activity. Am J Physiol 1974;226:1445-9.
7. Jahnberg T, Martinson J, Hultén L, Fasth S. Dynamic gastric response to expansion before and after vagotomy. Scand J Gastroenterol 1975;10:593-8.
8. Wilbur BG, Kelly KA. Effect of proximal gastric, complete gastric, and truncal vagotomy on canine gastric electric activity, motility and emptying. Ann Surg 1973;178:295-303.
9. Aune S. Intragastric pressure after vagotomy in man. Scand J Gastroenterol 1969;4:447-52.
10. Strunz UT, Grossman MI. Effect of intragastric pressure on gastric emptying and secretion. Am J Physiol 1978;235:E552-5.
11. Okike N, Kelly KA. Vagotomy impairs pentagastrin-induced relaxation of canine gastric fundus. Am J Physiol 1977;232:E504-9.
12. Valenzuela JE, Grossman MI. Effect of pentagastrin and caerulein on intragastric pressure in the dog. Gastroenterology 1975;69:1383-4.
13. Wilbur BG, Kelly KA. Gastrin pentapeptide decreases canine gastric transmural pressure. Gastroenterology 1974;67:1139-42.
14. Cooke AR, Chvasta TE, Weisbrodt NW. Effect of pentagastrin on emptying and electrical and motor activity of the dog stomach. Am J Physiol 1972;223:934-8.
15. Dozois RR, Kelly KA. Effect of a gastrin pentapeptide on canine gastric emptying of liquids. Am J Physiol 1971;221:113-7.
16. Hunt JN, Ramsbottom N. Effect of gastrin II on gastric emptying and secretion during a test meal. Br Med J 1967;4:386-7.
17. Valenzuela JE. Effect of intestinal hormones and peptides on intragastric pressure in dogs. Gastroenterology 1976;71:766-9.
18. Debas HT, Farooq O, Grossman MI. Inhibition of gastric emptying is a physiological action of cholecystokinin. Gastroenterology 1975;68:1211-7.
19. Yamagishi T, Debas HT. Cholecystokinin inhibits gastric emptying by acting on both proximal stomach and pylorus. Am J Physiol 1978;234:E375-8.
20. Debas HT, Yamagishi T, Dryburgh JR. Motilin enhances gastric emptying of liquids in dogs. Gastroenterology 1977;73:777-80.
21. Moragas G, Azpiroz F, Malagelada JR. Relationship between gastric tone and gastric emptying measured simultaneously in humans. Gastroenterology 1988;94:A309(abstr).
22. Azpiroz F, Malagelada JR. Physiological variations in canine gastric tone measured by an electronic barostat. Am J Physiol 1985;248:G229-37.
23. Azpiroz F, Malagelada JR. Gastric tone measured by an electronic barostat in health and postsurgical gastroparesis. Gastroenterology 1987;92:934-43.
24. Jacobs F, Akkermans LMA, Yoe OH, Hoekstra A, Wittebol P. A radioisotope method to quantify the function of fundus, antrum, and their contractile activity in gastric emptying of a semi-solid meal. In: Wienbeck M, ed. *Motility of a Digestive Tract*. New York: Raven Press, 1982:233-40.
25. Collins PJ, Horowitz M, Chatterton BE. Proximal, distal and total stomach emptying of a digestible solid meal in normal subjects. Br J Radiol 1988;61:12-8.
26. Azpiroz F, Malagelada JR. Intestinal control of gastric tone. Am J Physiol 1985;249:G501-9.

27. Heddle R, Collins PJ, Dent J, Horowitz M, Read NW, Chatterton B, Houghton LA. Motor mechanisms associated with slowing of the gastric emptying of a solid meal by an intraduodenal lipid infusion. J Gastroenterol Hepatol 1989;4:437-47.
28. Sonnenberg A, Müller-Lissner SA, Schattenmann G, Siewert JR, Blum AL. Duodenogastric reflux in the dog. Am J Physiol 1982;242:G603-7.
29. Clain JE, Go VL, Malagelada JR. Inhibitory role of the distal small intestine on the gastric secretory response to meals in man. Gastroenterology 1978;74:704-7.
30. Miller LJ, Malagelada JR, Taylor WF, Go VL. Intestinal control of human postprandial gastric function: the role of components of jejunoileal chyme in regulating gastric secretion and gastric emptying. Gastroenterology 1981;80:763-9.
31. Layer P, Zinsmeister AR, Di Magno EP. Effects of decreasing intraluminal amylase activity on starch digestion and postprandial gastrointestinal function in humans. Gastroenterology 1986;91:41-8.
32. Miolan JP, Roman C. The role of oesophageal and intestinal receptors in the control of gastric motility. J Auton Nerv Syst 1984;10:235-41.
33. Roman C, Gonella J. Extrinsic control of digestive tract motility. In: Johnson LR, ed. *Physiology of the Gastrointestinal Tract*. Volume 1. New York: Raven Press, 1981:289-334.
34. Andrews PL, Lawes IN. The role of vagal and intramural inhibitory reflexes in the regulation of intragastric pressure in the ferret. J Physiol (Lond) 1982;326:435-51.
35. Andrews PL, Lawes IN. Interactions between splanchnic and vagus nerves in the control of mean intragastric pressure in the ferret. J Physiol (Lond) 1984;351:473-90.
36. Harper AA, Kidd C, Scratcherd T. Vago-vagal reflex effects on gastric and pancreatic secretion and gastrointestinal motility. J Physiol (Lond) 1959;148:417-36.
37. Jahnberg T. Gastric adaptive relaxation. Effects of vagal activation and vagotomy. An experimental study in dogs and in man. Scand J Gastroenterol 1977; 12(suppl 46):1-32.
38. Jansson G. Extrinsic nervous control of gastric motility. An experimental study in the cat. Acta Physiol Scand 1969;75(suppl 326): 1-42.
39. Lundgren O. Vagal control of the motor functions of the lower oesophageal sphincter and the stomach. J Auton Nerv Syst 1983;9:185-97.
40. Martinson J. Studies on the efferent vagal control of the stomach. Acta Physiol Scand 1965;65(suppl 255):1-24.
41. Martinson J. Nervous control of gastroduodenal motility and emptying. Scand J Gastroenterol 1975;10(suppl 35):31-44.
42. Andrews PL, Grundy D, Lawes IN. The role of the vagus and splanchnic nerves in the regulation of intragastric pressure in the ferret. J Physiol (Lond) 1980;307:401-11.
43. Azpiroz F, Malagelada JR. Pressure activity patterns in the canine proximal stomach: response to distension. Am J Physiol 1984;247:G265-72.
44. Glise H, Abrahamson H. Reflex inhibition of gastric motility: pathophysiological aspects. Scand J Gastroenterol 1984;19(suppl 89):77-82.
45. Hakanson R, Vallgren S, Ekelund M, Rehfeld JF, Sundler F. The vagus exerts trophic control of the stomach in the rat. Gastroenterology 1984;86:28-32.
46. Hall KE, El-Sharkawy TY, Diamant NE. Vagal control of migrating motor complex in the dog. Am J Physiol 1982;243:G276-84.
47. Ahlman BH, Larson GM, Bombeck CT, Nyhus LM. Origin of the adrenergic nerve fibres in the subdiaphragmatic vagus in the dog. Am J Surg 1979;137:116-22.
48. Cohen S, Kravitz JJ, Snape WJ. Vagal control of lower esophageal sphincter function. In: Duthie HL, ed. *Gastrointestinal Motility in Health and Disease*. Baltimore: University Park Press, 1978:505-10.
49. Douglas WW, Malcolm JL. The effect of localized cooling on conduction in cat nerves. J Physiol (Lond) 1955;130:53-71.
50. Paintal AS. Block of conduction in mammalian myelinated nerve fibres by low temperatures. J Physiol (Lond) 1965;180:1-19.

51. Azpiroz F, Malagelada JR. Importance of vagal input in maintaining gastric tone in the dog. J Physiol (Lond) 1987;384:511-24.
52. Stanghellini V, Malagelada JR, Zinsmeister AR, Go VL, Kao PC. Stress-induced gastroduodenal motor disturbances in humans: possible humoral mechanisms. Gastroenterology 1983;85:83-91.
53. Azpiroz F, Malagelada JR. Vagally mediated gastric relaxation induced by intestinal nutrients in the dog. Am J Physiol 1986;251:G727-35.
54. Miolan JP, Roman C. Décharge unitaire des fibres vagales efférentes lors de la relaxation réceptive de l'estomac du chien. J Physiol (Paris) 1974;68:692-704.
55. Andrews PL, Lawes IN. Characteristics of the vagally driven non-adrenergic, non-cholinergic inhibitory innervation of ferret gastric corpus. J Physiol (Lond) 1985;363:1-20.
56. Valenzuela JE. Dopamine as a possible neurotransmitter in gastric relaxation. Gastroenterology 1976;71:1019-22.
57. Grider JR, Cable MB, Said SI, Makhlouf GM. Vasoactive intestinal peptide as a neural mediator of gastric relaxation. Am J Physiol 1985;248:G73-8.
58. Gershon MD, Dreyfus CF. Serotoninergic neurones in the mammalian gut. In: Brooks FP, Evers PL, eds. *Nerves and the Gut*. Thorofare: Slack, 1977:197-205.
59. Notivol R, Mearin F, Azpiroz F, Malagelada JR. Epigastric symptoms are elicited by selective stimulation of "in series" and "in parallel" gastric mechanoreceptors. Gastroenterology 1990;98:A377(abstr).
60. Moragas G, Azpiroz F, Malagelada JR. Strain on gastric accommodation after a meal spares emptying but produces symptoms. Gastroenterology 1990;98:A376(abstr).
61. Miller J, Kauffman G, Elashoff J, Ohashi H, Carter D, Meyer JH. Search for resistances controlling canine gastric emptying of liquid meals. Am J Physiol 1981;241:G403-15.
62. De Ponti F, Azpiroz F, Malagelada JR. Reflex gastric relaxation in response to distension of the duodenum. Am J Physiol 1987;252:G595-601.
63. Ray BS, Neill CL. Abdominal visceral sensation in man. Ann Surg 1947;126:709-24.
64. Azpiroz F, Malagelada JR. Perception and reflex relaxation of the stomach in response to gut distension. Gastroenterology 1990;98:1193-8.
65. Azpiroz F, Malagelada JR. Isobaric intestinal distension in humans: sensorial relay and reflex gastric relaxation. Am J Physiol 1990;258:G202-7.
66. Coffin B, Azpiroz F, Malagelada JR. Selective gastric hypersensitivity and reflex hyporeactivity in functional dyspepsia. Gastroenterology 1991;100:A431(abstr).
67. Camilleri M, Malagelada JR, Kao PC, Zinsmeister AR. Effect of somatovisceral reflexes and selective dermatomal stimulation on postcibal antral pressure activity. Am J Physiol 1984;247:G703-8.
68. Mearin F, Cucala M, Azpiroz F, Malagelada JR. Origin of gastric symptoms in functional dyspepsia. Gastroenterology 1989;96:A337(abstr).
69. Coffin B, Azpiroz F, Malagelada JR. Somatosensory modulation of gastrointestinal sensitivity in humans. Gastroenterology 1991;100:A431(abstr).
70. Lemann M, Dederding JP, Jian R, Flourié B, Franchisseur C, Rambaud JC. Abnormal sensory perception to gastric distension in patients with chronic idiopathic dyspepsia. The irritable stomach. Gastroenterology 1989;96:A294(abstr).
71. Jian R, Ducrot F, Ruskoné A, Chaussade S, Rambaud JC, Modigliani R, Rain JD, Bernier JJ. Symptomatic, radionuclide and therapeutic assessment of chronic idiopathic dyspepsia. A double-blind placebo-controlled evaluation of cisapride. Dig Dis Sci 1989;34:657-64.

# 6

# Stress and upper gut motility disorders: mechanisms involved

L. BUÉNO

*Department of Pharmacology INRA, 180 chemin de Tournefeuille, B.P. 3, 31931 Toulouse, France*

## Introduction

The relationships between stress and gastrointestinal disorders have been known for many centuries. Nevertheless it was only in 1936 that Selye [1] described the presence of gastric ulcer as one of the three patho-anatomical entities corresponding to the stress syndrome.

Following this pioneering concept, it was shown in humans that experimental stress is accompanied by motor disorders of both the upper and the lower digestive tract. In 1982, Thompson *et al.* showed that hand immersion in cold water is accompanied by a slowing of gastric emptying corresponding to alterations in duodenal motility [2]. Subsequently numerous experimental data have confirmed that stress alters gastric emptying in humans (Table I). More recently, it was confirmed that other stresses, such as labyrinthine stimulation, noise, driving in traffic, arcade games, etc., are accompanied by changes in gastric and/or intestinal motility in fed [2, 4] and fasted man [5, 6].

Following the findings of Stacher [7], which showed that acoustic stimuli invoke spontaneous synchronous oesophageal contractions in healthy persons, it was more recently shown that caloric labyrinthine stimulation causes a reduction in basal lower oesophageal sphincter (LOS) relaxation [8].

Accordingly experiments were performed in animals using various experimental models of acute and chronic stress, such as cold restraint, wrap restraint, water immersion, surgery, trephination, acoustic stress and more recently psychic stress based on passive avoidance or fear-conditioned reaction.

**Table I.** Comparative influence of different stressors on motility of the upper gut in man.

|  | Stressor | Effects | References |
|---|---|---|---|
| Oesophagus | A.S. | Cluster contractions | Stacher et al., 1979 |
|  | P.S. | Amplitude | Young et al., 1987 |
|  | L.Stim. | LOS pressure | Cook et al., 1987 |
| Stomach | C.W.S. | Inhibition | McRae et al., 1980 |
|  |  |  | Thompson et al., 1982 |
|  | M.S. | No effect | McRae et al., 1983 |
|  | I.S.M. | Tachygastria | Koch et al., 1990 |
|  | C.P.T. |  |  |
|  | L.Stim. | Inhibition | Stanghellini et al., 1983 |
| Duodenum | P.S. | MMC inhibition | Valori et al., 1986 |
|  | Noise | No effect | Erckenbrecht et al., 1988 |
|  | L.Stim. | Induced phase III | Stanghellini et al., 1983-84 |
|  | M.S. | MMC cycle | Holtmann et al.,1989 |

A.S.: acoustic stress; P.S.: psychological stress; L.Stim.: labyrinthine stimulation; M.S.: mental stress; C.P.T.: cold pressure test; I.S.M.: illusory self-motion; MMC, migrating motor complex; LOS, lower oesophageal sphincter; C.W.S.: cold water stress.

**Table II.** Effect of different stressful stimuli on gastric emptying in animals.

| Stressors | Species | Meal | Gastric emptying | References |
|---|---|---|---|---|
| Operant avoidance | Monkey | Water | Delay | Dubois, Natelson, 1978 |
| Radiation | Monkey | Water | Delay | Dorval et al., 1985 |
| Handling, noise | Guinea pig | Non cal. | Delay | Costall et al., 1983 |
| Passive avoidance | Rat | Food-water | Delay | Enck et al., 1988 |
| Haemorrhage | Rat | Liq. non cal. | Delay | Limlomwongse et al., 1988 |
| Cold, 2-3 h | Rat | Liq. non cal. | Delay | Koo et al., 1985 |
| Tail shocks | Rat | Liq. non cal. | Delay | Taché et al., 1989b |
| Surgery | Rat | Liq. non cal. | Delay | Taché et al., 1989b |
| Trunk clamping | Rat | Liq. non cal. | Delay | Lenz et al., 1988b |
| Wrap restraint | Rat | Liq. non cal. | No change | Taché et al., 1988b |
|  |  |  |  | Williams et al., 1987, 1988 |
| Cold, 30-80 min | Rat | Liq. non cal. | Increase | Koo et al., 1985 |
|  |  |  |  | Taché et al., 1988b |
| Cold, 20 min | Mice | Milk | Increase | Buéno, Gué, 1988 |
| Acoustic (≤90 dB) { Mice | Mice | Milk | Increase | Buéno, Gué, 1988 |
| Dog | Dog | Cal. | Decrease | Gué et al., 1989 |

(from Taché et al., 1989)

## Physiological basis

In 1936, Selye discovered that toxic doses of drugs and other noxious treatments (stressful stimuli) produced hypertrophy of the adrenal cortex in intact but not in hypophysectomised rats, suggesting that these effects are related to enhanced adrenocorticotrophic hormone (ACTH) secretion. This resulted in enormous interest in the mechanisms controlling ACTH secretion, particularly to confirm Harris's hypothesis [9] that the secretory activity of the adenohypophysis may be controlled by a chemical transmitter substance from the hypothalamus. This substance was later named corticotropin releasing factor (CRF) by Saffran et al. [10] and 26 years later CRF was structurally characterized in sheep as a 41 amino acid peptide [11]. This peptide was shown to act primarily as a physiological regulator of pituitary ACTH secretion [12] but the widespread distribution of CRF and CRF receptors throughout the central nervous system supports the concept that this peptide may subserve functions apart from its hypophysiotropic role [13, 14]. Indeed, intracerebroventricular (ICV) administration of CRF produces multiple autonomical, behavioural and visceral effects that are characteristic of stress reactions [15, 16].

Consequently, CRF was hypothesized to be an important mediator of the coordinated and integrated endocrine and autonomic responses to stress, suggesting that it might have a role in the genesis of gastrointestinal secretory and motor alterations. Furthermore CRF is present in hypothalamic and medullary nuclei regulating visceral functions and particularly gastrointestinal motility [13, 14].

## Role of corticotropin releasing hormone

### Influence of CRF on gastrointestinal motility and transit

Several oligopeptides present in the brain and affecting gastric acid secretion are also able to affect the muscular activity of the gut when administered centrally in rats at picomolar doses [17]. These results have suggested that CRF may also play a role in the control of digestive motility.

The first evidence that CRF injected centrally affects gastrointestinal motility was obtained in dogs [18]. In fasted dogs, as in other species including humans, the motility of the gastric corpus and antrum is characterized by cyclic phases of grouped high amplitude contractions, also called "activity front" or gastric migrating motor complex (MMC). These phases, which last about 20 min and occur at 90-120 min intervals, are propagated to the duodenum and then migrate to the terminal ileum. In the dog, ICV administration of ovine CRF (oCRF, 20 to 100 ng/kg) suppresses these gastric cyclic MMCs, which are replaced by small amplitude irregular contractions over several hours without affecting the cyclic motility of the jejunum. The lack of effects of ICV or intravenous infusion of ACTH or cortisol have suggested that in dogs CRF may be involved in the central control of the interdigestive gastric motility and that these effects are not related to the stimulation of the hypothalamo-pituitary-adrenocortical (HPA) axis. These effects depend on the digestive state, and similar ICV picomolar doses of CRF injected postprandially in dogs do not affect phase III activity of antral contractions while they increase both the amplitude and frequency of jejunal contractions [19].

Similarly in rats, Garrick et al. [19] have shown that intracisternal (IC) administration of CRF inhibits the antral motor response to administration of the TRH analogue RX77368 by the same route, but in contrast, at similar doses ICV, it enhances the late phase-II-like activity associated with the postprandial state when injected 1 to 2 hours after the meal. The neurohumoral mechanisms through which central CRF alters gastrointestinal contractility are unknown although they may involve the parasympathetic outflow in rats and dogs since they are respectively blocked by atropine and are suppressed after vagotomy [18, 19].

Gastric emptying and intestinal transit are altered by central administration of CRF in rats, mice and dogs. In rats intracisternal or intracerebroventricular injection of CRF and related peptides such as sauvagine reduces gastric emptying of a non-nutritive liquid meal associated with a decrease in small bowel transit and an enhanced colonic transit and faecal output [20-23]. Similarly in dogs, CRF injected into the IIIrd ventricle also delays gastric emptying of a liquid protein meal while in contrast in mice ICV injection of CRF increases gastric emptying of a milk meal [24, 25].

Pretreatment with a ganglionic or noradrenergic blocker [16, 20], as well as vagotomy, suppresses the CRF-induced delay in gastric emptying and intestinal transit while only vagotomy is able to prevent the effects of CRF on colonic transit [16].

## Evidence of CRF involvement in stress-induced GI motor alterations

In animals, stress-induced alterations in intestinal motility have been known since the beginning of the century, when Cannon in 1902 [26] noted changes in the contour and flow of intestinal contents in cats confronted by a growling dog.

In 1980, Fioramonti et al. [27] showed that in fasted rats submitted to cold restraint stress gastric motility was transiently increased (1-2 hours) and then was dramatically inhibited, such hypomotility preceding the macroscopic evidence of gastric ulceration.

In conscious dogs, acoustic stress produced by a 1 hour exposure to intense music through earpieces (comprised between 70 and 90 dB) inhibits the succeeding gastric MMC in the same way as oCRF injected ICV [28] without affecting intestinal motility. These motor effects, which are associated with a significant rise in plasma cortisol level, are not blocked by previous treatment with opiate antagonists and adrenergic blockers. The fact that such effects of acoustic stress on one hand are prevented by treatment with diazepam, a benzodiazepine, or muscimol, a GABAergic agonist, both affecting the CNS release of CRF [29, 30] and on other hand that they are suppressed after vagotomy strongly suggests that they are related to the central release of CRF.

In mice, both acoustic (AS) and cold exposure (CS) stress increase gastric emptying of a nutritive (milk) meal, an effect mimicked by ICV administration of oCRF [24]. Similarly most of the stressors associated with the release of CRF, such as noise, wrap restrain, ether exposure, water swim or psychic stress [31, 32], decrease gastric emptying of a non-nutritive meal and intestinal transit corresponding to fasted state in rats and dogs [23, 26, 33]. In contrast, cold restraint stress has been shown in rats to have a biphasic effect on gastric emptying, increasing the rate of flow during about 60 min, followed by a strong slowing associated with hypothermia [34]. These alterations in gastrointestinal transit observed in rats are similar to those elicited by intracerebroventricular administration of CRF, i.e. a decrease in gastric emptying of a non-nutritive meal [20, 21], a slowing of intestinal transit and an increase in colonic transit [20, 35].

Finally, the evidence that CNS release of CRF is directly involved in the initiation of digestive motor disturbances induced by different stressors was obtained firstly in rats [35] and then in mice [25] (Table III). In this last species, pretreatment with ICV administration of antiserum against rat CRF, as well as α-helical $CRF_{9-41}$ [36], considered to be a CRF antagonist [37], is able to prevent the increase in gastric emptying of a milk meal induced by acoustic and cold stress at doses that block the effects produced by ICV administration of CRF.

This result was confirmed in rats [38] on which cerebroventricular administration of α helical $CRF_{9-41}$, but not of the CRF fragment $CRF_{1-20}$, prevents the gastrointestinal secretory and motor (transit) responses elicited by partial body restraint. Moreover α-helical $CRF_{9-41}$ prevents the abdominal-surgery-induced inhibition of gastric emptying [33].

## Mechanisms and pathways involved

A cascade of hormonal releases and subsequent activation of autonomic nervous system is related to CRF release. Numerous results suggest that some effects are related to peripheral adrenergic activation [16, 39] or to the peripheral release of β endorphin [4]. However, most studies suggest that CRF released by stressful stimuli acts directly on the supraspinal structures controlling gastric and intestinal motility and not through a stimulation of the HPA system. In agreement with such hypothesis, systemic administration of ACTH or corticosteroids at doses which mimic plasma increases in stress conditions does not affect gastric emptying in mice [24] or gastrointestinal motility in dogs [18], and ACTH and β endorphin do not affect intestinal transit in rats [23]. Furthermore neither adrenalectomy nor hypophysectomy prevent the slowing of intestinal transit induced by wrapping-restraint stress [23]. In acoustic stress in dogs, opiate antagonists as well as α and β adrenergic blockers are unable to prevent the alterations in gastric motility [40]; similarly in rats neither naloxone nor phentolamine prevent alterations in gastric emptying induced by acoustic and cold stress, but propranolol is efficient, suggesting the involvement of central and(or) peripheral β adrenergic receptors and(or) pathways in their induction. Such a

**Table III.** Evidence for CRF involvement in stress-induced alterations of transit.

| Species | Stressful stimulus | Method | Route | Gastric emptying | Intestinal transit | Colonic transit | References |
|---|---|---|---|---|---|---|---|
| Rat | W.R.S. | α-helical | IV/ICV | — | unblocked | blocked | Williams et al., 1987 |
| Mice | A.S.+A.S. | Antiserum | ICV/IV | blocked | blocked | — | Buéno et al., 1988 |
| | A.S.+C.S. | α-helical | ICV | blocked | blocked | — | Gué et al., 1988 |
| Rat | P.R.S. | α-helical | ICV | blocked | blocked | blocked | Lenz et al., 1988 |
| Rat | S.S. | α-helical | ICV | blocked | — | — | Taché et al., 1988 |

A.S.: acoustic stress; C.S.: cold stress; W.R.S.: wrapping restraint stress;
P.R.S.: partial restraint stress; S.S.: surgical stress.
I.C.V.: intracerebroventricular; IV: intravenous.

hypothesis is supported by observations showing that a β adrenergic antagonist atenolol, but not α blockers, reduces the CS-induced acceleration of the orocaecal transit in humans [39].

Blockade of the effects of stress on gastric motility after vagotomy in dogs [28], as well as the inefficiency of central CRF to alter gastric emptying in vagotomized rats, strongly suggests that the vagus is involved. Central administration of CRF modulates the parasympathetic outflow from the brain regulating gastric functions [41] and similarly stressful stimuli are known to produce vagal excitation, but the lack of preventing effects of CNS administration of atropine or pirenzepine on acoustic-stress-induced gastric motor inhibition (unpublished observations) is not in agreement with this hypothesis.

Finally, if it is well established that CRF released at CNS level plays a major role in the genesis of stress-induced gastrointestinal and colonic motor alterations induced by stressful stimuli, the effects observed are not univocal and mostly depend on the digestive status, suggesting that they are mediated through different neural or hormonal pathways which remain to be elucidated.

## References

1. Selye M. Syndrome produced by diverse nocuous agents. Nature 1936;138:32-4.
2. Thompson DG, Richelson E, Malagelada JR. Perturbation of gastric emptying and duodenal motility through the central nervous system. Gastroenterology 1982;83:1200-6.
3. Stanghellini V, Malagelada JR, Zinsmeister AR, Go VL, Kao PC. Stress-induced gastroduodenal motor disturbances in humans: possible humoral mechanisms. Gastroenterology 1983;85:83-91.
4. Stanghellini V, Malagelada JR, Zinsmeister AR, Go VL, Kao PC. Effect of opiate and adrenergic blockers on the gut motor response to centrally acting stimuli. Gastroenterology 1984;87:1104-13.
5. McRae S, Thompson DG, Wingate DL, Youger K. Changes in the pattern of fasting jejunal activity during mental stress. J Physiol (Lond) 1980;308:25P(abstr).
6. Valori RM, Kumar D, Wingate DL. Effects of different types of stress and of "prokinetic" drugs on the control of the fasting motor complex in humans. Gastroenterology 1986,90:1890-900.
7. Stacher G. The responsiveness of the oesophagus to environmental stimuli. In: Holzl R., Whitehead WR, eds. *Psychophysiology of the Gastrointestinal Tract*. New York: Plenum, 1983:21-31.
8. Cook IJ, Collins SM. Influence of acute mental stress on the frequency and duration of gastroesophageal reflux in normal volunteers. Can J Gastroenterol 1987;1:7-10.
9. Harris GW. The induction of ovulation in the rabbit, by electrical stimulation of the hypothalamo-hypophysial mechanism. Proc R Soc Biol Sci 1937;122:374-94.
10. Saffran M, Schally AV, Benfey BG. Stimulation of the release of corticotropin from the adenohypophysis by a neurohypophysial factor. Endocrinology 1955;57:439-44.
11. Vale W, Spiess J, Rivier C, Rivier J. Characterization of a 41-residue ovine hypothalamic peptide that stimulates secretion of corticotropin and β-endorphin. Science 1981:213:1394-7.
12. Rivier C, Rivier J, Vale W. Inhibition of adrenocorticotropic hormone secretion in the rat by immunoneutralization of corticotropin-releasing factor. Science 1982;218:377-9.
13. Swanson LW, Sawchenko PE, Rivier J, Vale WW. Organization of ovine CRF immunoreactive cells and fibres in the rat brain: an immunohistochemical study. Neuroendocrinology 1983;36:165-86.

14. De Souza EB. Corticotropin-releasing factor receptors in the rat central nervous system: characterization and regional distribution. J Neurosci 1987;7:88-100.
15. Brown MR, Fisher LA, Webb V, Vale WW, Rivier JE. Corticotropin-releasing factor: a physiologic regulator of adrenal epinephrine secretion. Brain Res 1985;328:355-7.
16. Lenz HJ, Readler A, Greten H, Brown MR. CRF initiates biological actions within the brain that are observed in response to stress. Am J Physiol 1987;252:R34-9.
17. Buéno L, Ferre JP. Central regulation of intestinal motility by somatostatin and cholecystokinin octapeptide. Science 1982;216:1427-9.
18. Buéno L, Fargeas MJ, Gué M, Peeters TL, Bormans V, Fioramonti J. Effects of corticotropin-releasing factor on plasma motilin and somatostatin levels and gastrointestinal motility in dogs. Gastroenterology 1986;91:884-9.
19. Garrick T, Veiseh A, Sierra A, Weiner H, Taché Y. Corticotropin-releasing factor acts centrally to suppress stimulated gastric contractility in the rat. Regul Pept 1988;21:173-81.
20. Lenz HJ, Burlage M, Raedler A, Greten H. Central nervous system effects of corticotropin-releasing factor on gastrointestinal transit in the rat. Gastroenterology 1988;94:598-602.
21. Taché Y, Maeda-Hagiwara M, Turkelson CM. Central nervous system action of corticotropin-releasing factor to inhibit gastric emptying in rats. Am J Physiol 1987,253:G241-5.
22. Broccardo M, Improta G, Melchiorri P. Effect of sauvagine on gastric emptying in conscious rats. Eur J Pharmacol 1982;85:111-4.
23. Williams CL, Villar RG, Peterson JM, Burks TF. Stress-induced changes in intestinal transit in the rat: a model for irritable bowel syndrome. Gastroenterology 1988;84:611-21.
24. Gué M, Fioramonti J, Buéno L. Comparative influences of acoustic and cold stress on gastrointestinal transit in mice. Am J Physiol 1987;253:G124-8.
25. Buéno L, Gué M. Evidence for the involvement of corticotropin-releasing factor in the gastrointestinal disturbances induced by acoustic and cold stress in mice. Brain Res 1988;441:1-4.
26. Cannon WB. The movements of the intestines studied by means of the Roentgen rays. Am J Physiol 1902;6:251-77.
27. Fioramonti J, Buéno L. Gastrointestinal myoelectric activity disturbances in gastric ulcer disease in rats and dogs. Dig Dis Sci 1980;25:575-80.
28. Gué M, Fioramonti J, Frexinos J, Alvinerie M, Buéno L. Influence of acoustic stress by noise on gastrointestinal motility in dogs. Dig Dis Sci 1987;32:1411-7.
29. Makara GB, Stark E. Effects of gamma-aminobutyric acid (GABA) and GABA antagonist drugs on ACTH release. Neuroendocrinology 1974;16:178-90.
30. Ninan PT, Insel TM, Cohen RM, Cook JM, Skolnick P, Paul SM, Benzodiazepine receptor-mediated experimental "anxiety" in primates. Science 1982;218:1332-4.
31. Nakane T, Audhya T, Kanie N, Hollander CS. Evidence for a role of endogenous corticotropin-releasing factor in cold, ether, immobilization and traumatic stress. Proc Natl Acad Sci (USA) 1985;82:1247-51.
32. Hashimoto K, Suemaru S, Takao T, Sugawara M, Makino S, Ota Z. Corticotropin-releasing hormone and pituitary-adrenocortical responses in chronically stressed rats. Regul Pept 1988;23:117-26.
33. Taché Y, Kolve E, Stephens R, Rivier J. Role of brain CRF in mediating surgical stress induced inhibition of gastric function in the rat. 7th International symposium on gastrointestinal hormones. Shizuoka, 1988.
34. Koo MW, Ogle CW, Cho CH. The effect of cold-restrain stress on gastric emptying in rats. Pharmacol Biochem Behav 1985;23:969-72.
35. Williams CL, Peterson JM, Villar RG, Burks TF. Corticotropin-releasing factor directly mediates colonic responses to stress. Am J Physiol 1987;253:G582-6.
36. Gué M, Buéno L. Involvement of CNS corticotropin-releasing factor in the genesis of stress-induced gastric motor alterations in nerves and the gastrointestinal tract. Singer, Goebell eds. 1988:217-25.

37. Rivier J, Rivier C, Vale W. Synthetic competitive antagonists of corticotropin-releasing factor: effect on ACTH secretion in the rat. Science 1984;224:889-91.
38. Lenz HJ, Raedler A, Greten H, Vale WW, Rivier JE. Stress-induced gastrointestinal secretory and motor responses in rats are mediated by endogenous corticotropin-releasing factor. Gastroenterology 1988;95:1510-7.
39. O'Brien JD, Thompson DG, Day S, Burnham WR, Walker E. Stress induced disturbances of human postprandial antroduodenal motility and orocaecal transit. The contribution of adrenergic pathways. Dig Dis Sci 1985;30:785(abstr).
40. Gué M, Buéno L. Diazepam and muscimol blockade of the gastrointestinal motor disturbances induced by acoustic stress in dogs. Eur J Pharmacol 1986;131:123-7.
41. Brown MR, Fischer LA, Rivier J, Spiess J, Rivier C, Vale W. Corticotropin-releasing factor: effects on the sympathetic nervous system and oxygen consumption. Life Sci 1982;30:207-10.

# 7

# Control of appetite and satiety

D. RIGAUD

*Hôpital Bichat, 46 rue Henri Huchard, 75018 Paris, France*

Experimental and human studies on the regulation of food intake have shifted their focus markedly during the past 10 years. If the theory of the "dual-centre" in the brain, i.e. a lateral hypothalamic feeding centre and a medial hypothalamic satiety centre, remains acceptable [1-5], it has been largely reinterpreted in light of observations which did not fit with the initial results [4]. More recent studies have emphasized the role of metabolic and humoral factors originating in peripheral organs, in addition to the brain and its dual centre [6]. It now appears that the periphery, namely the gut and the liver, plays an important role in the control of food intake. Signals such as hormones or neuromediators originating mostly from the gut modulate hunger feeling, satiation and satiety.

**The brain**

The dual centre theory is based on investigations in which the putative centres which control food intake were defined using gross destructions of brain's area by stereotaxic lesions [1, 2]. Destroying the lateral hypothalamic area (LHA) induced a dramatic decrease in food intake (hypo- or aphagia) and weight loss, while destructions of the ventro-medial hypothalamic area (VMHA) was responsible for a syndrome of hyperphagia and obesity.

It is now well-known that the prolonged period of aphagia observed after LHA destruction is the result of destruction of the ascending dopamine neurones (passing through LHA) which are in charge of most arousal sensations (and not only of eating behaviour). Similarly hyperphagia after VMHA lesions also derives from associated hyperinsulinism related to the decrease in sympathetic tone.

# Factors modulating food intake

## Definitions

Food intake is only one of the phases of eating behaviour (Table I). There is first a pre-ingestive phase which is initiated by arousal to eat, i.e. hunger feeling. This pre-ingestive phase depends in animals on external and internal factors as different from each other as social and familial environment, personal life experience, the time of day, present occupations, and mood.

Eating is one of the components of the ingestive phase: it is clearly related to the pre-ingestive phase, in particular the feeling of hunger. The feeling of hunger can be defined as the overall sensations caused by a need for food: arousal caused by the image of food, desire (or craving), and also weakness and abdominal discomfort (or pain). The general tendency, i.e. the positive (or negative) power, is mostly related to previous personal experience relating to foods and meals: it is not impossible that in patients with non-ulcer dyspepsia, the abdominal and central sensations associated with hunger are bound up with bad experiences and are thus negatively perceived or reinterpreted. From a physiological point of view, hunger feeling is related to energy needs: a meal is taken when energy (and not only glucose) is required [7].

Appetite is the overall positive (pleasant) sensation related to food images (and not only to hunger). In other words, animals and humans have only one hunger feeling (which may be unpleasant) and several selective, food-item-related, appetite sensations (which are in the field of desire).

Satiation is defined as the progressive suppression of all sensations related to hunger and appetite: at this time food intake is decreasing, and is then discontinued.

**Table I.** The 3 phases of food intake.

|  |  | Food Intake |
|---|---|---|
| Pre-ingestive phase | Arousal (brain, gut) | Increase |
| Ingestive phase | • Peripheral sensory system<br>• Gastric filling | Increase (decrease)<br>Decrease |
| Post-ingestive phase | • Gastric emptying<br>• Small bowel filling<br>• Digestion, absorption<br>• Nutrient systemic circulation (portal vein, brain)<br>• Colon filling | Influx regulation<br>?<br>?<br>Negative<br>?<br>(Negative) |

Satiety is defined as the absence of arousal for foods and meals: there is no image of foods in mind. At this time, inhibitory stimuli generated by the previous meal exert a maximal influence on central inhibitory systems regulating food intake [5, 6].

**Environmental and individual factors**

Schematic representations of environmental and individual factors that might control food intake are shown in Table II.

Environmental factors include culture, society, and psychological stress which have either negative or positive influences on food intake. Two major factors, i.e. conditioning and availability, positively modulate food intake in western societies. The last but not the least factor is the palatability of foods, i.e. the organoleptic properties of foods which are responsible for their flavour, savour, and consistency. Food palatability is related to macronutrient and also to micronutrient components of the foods.

Individual factors play a major influence in the control of food intake. Some concern the brain, but others are of digestive origin (Table I). Both have positive and/or negative influences on food intake. There is no doubt that several of these factors are genetically determined; others are related to or associated with previous pleasant or unpleasant experiences. For new food items of unusual aspect or taste, the subject may feel neophobia, i.e. aversion for food of suspicious nature, when it is offered for the first time. Among the factors modulating food intake, the brain factors may act as promoting factors as well as inhibitory ones: habits, conscious self-control of body weight. The most important non-brain factors are of gut origin or are peripheral to the brain. Palatability of food is quantified by the peripheral sensory system, i.e. vision, taste and smell. These senses are controlled by central factors such as attention and memory. Sensory capacity varies greatly from one individual to another. Concerning sensations related to foods, several assertions are pure misconceptions: the loss of one sense is not necessarily compensated for by more effective functioning of the other senses; aging is not systematically associated with a dramatic decrease in sensory sensitivity; pregnant women are not unusually hypersensitive to odours.

**Table II.** Negative and positive factors modulating food intake.

| \<Surrounding\> | | | \<Subject\> | | |
|---|---|---|---|---|---|
| Negative | | Positive | Negative | | Positive |
| + | Culture | +++ | + | Genetics | + |
| + | Society | + | + | Experience | + |
| ++ | Stress | (+) | + | Neophobia | 0 |
| ? | Conditioning | ++ | + | CNS | + |
| 0 | Availability | ++ | (+) | PSS | ++ |
| + | Palatability | ++ | ++ | Gut | (+) |
| | | | +++ | Energy flux (Gut, brain) | (+) |

CNS: central nervous system; PSS: peripheral senses system (taste, smell, ...).

## Peripheral factors

Chemical senses are of great importance in the regulation of gut function. It is well established that the overall response to the chemical properties of food modify gastric and pancreatic functions as well as gut motility. During sham feeding a two-or threefold increase in gastric acid and exocrine pancreatic secretions is observed. These responses can reach one third or even one half (in "high responder" subjects) of the maximal response of the stomach or the pancreas. But sham feeding may also release some gut hormones such as gastrin (in dogs), pancreatic polypeptide (in animals and man), or insulin. In normal volunteers we have shown that a "double max meal", i.e.

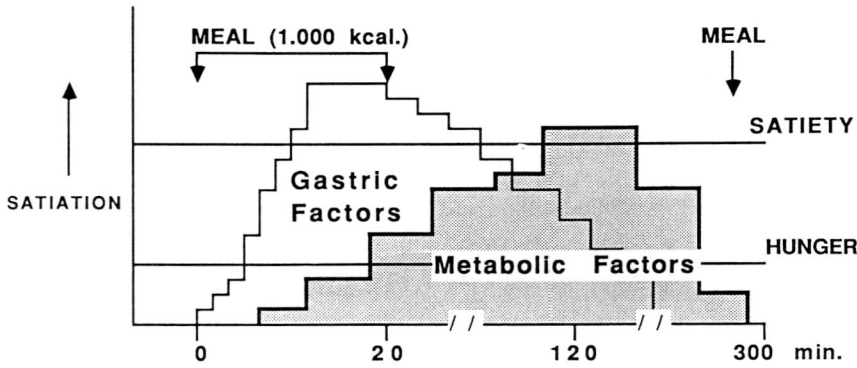

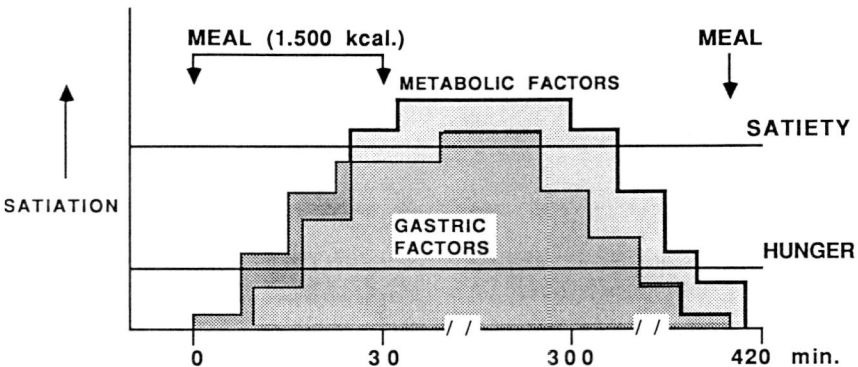

**Figure 1.** Effects of gastric and metabolic factors on food intake: the figure shows two types of satiation: in example **A,** the gastric pressure increases markedly inducing prompt satiation, which decreases rapidly together with gastric emptying. Finally the subject ingested only 1000 kcal. In example **B,** ingestion lasts 30 min and the subject can ingest 1500 kcal: satiety is longer than in example A.

a very appetizing and high energy (>1500 kcal) meal, induced a large integrated response of pancreatic polypeptide, CCK, and neurotensin. When the subjects were offered the same meal in less pleasant conditions, the hormonal responses (in particular the early phase of the hormonal responses) was decreased.

**Gut factors**

Perhaps the most well-known inhibitory signal of food intake results from gastric distension. It appears, however, that many other signals originating from the gut have a role in the control of food intake: gastric emptying, small bowel filling and motility, delivery of energy by digestion and absorption processes, colonic motility (and its luminal bacterial content?). After ingestion of a meal the sequence of these gut factors promotes satiety. The meal generates inhibitory signals which provoke satiation. The quality, intensity and duration of these inhibitory signals may be different from one subject to another (Fig. 1A and 1B). These signals could be modified by diseases such as non-ulcer dyspepsia and irritable bowel syndrome, two conditions where gut sensations related to food are perceived as unpleasant or noxious.

*Gastric factors.* There is no doubt that feeling the stomach "full", i.e. gastric distension, stops food intake (Fig. 2) [8, 9]. Further food intake can induce discomfort, nausea or vomiting. But these symptoms occur only with abnormally large or abnormally fast food intake, which does not permit the stomach muscle to relax. Indeed increasing the volume of the stomach has been shown to produce a cascade of events: (1) conscious but labile perception of a foreign body at a threshold intragastric pressure;

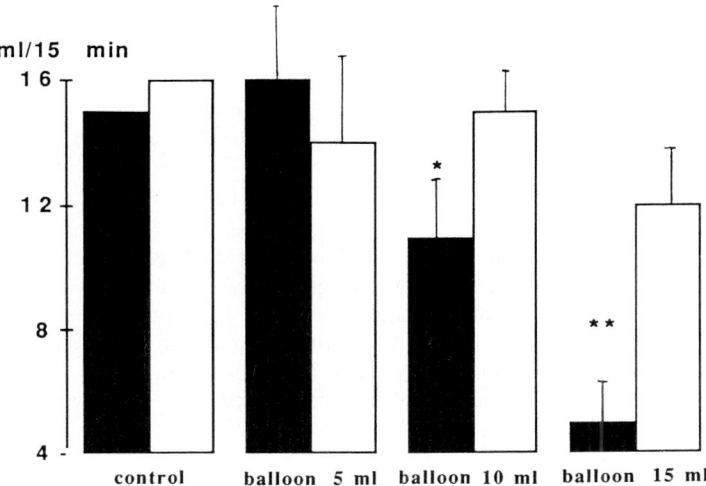

**Figure 2.** Effect of gastric distension by a balloon on food intake in rat. Note that the inhibitory effect occurs for a large distension (10 ml or more). After a truncal vagotomy (white columns) the inhibitory effect of gastric distension on food intake is blunt, as compared with sham operation (black columns). *$p<0.05$ *vs* controls or truncal vagotomy; **$p<0.01$ *vs* controls or truncal vagotomy.

(2) conscious and permanent perception at a higher pressure; (3) conscious and painful sensation at a higher pressure obtained for supraphysiological volumes. These data, similar to those obtained for the rectum, clearly suggest a pressure-related relaxation of gastric muscle. These three steps of gastric muscle response are related to the reflex relaxation of smooth muscle fibres when the meal is arriving in the stomach. The velocity of relaxation and the capacity of the stomach to relax are extremely variable from one subject to another (and probably from one day to another in the same subject), and condition feelings of fullness or pain in response to the meal. Another important factor is the ability of the gastric muscle to adapt. This is clearly supported by the disappearance (within a few weeks) of any perception of the gastric distension provoked by the intragastric placement of a 600 ml chronically inflated balloon in obese patients (personal communication). This progressive disappearance of feelings of distension was shown to be associated with progressive reappearance of the hunger feeling before each meal. These data indicate that both satiation and satiety are partly related to intragastric pressure and not only to intragastric volume.

The last but not the least gastric factor which modulates food intake and satiation is gastric emptying [10]. Several studies indicated that the stomach acts as an energy jet regulator which allows delivery of relatively similar energy boluses to the duodenum around the clock, whatever the nature of the meal eaten. Liquid mixtures (with thus low energy densities) leave the stomach faster than solid meals of higher energy density; lipids (9 kcal/g) leave the stomach slower than carbohydrates or proteins (4 kcal/g). Some authors estimate the mean energy gastric output at 5-6 kcal/min.

*Post-gastric and metabolic factors.* Energy *influx* is the result of digestion and absorption processes. In animals as well as in man, satiation is clearly related to energy influx [6, 11]. In rats, food intake inhibition by duodenal energy load is dose-dependent. But the effect can be different for meals of different palatability (Fig. 3).

As the meal enters the duodenum, it promotes and then maintains for a couple of hours several central inhibitory signals. The meal can only be initiated spontaneously when most of these inhibitory stimuli generated by the previous meal dissipate. These signals are both endocrine and neurocrine messengers, reaching the brain through different pathways via the vagus nerves and the blood.

It must be kept in mind that different duodenal energy contents produce qualitatively and quantitatively different releases of gut hormones such as cholecystokinin (CCK), insulin, and pancreatic polypeptide (PP), three hormones well recognized to control food intake. Concerning insulin, we also know that in hyperglycaemic states gastric inhibitory polypeptide (GIP) increases insulin release and thus may participate in satiation. The fast insulin response to the meal (namely its cephalic phase) can however be responsible for the well established "aperitif effect" of some foods taken before the normal meal.

Two to three hours after ingestion, a large part of the meal (most of the lipids) has not left the stomach, whereas another part (liquids and water-soluble nutrients) has reached the ileum, promoting the release of enteroglucagon and polypeptide YY. Thus for every time point after the first bolus arriving in the duodenum, both inhibitory (CCK, insulin) and stimulatory (PP, PYY, insulin?) signals originate from the gut and are sent to the brain [12]. It is not clear how the brain, and dual centre of food intake, integrates these opposite signals.

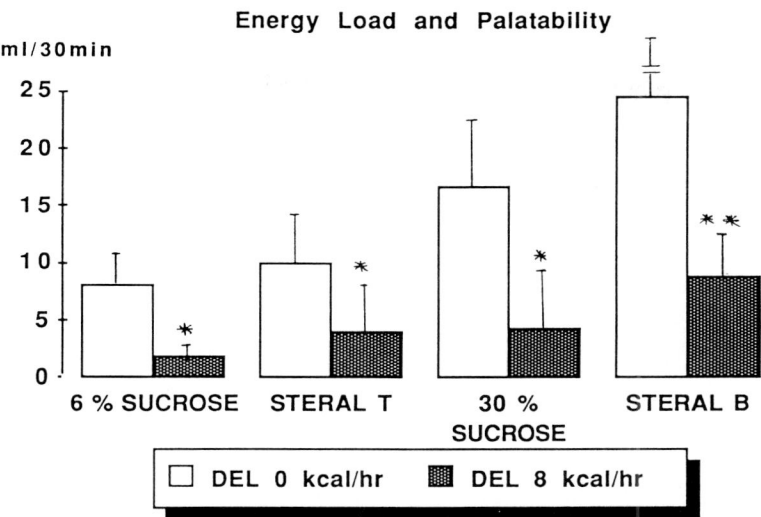

**Figure 3.** Effect of palatability and duodenal energy load (DEL) on food intake during sham feeding in rat. 30% sucrose and Steral B are two highly palatable diets, whereas 6% sucrose and Steral T are not very palatable. Note that duodenal 8 kcal/h load decreases food intake for all liquid meals. *$p<0.02$; **$p<0.0001$.

But gut and metabolic regulation of feeding also results from a variety of signals which reached the brain via the vagus: the satiety effect of CCK [13-16] is blocked by abdominal vagotomy in rats [17]; the satiation effect of gastric distension is also abolished by vagotomy [18]; and selective hepatic vagotomy eliminates the satiation effect of glucose, pyruvate, insulin or glucagon [19-23]. The role of the vagus in the control of food intake is probably the result of the presence of CCK fibres and of the vagal firing-rate-dependence on sodium-potassium ATPase [24]. Indeed, in states where energy is lacking, oxidations are at their minimal level; consequently membranes are partly depolarized, which results in high vagal firing rate [24]. With the energy influx (via the gut, and through the liver), the oxidation step increases and, through the ATP yielded, is thought to activate sodium-potassium ATPase, to hyperpolarize membranes, to decrease vagal firing rate, and consequently to induce satiety [24].

## Conclusions

Like the initiation of feeding, satiation and satiety cannot be attributed to a single afferent peripheral signal. Indeed it is the combination of different influences originating from the different nutrients and gut functions which is needed to suppress feeding in man. We can hypothesize that both metabolic and neuroendocrine signals arising either from eating the meal or from the changing pattern of substrate utilization and gut hormone secretions are monitored centrally to terminate (and, afterwards, initiate) food intake [25, 26]. The afferent fibres of the vagus carry this information. Hypothalamic centres and other brain centres integrate both blood-borne and cerebrospinal-fluid-borne nutrient-related signals [27]. They also receive information from sensory inputs and from higher centres, and then modulate responses according to the local (central) secretion of neuropeptides.

In this complex regulation, the gut acts both as a promoting factor of feeding, and as a limiting factor, but only in unusual conditions such as very large meals or very rapid ingestion. In disease, the inhibitory influence of the gut on food intake could be related to an abnormal motility response to ingested foods.

## References

1. Anand BK, Brobeck JR. Hypothalamic control of food intake in rats and cats. Yale J Biol Med 1951;24:123-40.
2. Brobeck JR, Tepperman J, Long CNH. Experimental hypothalamic hyperphagia in the albinos rat. Yale J Biol Med 1943;15:831-53.
3. Powley TL. The ventromedial hypothalamic syndrome, satiety, and a cephalic phase hypothesis. Psychol Rev 1977;84:89-126.
4. Le Magnen J. Body energy balance and food intake: a neuroendocrine regulatory mechanism. Physiol Rev 1983;63:314-36.
5. Stricker EM. Biological bases of hunger and satiety: therapeutic implications. Nutr Rev 1984;42:333-40.
6. Friedman MI, Tordoff MG, Ramirez I. Integrated metabolic control of food intake. Brain Res Bull 1986;17:855-9.
7. Even P, Nicolaidis S. Short-term control of feeding: limitation of the glucostatic theory. Brain Res Bull 1986;17:621-6.
8. Deutsch JA, Gonzalez MF. Gastric fat content and satiety. Physiol Behav 1981;26:673-6.
9. Renaud LP, Tang M, McCann MJ, Stricker EM, Verbalis JG. Cholecystokinin and gastric distension activate oxytocinergic cells in rat hypothalamus. Am J Physiol 1987;253:R661-5.
10. Mc Cann MJ, Stricker EM. Gastric emptying of glucose loads in rats: effects of insulin-induced hypoglycemia. Am J Physiol 1986;251:R609-13.
11. Oomura Y. Contributions of endogenous substances to control of feeding. In: Björntorp P, Rössner S, eds. *Obesity in Europe 88*. Proceedings of the 1st European Congress on Obesity. London: John Libbey,1988:101-8.
12. Flanagan LM, Verbalis JG, Stricker EM. Naloxone potentiation of effects of cholecystokinin and lithium chloride on oxytocin secretion, gastric motility and feeding. Neuroendocrinology 1988;48:668-73.
13. Gibbs J, Young RC, Smith GP. Cholecystokinin elicits satiety in rats with open gastric fistulas. Nature 1973;245:323-5.
14. Gibbs J, Young RC, Smith GP. Cholecystokinin decreases food intake in rats. J Comp Physiol Psychol 1973;84:488-95.
15. Antin J, Gibbs J, Holt J, Young RC, Smith GP. Cholecystokinin elicits the complete behavioural sequence of satiety in rats. J Comp Psychol 1975;89:784-90.
16. Hewson G, Leighton GE, Hill RG, Hughes J. The cholecystokinin receptor antagonist L364, 718 increases food intake in the rat by attenuation of the action of endogenous cholecystokinin. Br J Pharmacol 1988;93:79-84.
17. Smith GP, Jerome C, Cushin BJ, Eterno R, Simansky KJ. Abdominal vagotomy blocks the satiety effect of cholecystokinin in the rat. Science 1981;213:1036-7.

18. Gonzalez MF, Deutsch JA. Vagotomy abolishes cues of satiety produced by gastric distension. Science 1981;212:1283-4.
19. Geary N, Smith GP. Selective hepatic vagotomy blocks pancreatic glucagon's satiety effect. Physiol Behav 1983; 31: 391-4.
20. Granneman J, Friedman MI. Effect of hepatic vagotomy and/or coeliac ganglionectomy on the delayed eating response to insulin and 2DG injection in rats. Physiol Behav 1984;33:495-7.
21. Langhans W, Egli G, Scharrer E. Selective hepatic vagotomy eliminates the hypophagic effect of different metabolites. J Auton Nerv Syst 1985; 13:255-62.
22. Niijima A. Visceral afferents and metabolic function. Diabetologia 1981;20(suppl):325-30.
23. Niijima A. Glucose-sensitive afferent nerve fibers in the liver and their role in food intake and blood glucose regulation. J Auton Nerv Syst 1983;9:207-20.
24. Langhans W, Scharrer E. Evidence for a role for the sodium pump of hepatocytes in the control of food intake. J Auton Nerv Syst 1987;20:199-205.
25. Uvnäs-Moberg K. Neuroendocrine regulation of hunger and satiety. In: Björntorp P, Rössner S, eds. *Obesity in Europe*. Volume 1. London: John Libbey, 1989:1-13.
26. Woods SC, Porte D Jr. The central nervous system, pancreatic hormones, feeding and obesity. In: Levine R, Luft ER, eds. *Advances in Metabolic Disorders*. Volume 9. New York: Academic Press, 1978:283-312.
27. Davis JD, Wirtshafter D, Asin KE, Brief D. Sustained intracerebroventricular infusion of brain fuels reduces body weight and food intake in rats. Science 1981;212:81-3.

# SESSION II
# Pathophysiology

Chairman: J. FOURNET

# 8

# Motor disturbances:
# 1. Manometry

V. STANGHELLINI, M. RICCI MACCARINI, C. GHIDINI, R. CORINALDESI, L. BARBARA

*Institute of Medical Clinic and Gastroenterology, University of Bologna, Bologna, Italy*

## Introduction

Idiopathic (or non-ulcer) dyspepsia is a syndrome which is the cause of approximately one third of all gastroenterological consultations in general practice (seven times more frequent than peptic ulcer!) [1]. Despite this great frequency and the relative economic relevance, the syndrome still defies a definition and its pathogenesis and therapy are far from being identified. Some of the definitions so far adopted probably indicate subgroups of patients with different underlying pathogenic mechanisms. Thompson [2] coined the term non-ulcer dyspepsia to indicate symptoms suggestive of peptic ulcer in the absence of focal lesions of the mucosa of the gut. Others hybridized dyspepsia and irritable bowel syndrome (IBS) [3]. More recently a certain consensus has developed in defining idiopathic dyspepsia as a set of symptoms (syndrome) referable to the proximal portions of the gut in the absence of detectable disease [4, 5]. This remains a very vague definition, but has the advantage of differentiating dyspepsia from IBS, which is already recognized as a separate nosological entity [6]. The clinical application of this definition is complicated by the frequent coexistence of dyspepsia and IBS in the same patient [7]. A precise description of the patients' complaints has not been included in the majority of papers so far published on idiopathic dyspepsia. We shall try to take these possible sources of error into consideration while reviewing the published reports on manometric findings in patients with idiopathic dyspepsia.

## Gastrointestinal manometric techniques

Different contractile activities are exerted by the various segments of the gut. The development of reliable techniques has recently resulted in a rapid growth of our knowledge of the physiology of gastrointestinal motility and the application of these techniques in clinical studies has led to the recognition of abnormal motor patterns in a number of pathological conditions including idiopathic dyspepsia. A review on the technical aspects of gastrointestinal manometry has recently been published [8]. Recording systems invariably include a pressure sensor and/or a transducer, an amplifier and a recorder. The first recordings of pressure changes were obtained by intragastric flaccid balloons filled with water or air and attached to an external transducer. Recordings, however, were influenced by the pressure variations of the plastic wall [9]. The electronic barostat developed by Azpiroz et al. [10] has overcome these problems, allowing recording of both positive and negative pressures. It has been successfully employed for measuring tonic and phasic pressure changes in the gastric fundus and is described in detail in another chapter of this book. Phasic contractions of the gastric antrum and small bowel can be recorded in humans by miniature transducers or perfused catheters attached to external transducers. The sensitivity and recording quality of perfused catheters and intraluminal miniature transducers were compared in an animal model by Valori et al. [11]. The standard was represented by serosal strain gauges sewn parallel to the circular smooth muscle layer. Open-tipped perfused catheters were significantly more sensitive in recording antral contractions than intraluminal transducers. The two systems displayed similar sensitivities in the small bowel, but the quality of the tracings was superior in recordings obtained using perfused catheters. Pyloric motility can be recorded both by perfused catheters with a series of 5 to 10 closely-spaced (<1 cm) recording sites or by 4-5 cm long rubber sleeve sensors, which are positioned at the gastroduodenal junction. Both techniques have advantages and disadvantages in recording pressure changes at sphincteric regions, as demonstrated by a comparative study in the canine ileocolonic junction [12]. The sleeve sensor was superior to the multiple perfused catheters in recording tonic pressure activities and allowed a continuous recording of the sphincteric zone with only sporadic repositioning. On the other hand, it displayed a low fidelity for recording amplitude, duration, localization and propagation of phasic contractions. Modern manometric perfused catheters (with or without a pyloric sleeve) are soft, can be introduced through the nose and are generally well accepted for prolonged periods of time as well.

## Gastrointestinal manometry in dyspepsia

Symptoms such as postprandial fullness, nausea and vomiting are strongly suggestive of abnormal gastrointestinal motility, and several manometric studies have been carried out over the last decade to investigate this important digestive function in patients with idiopathic dyspepsia [13-21]. Tables I and II summarize the main findings reported in these studies, using gastric and intestinal recordings. With the exception of the study carried out at the Mayo Clinic [15], relatively small groups of patients were studied and the presence of patients with associated IBS was clearly reported in two studies [18, 20]. Interdigestive antral hypomotility was reported in all studies

## Manometry

**Table I.** Antral manometry in patients with idiopathic dyspepsia.

| Reference | | No. pts | IBS (No. pts) | Fasting | Postprandial |
|---|---|---|---|---|---|
| Rees et al. [13] | 1980 | 1 | ± | Absence A III (67% III) | Decreased amplitude |
| Reboa et al. [14] | 1984 | 7 | ? | — | Normal mean MI |
| Malagelada and Stanghellini [15] | 1985 | 104 | + (?) | Constant antral motility (3% pts) | Decreased MI (72% pts) |
| Narducci et al. [16] | 1986 | 18 | ? | Absence A III (75% III) | — |
| Labò et al. [17] | 1986 | 22 | ? | Absence A III (78% III) | — |
| Camilleri et al. [18] | 1986 | 16 | + (4) | — | Decreased MI (50% pts) |
| Abell et al. [19] | 1988 | 8 | ? | — | Decreased MI (63% pts) |
| Kerlin et al. [20] | 1989 | 20 | + (8) | Normal | Decreased MI (70% pts) |

Abbreviations: No. = number; pts = patients; IBS = irritable bowel syndrome; A = antral; III = phase III of the interdigestive migrating motor complex; MI = motility index.

**Table II.** Intestinal manometry in patients with idiopathic dyspepsia.

| Reference | | No. pts | IBS (No. pts) | Intestinal motor patterns (No. pts) |
|---|---|---|---|---|
| Rees et al. [13] | 1980 | 1 | ± | Normal |
| Reboa et al. [14] | 1984 | 7 | ? | Normal |
| Malagelada and Stanghellini [15] | 1985 | 104 | + (?) | Abnormal III (13), Bursts (13), No Fed (6) |
| Narducci et al. [16] | 1986 | 18 | ? | Hyperdyskinesia (8), Abnormal III (27% III) |
| Labò et al. [17] | 1986 | 22 | ? | Absence of III (11) |
| Abell et al. [19] | 1988 | 8 | ? | Bursts (4), sustained incoordinated contractions (1) Hypomotility (1), No Fed (1) |
| Kerlin [20] | 1989 | 20 | + (8) | Bursts (1), No Fed (1) |
| Bassotti et al. [21] | 1990 | 33 | ? | Abnormal III (15) |

Abbreviations: No. = number; pts = patients; III = phase III of the interdigestive migrating motor complex; No Fed = inability of meal ingestion to convert fasting into fed motor pattern.

where it was directly quantified [13, 16, 17], except one [20]. In healthy individuals, activity fronts (phase III of the interdigestive migrating motor complex) present an antral component in over 80% of the cases [8], while activity fronts starting in the antrum are recorded only in 22 to 33% of the cases in patients with idiopathic dyspepsia [13, 18]. Antral activity fronts are responsible for clearing the stomach during fasting of digestive secretions, exfoliated cells and large indigestible solid particles [22], which tend to accumulate in their absence. Thus the majority of dyspeptic patients certainly have impaired gastric clearing activity during fasting, but the clinical relevance of this abnormality is unclear. Postprandially, antral contractions accomplish two important functions: (1) they discriminate gastric contents with different physical properties [23]; (2) they push gastric contents against the pylorus, thus breaking digestible solids into tiny particles (1-3 mm) that are then emptied from the stomach suspended in the liquid contents [24]. With the exception of the paper by Reboa et al. [14], decreased postprandial antral contractility was invariably reported in the studies evaluating this variable [13, 15, 18-20]. Specifically, 50 to 70% of patients with idiopathic dyspepsia presented contractile activities lower than the respective normal values [18, 20]. This motor abnormality may contribute to determining the delayed gastric emptying of solids that is found in dyspeptic patients [25, 26].

Intestinal manometry, on the other hand, has given more conflicting results in patients with chronic idiopathic dyspepsia (Table II). In the largest study published so far, 104 patients consecutively underwent gastrointestinal manometry [15]. Abnormal small bowel motor patterns were recorded in 32 patients: ingestion of the test meal did not modify the interdigestive motor patterns in six, activity fronts for propagation and/or configuration were recorded in 13, and bursts (defined as groups of contractions with increased intensity and frequency which, unlike activity fronts, are not propagated and not followed by motor quiescence) in the remaining 13. This study, however, does not strictly reflect the manometric picture of chronic idiopathic dyspepsia, since patients with altered bowel habits and with associated diseases (autonomic neuropathies, diabetes) were also included. Small bowel dysmotility is relatively frequent among patients with both IBS [26, 27] and autonomic neuropathies [28], regardless of the presence of dyspeptic symptoms. In a smaller but more homogeneous group of patients, Kerlin [20] recently detected intestinal motor abnormalities only in three out of 20 cases: bursts in one, and inability of meal ingestion to induce a fed motor pattern in two. Interestingly, the three dyspeptic patients with intestinal dysmotility also had IBS. The majority of the studies exploring intestinal motility in idiopathic dyspepsia have detected abnormal patterns, but have failed to specify whether or not patients had associated IBS, and interpretation of the results is thus difficult.

## Causes of gastrointestinal motor disorders in dyspeptic patients

It has been claimed that both endocrine and neural abnormalities are involved in determining gut dysmotility in patients with idiopathic dyspepsia.

Narducci et al. [16] reported that infusion of naloxone accelerates gastric emptying in dyspeptic patients with duodenal hyperdyskinesia, thus suggesting that intestinal motor abnormalities may be due to either abnormal release of endorphins and/or enkephalins or to abnormal sensitivity of the smooth muscle cells to endogenous opioids. Labò et al. [17] found a reduction in interdigestive motilin peaks in patients who had activity fronts without an antral component (20/22) or complete absence of activity fronts (11/22). Cholecystokinin reduces food intake and induces satiety, by acting both in the central nervous system and peripherally in the gut via afferent vagal fibres [29]. Basal, but not postprandial, circulating gastrin levels were found to be abnormally raised in patients with "non-ulcer dyspepsia" [30]. Sex hormones may also play a conditioning role in idiopathic dyspepsia. The syndrome is more frequent among women and experimental data demonstrate that progesterone, oestradiol and prolactin can markedly affect smooth muscle contractility and also influence gastrointestinal transit times [31, 32].

Infective and idiopathic neuropathies may be the cause of gastrointestinal motor abnormalities. Viral infections have been indicated as putative causes of gut dysmotility in a variety of case reports [33-37]. Possible viral agents of "infectious dyspepsia" are herpes zoster [33] and Epstein Barr viruses [34]. Oh and Kim [38] described five cases seen at the Mayo Clinic between 1977 and 1988 who developed gastroparesis shortly after a viral infection. Gastroparesis was scintigraphically and manometrically documented in 103 patients in that period, but no relationship to viral infections could be retrospectively documented in 96. In two patients with suspected viral infection, manometry was not performed. Among the five patients studied, three also underwent autonomic function tests which demonstrated the presence of autonomic neuropathy. Gastrointestinal motility was invariably found to be abnormal, with antral hypomotility in four patients and intestinal dysmotility in two. Symptoms disappeared, on average, within three years. The authors concluded that postviral gastroparesis is a rare, benign syndrome often associated with autonomic dysfunction. Preliminary data indicate that viral infections may be involved in the pathogenesis of long lasting dyspepsia in a significant number of cases [39]. Patients with chronic idiopathic dyspepsia in fact were found to present an average increase of antibody titre against cytomegalovirus. Gastrointestinal dysautonomias are responsible for severe motor disturbances and may be associated with digestive symptoms as demonstrated in patients with idiopathic orthostatic hypotension [28]. Whether milder forms of abnormality of the autonomic neural supply to the gut are present in the average dyspeptic patient has not been systematically investigated.

Endocrine and neuroendocrine disturbances may potentiate each other in determining gastrointestinal disorders and in eliciting perception of dyspeptic symptoms [40, 41]. These observations have not yet been clinically confirmed and must still be regarded as attractive hypotheses for future research.

## Clinical application of gastrointestinal manometry

A compendium of experiences obtained by clinical applications of gastrointestinal manometry has recently been published [42]. Manometry allows an objective evaluation of gut motor abnormalities that cannot reliably be predicted by the analysis of the symptoms alone [15]. Specificity and sensitivity of the results of the technique, however, have never been directly investigated. Antral hypomotility is not a specific finding since it has been detected in a variety of clinical conditions which, as well as idiopathic dyspepsia, include insulin-dependent diabetes [43, 44], postvagotomy dyspeptic syndrome [43], postfundoplication dyspeptic syndrome [45], spinal cord transection [46], orthostatic hypotension [28], gastric ulcer [47], and anorexia nervosa [48] (Table III). On the other hand, manometric small bowel abnormalities can give some clue to the underlying pathogenic mechanisms. Diseases affecting the smooth muscle cells but not the neural supply to the alimentary canal give rise to manometric tracings characterized by the absence of contractility or the presence of pressure waves which, while having normal coordination, are markedly reduced in amplitude [42]. Neurogenic disorders of gastrointestinal motility, on the other hand, are characterized

**Table III.** Diseases associated with antral hypomotility.

| Reference | | No. pts | Associated disease | Fasting | Postprandial |
|---|---|---|---|---|---|
| Malagelada et al. [43] | 1980 | 7 | Insulin-dependent diabetes | Absence A III (86% pts) | — |
| Stanghellini & Malagelada [45] | 1983 | 6 | Post-fundoplication | Absence A III (83% pts) | Decreased contractility (85% pts) |
| Fealey et al. [46] | 1984 | 5 | Spinal cord transection | Absence A III (60% III) Constant A Mot (20% pts) | Increased contractility (40% pts) (liquid meal) |
| Camilleri et al. [28] | 1985 | 9 | Orthostatic hypotension | Absence A III (100% III) | Decreased contractility (56% pts) |
| Miranda et al. [47] | 1985 | 17 | Gastric ulcer | Absence A III (91% III) | — |
| Mearin et al. [44] | 1986 | 24 | Insulin-dependent diabetes | Absence A III (88% III) | Decreased mean MI |
| Abell et al. [48] | 1987 | 8 | Anorexia nervosa | — | Decreased MI (100% pts) |

Abbreviations: No. = number; pts = patients; A = antral; III = phase III of the interdigestive migrating motor complex; MI = motility index.

by incoordinated, high amplitude contractions [28, 42]. In some cases, intestinal manometry can also help to differentiate mechanical from functional obstruction of the small bowel [42, 49]. Indirect data suggest that manometry has good sensitivity. The technique invariably detects intestinal motor abnormalities in patients with severe syndromes such as chronic intestinal pseudo-obstruction [50] and therefore the normal manometric tracings obtained in 30 to 50% of dyspeptic patients are unlikely to be false negative results. The observation that psychogenic disorders are particularly frequent among patients complaining of digestive symptoms without evidence of manometric abnormalities [15] further substantiates the reliability of the technique. Other studies confirm that the relationship between gut dysmotility and symptoms is not a direct one. Abell *et al.* [19] described eight patients with cyclic nausea and vomiting in whom gastrointestinal motor abnormalities could also be detected during asymptomatic periods, suggesting that dysmotility represents a substrate which, in certain individuals exposed to unknown precipitating factors, facilitates the development of a dyspeptic syndrome. Because of the uncertainties still existing on the relationship between gut dysmotility and clinical syndromes and because of the discrepancy between the availability of centres with manometric facilities and the number of potentially affected individuals, measurement of gastrointestinal motility is limited to a restricted number of patients. After having excluded organic, metabolic and systemic diseases, a short-term course of treatment (4-8 weeks) with prokinetic drugs should be attempted in all symptomatic patients. If symptoms do not respond favourably to therapy, patients should be referred to a specialist centre for quantitative measurement of gastric emptying (by scintigraphy) and/or gastrointestinal motility (by manometric techniques). Gastric emptying tests have the major advantage of being non-invasive, but manometry provides information on the nature of the underlying pathogenic mechanisms and can help to identify the nature of the motor disorders that are responsible for the derangement of gastric emptying: abnormal fundal tone, decreased antral motility, increased pyloric and/or intestinal resistance to flow, and antroduodenal incoordination. The effect of pharmacological agents on gut motility can also be quantified so that therapeutic decisions do not exclusively rely on symptoms, and drugs that favourably affect motility can be continued to encourage the digestive processes and maintain adequate nutrition.

In conclusion, gastrointestinal manometric techniques are reliable tools for physiological, pathophysiological and pharmacological research. Their clinical utility is at present limited to some selected cases. Their broader clinical application depends on the recognition of groups of patients with a correlation between motor disorders and clinical features, as well as on the development of more efficient and selective drugs for these disorders.

# References

1. Loof L, Adami HO, Agenas I, Gustavsson S, Nyberg A, Nyrén O. The Diagnosis and Therapy Survey, October 1978-March 1983, health care consumption and current drug therapy in Sweden with respect to the clinical diagnosis of gastritis. Scand J Gastroenterol 1985;20(suppl 109):35-9.
2. Thompson WG. Non-ulcer dyspepsia. Can Med Assoc J 1984;130:565-9.
3. Rind JA, Watson L. Gallstone dyspepsia. Br Med J 1968;1:32.

4. Colin-Jones DG, Bloom B, Bodemar G, Crean G, Freston J, Gugler R, Malagelada J, Nyrén O, Petersen H, Piper D. Management of dyspepsia: report of a working party. Lancet 1988;1:576-9.
5. Barbara L, Camilleri M, Corinaldesi R, Crean GP, Heading RO, Johnson AG, Malagelada JR, Stanghellini V, Wienbeck M. Definition and investigation of dyspepsia. Consensus of an international *ad hoc* working party. Dig Dis Sci 1989;34:1272-6.
6. Manning AP, Thompson WG, Heaton KW, Morris AF. Towards positive diagnosis of the irritable bowel. Br Med J 1978;2:653-4.
7. Talley NJ, Phillips SF. Non-ulcer dyspepsia: potential causes and pathophysiology. Ann Intern Med 1988;108:865-79.
8. Stanghellini V, Corinaldesi R, Ghidini C, Ricci Maccarini M, Barbara L. Methodology of gastroduodenal manometry. In: Scarpignato C, Bianchi Porro G, eds. *Clinical Investigation of Gastric Function*. Volume 17. Basel: Karger, 1990, 258-73.
9. Wolf S. The relationship to nausea in man. J Clin Invest 1943;22:877-82.
10. Azpiroz F, Malagelada JR. Gastric tone measured by an electronic barostat in health and postsurgical gastroparesis. Gastroenterology 1987;92:934-43.
11. Valori RM, Collins SM, Daniel EE, Reddy SN, Shannon S, Jury J. Comparison of methodologies for the measurement of antroduodenal motor activity in the dog. Gastroenterology 1986;91:546-53.
12. Quigley EM, Dent J, Phillips SF. Manometry of canine ileo-colonic sphincter: comparison of sleeve method to point sensors. Am J Physiol 1987;262:G585-91.
13. Rees WD, Miller LJ, Malagelada JR. Dyspepsia, antral motor dysfunction, and gastric stasis of solids. Gastroenterology 1980;78:360-5.
14. Reboa G, Arnulfo G, Di Somma C, et al. Prokinetic effects of cisapride on normal and reduced antroduodenal motility and reflexes. Curr Ther Res 1984;36:18-23.
15. Malagelada JR, Stanghellini V. Manometric evaluation of functional upper gut symptoms. Gastroenterology 1985;88:1223-31.
16. Narducci F, Bassotti G, Granata MT, Gaburri M, Farroni F, Palumbo R, Morelli A. Functional dyspepsia and chronic idiopathic gastric stasis. Role of endogenous opiates. Arch Intern Med 1986;146:716-20.
17. Labò G, Bortolotti M, Vezzadini P, Bonora G, Bersani G. Interdigestive gastroduodenal motility and serum motilin levels in patients with idiopathic delay in gastric emptying. Gastroenterology 1986;90:20-6.
18. Camilleri M, Malagelada JR, Kao PC, Zinsmeister AR. Gastric and autonomic responses to stress in functional dyspepsia. Dig Dis Sci 1986; 31:1169-77.
19. Abell TL, Kim CH, Malagelada JR. Idiopathic cyclic nausea and vomiting — a disorder of gastrointestinal motility? Mayo Clin Proc 1988;63:1169-75.
20. Kerlin P. Postprandial antral hypomotility in patients with idiopathic nausea and vomiting. Gut 1989;30:54-9.
21. Bassotti G, Pelli MA, Morelli A. Duodenojejunal motor activity in patients with chronic dyspeptic symptoms. J Clin Gastroenterol 1990;12:17-21.
22. Kelly KA. Gastric emptying of liquids and solids: roles of proximal and distal stomach. Am J Physiol 1980;239:G71-6.
23. Hinder RA, Kelly KA. Canine gastric emptying of solids and liquids. Am J Physiol 1977;233:E335-40.
24. Meyer JH, Ohashi H, Jehn D, Thomson JB. Size of liver particles emptied from the human stomach. Gastroenterology 1981;80:1489-96.
25. Corinaldesi R, Stanghellini V, Raiti C, Rea E, Salgemini R, Paternico A, Paparo GF, Barbara L. Gastric acid secretion and gastric emptying (GE) of solids in patients with chronic idiopathic dyspepsia (CID), Dig Dis Sci 1986;31(suppl 10):343S(abstr).
26. Jian R, Ducrot F, Ruskoné A, Chaussade S, Rambaud JC, Modigliani R, Rain JD, Bernier JJ. Symptomatic, radionuclide and therapeutic assessment of chronic idiopathic dyspepsia. A double-blind placebo-controlled evaluation of cisapride. Dig Dis Sci 1989;34:657-64.

27. Kellow JE, Gill RC, Wingate DL. Prolonged ambulant recordings of small bowel motility demonstrate abnormalities in the irritable bowel syndrome. Gastroenterology 1990; 98:1208-18.
28. Camilleri M, Malagelada JR, Stanghellini V, Fealey RD, Sheps SG. Gastrointestinal motility disturbances in patients with orthostatic hypotension. Gastroenterology 1985; 88:1852-9.
29. Morley JE. Neuropeptide regulation of appetite and weight. Endocr Rev 1987;8:256-87.
30. Nyrén O, Adami HO, Bergstrom R, Gustavsson S, Loof L, Lundqvist G. Basal and food-stimulated levels of gastrin and pancreatic polypeptide in non-ulcer dyspepsia and duodenal ulcer. Scand J Gastroenterol 1986;21:471-7.
31. Wald A, Van Thiel DH, Hoechstetter L, Gavaler JS, Egler KM, Verm R, Scott L, Lester R. Gastrointestinal transit: the effect of the menstrual cycle. Gastroenterology 1981; 80:1497-500.
32. Gopalakrishnan V, Ramaswamy S, Pillai NP, Ghosh MN. Effect of prolactin and bromocriptine on intestinal transit in mice. Eur J Pharmacol 1981;74:369-72.
33. Chang AE, Young NA, Reddick RL, Orenstein JM, Hosea SW, Katz P, Brennan MF. Small bowel obstruction as a complication of disseminated varicella-zoster infection. Surgery 1978;83:371-4.
34. Yahr MD, Frontera AT. Acute autonomic neuropathy. Its occurrence in infectious mononucleosis. Arch Neurol 1975;32:132-3.
35. Meeroff JC, Schreiber DS, Trier JS, Blacklow NR. Abnormal gastric motor function in viral gastroenteritis. Ann Intern Med 1980;92:370-3.
36. Rhodes JB, Robinson RG, McBride N. Sudden onset of slow gastric emptying of food. Gastroenterology 1979;77:569-71.
37. Kebede D, Barthel JS, Singh A. Transient gastroparesis associated with cutaneous herpes zoster. Dig Dis Sci 1987;32:318-22.
38. Oh JJ, Kim CH. Gastroparesis after a presumed viral illness: clinical and laboratory features and natural history. Mayo Clin Proc 1990;65:636-42.
39. Bortolotti M, Bersanin G, Labò G. Association between chronic idiopathic gastroparesis and cytomegalovirus infection. Gastroenterology 1987;92:1324(abstr).
40. Notivol R, Mearin F, Azpiroz F, Malagelada JR. Epigastric symptoms are elicited by selective stimulation of "in series" and "in parallel" gastric mechanoreceptors. Gastroenterology 1990;98:A377(abstr).
41. Moragas G, Azpiroz F, Malagelada JR. Strain on gastric accommodation after a meal spares emptying but produces symptoms. Gastroenterology 1990;98:A376(abstr).
42. Malagelada JR, Camilleri M, Stanghellini V. Manometric diagnosis of gastrointestinal motility disorders. New York: Thieme, 1986.
43. Malagelada JR, Rees WD, Mazzotta LJ, Go VL. Gastric motor abnormalities in diabetic and postvagotomy gastroparesis: effect of metoclopramide and bethanechol. Gastroenterology 1980;78:286-93.
44. Mearin F, Camilleri M, Malagelada JR. Pyloric dysfunction in diabetics with recurrent nausea and vomiting. Gastroenterology 1986;90:1919-25.
45. Stanghellini V, Malagelada JR. Gastric manometric abnormalities in patients with dyspeptic symptoms after fundoplication. Gut 1983;24:790-7.
46. Fealey RD, Szurszewski JH, Merritt JL, Di Magno EP. Effect of traumatic spinal cord transection on human upper gastrointestinal motility and gastric emptying. Gastroenterology 1984;87:69-75.
47. Miranda M, Defilippi C, Valanzuela JE. Abnormalities of interdigestive motility complex and increased duodenogastric reflux in gastric ulcer patients. Dig Dis Sci 1985;30:16-21.
48. Abell TL, Malagelada JR, Lucas AR, Brown ML, Camilleri M, Go VL, Azpiroz F, Callaway CW, Kao PC, Zinsmeister AR, Huse DM. Gastric electromechanical and neurohormonal function in anorexia nervosa. Gastroenterology 1987;93:958-65.

49. Stanghellini V, Corinaldesi R, Barbara L. Pseudo-obstruction syndromes. In: Grundy D, Read NW, eds. *Gastrointestinal Neurophysiology*. Baillière's Clin Gastroenterol. London: Baillière Tindall, 1988:225-58.
50. Stanghellini V, Camilleri M, Malagelada JR. Chronic idiopathic intestinal pseudo-obstruction: clinical and intestinal manometric findings. Gut 1987;28:5-12.

# 9

# Motor disturbances:
# 2. Abnormalities of gastric myoelectrical activity

A.J.P.M. SMOUT, H.J.A. JEBBINK, P.P.M. BRUIJS, D.R. FONE

*Departments of Gastroenterology and Surgery, University Hospital Utrecht, The Netherlands*

## Introduction

The myoelectrical activity of the distal stomach forms one of the major mechanisms that control its motor activity. It is clear, therefore, that abnormal myoelectrical activity may lead to abnormal gastric motility and emptying. Since the myoelectrical activities of the stomach are even less accessible for study than the motor activities of this organ, our knowledge of normal and disordered gastric myoelectrical activity is rather limited. Much of what we do know is based on studies performed in laboratory animals, in particular dogs.

In this chapter an attempt will be made to give an overview of our present knowledge of gastric myoelectrical activities, of the available techniques to record these activities and the relationships between abnormalities of gastric myoelectrical activity and upper abdominal symptoms, especially those that occur in non-ulcer dyspepsia.

## Myoelectrical activity of the stomach

The smooth muscle cells in the wall of the distal stomach, the small intestine and colon generate rhythmic electrical activity. This rhythmic activity cannot be found in the most proximal part of the stomach (fundus and upper part of the corpus) [1, 2]. The source of the electrical activity is formed by rhythmic variations in cell membrane potential. When a microelectrode is introduced into a gastric smooth muscle cell, regularly recurring spontaneous depolarization and repolarization of the cell membrane can be recorded [3]. These rhythmic fluctuations give rise to extracellular potential variations than can be detected by extracellular electrodes. The signal then recorded is called "slow waves", "basic electrical rhythm" (BER) or "electrical control activity" (ECA) (Fig. 1). A single ECA pulse is also known as "control potential" (CP). An important difference with the electrical activities of other types of muscle cells is that ECA is always present, whether or not the organ is mechanically active.

Until recently it was held that the ECA is generated autonomously by the smooth muscle cells themselves. Recent evidence suggests, however, that the ECA rhythm is in fact generated by the interstitial cells of Cajal, a specialized type of neurone, located directly underneath the circular muscle layer.

The frequency of the ECA is organ-dependent. In the human stomach its frequency is 3 cycles per minute (cpm); in the small intestine a gradient from 12 cpm in the duodenum declining gradually to 7 cpm in the terminal ileum is observed. In the human colon multiple ECA frequencies are simultaneously present, leading to a rather chaotic pattern. The frequencies of gastrointestinal slow waves are also species-dependent. In the dog, a commonly used laboratory animal for this kind of study, the frequency of the gastric slow waves is about 5 cpm.

Gastric ECA appears to arise from a pacemaker area at the greater curvature in the orad corpus. From this pacemaker area the CPs first propagate circumferentially, so that a ring-shaped front of control potentials is generated. This ring propagates in the direction of the pylorus, at a rate increasing from 0.3 to 1.0 cm/sec.

Contractions of the gastric smooth muscle cell are preceded by a second type of electrical activity. When recorded intracellularly, this activity is characterized by a plateau phase on which fast potentials, also known as spike potentials or action potentials, are often superimposed. The extracellular manifestation of this is referred

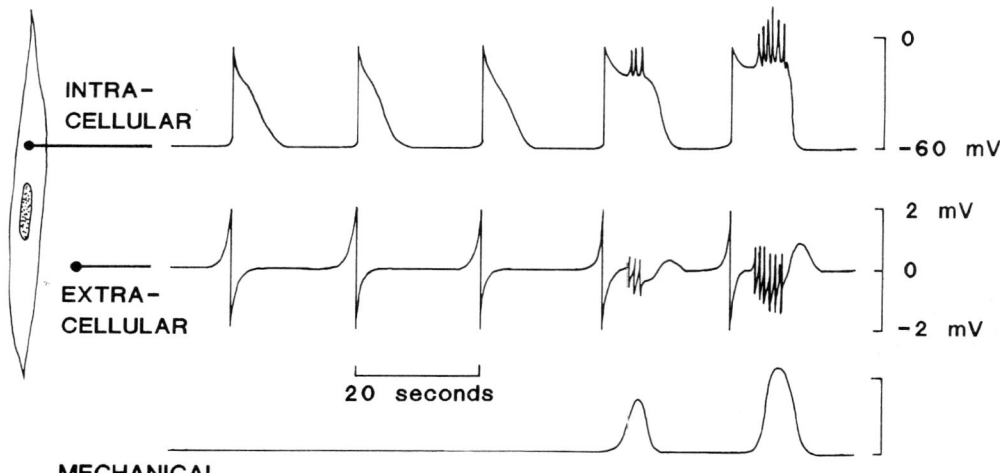

**Figure 1.** Relationships between intracellular and extracellular electrical activity and contractile activity of gastric smooth muscle (schematic).
First three cycles: mechanically quiescent cell; only ECA, no ERA present.
Fourth and fifth cycle: contracting cell; spike potentials (ERA) present.

to as "electrical response activity" (ERA) (Fig. 1). ERA (and thus phasic contractions) can only occur in the second quarter of an ECA cycle. In this way, ECA determines the moments at which phasic contractions of the distal stomach may occur, and determines the propagation direction and velocity of these contractions.

## Methods of recording gastric myoelectrical activity *in vivo*

**Mucosal electrodes**

There have been a number of studies in which the electrical activity of the human stomach has been recorded from intraluminal (mucosal) electrodes [1, 4-12]. Gastric ECA can only be recorded from mucosal electrodes by techniques which keep the electrode in close contact with the mucosa. Usually this is achieved by means of negative pressure (suction) cup electrodes (Fig. 2) [7, 8, 11, 12]. Suction electrodes cannot be used in the fed state. Another technique involves the use of a small internal and a large external magnet to press the intraluminal electrode to the mucosa [4, 5]. With this technique, longer periods of recording and studies in the postprandial state appear to be possible [13]. A disadvantage of all mucosal recording techniques is that the electrode can be easily dislodged, in particular during episodes of motor activity. For reasons unclear to us, most investigators who used a mucosal recording technique have confined themselves to describing the ECA, and did not describe the ERA.

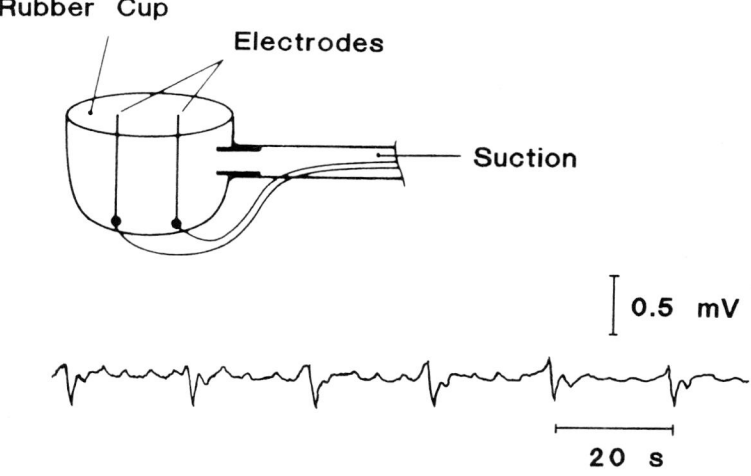

**Figure 2.** Mucosal electrode used by You and coworkers [11] and example of normal myoelectrical activity of the antrum recorded with the electrode. The cup with the electrodes is held in contact with the mucosa by means of suction. The recorded signal shows CPs at 20 sec intervals (ECA).

## Serosal electrodes

Surgically implanted serosal electrodes have been used in man to record gastric electrical activity, but on a very limited scale [6, 9, 10, 14]. In general, the quality of serosally recorded signals is superior to that of mucosal recordings. However, serosal recording in man is only possible for short periods, either peroperatively or in the first few days after operation. In laboratory animals, such as the dog, serosal electrodes form the gold standard for *in vivo* recording of extracellular electrical activity of the stomach.

## Cutaneous electrodes

Gastric myoelectrical activity can also be recorded from the body surface, using cutaneous electrodes. This technique is called electrogastrography (EGG). The first cutaneous EGG was recorded in 1921, by Walter Alvarez [15]. This first recording was made with a string galvanometer in an elderly woman with a large cicatricial hernia. The recorded signal was sinusoidal and had a frequency of 3 cpm. Despite considerable improvement in recording technology, EGG signals recorded nowadays still resemble the original recordings made by Alvarez (Fig. 3A).

Standard silver/silver chloride ECG electrodes can be used to record EGG signals, provided that their low frequency electrode noise is minimal. The signals must be filtered to discard very low frequency noise (below 0.01 Hz) and "high" frequency noise above 0.5 Hz. Electrogastrographic signals can be recorded from electrodes placed anywhere on the body, but the best recordings are obtained with electrodes placed on the upper abdomen. Usually a bipolar technique is used, in which the potential difference between two adjacent electrodes is recorded. The optimal position of the electrodes varies from subject to subject and even within subjects, so that simultaneous recording from a number of sites is advised [2, 16].

Since visual inspection of the time signals is often difficult and prone to observer bias, automated quantitative analysis techniques have been developed. The most frequently used method is fast Fourier transform (FFT), which transforms the signal from the time domain to the frequency domain. This procedure results in the generation of a spectrum in which, under normal circumstances, a peak at 3 cpm can be distinguished. An extension of the FFT technique is the so-called running spectrum analysis. In running spectrum analysis, spectra of short overlapping stretches of EGG signals are computed [17]. In our laboratory, signal stretches of 256 sec, overlapping for 192 sec, are used routinely, so that a new spectral line is begun every 64 sec. The result of running spectrum analysis can be displayed either in a pseudo-3-dimensional manner (Fig. 3B) or as a grey-scale plot (Fig. 3C). Other signal enhancement techniques are being developed [18].

EGGs recorded from fasting healthy volunteers characteristically show a gastric peak (frequency $3.0 \pm 0.15$ cpm) with low amplitude. Detection of the interdigestive migrating complex by means of surface recording appears to be cumbersome and provides inconsistent results [19]. After ingestion of a meal, the amplitude of the EGG signal increases (Fig. 3B and 3C) [7, 20]. In the first 5 to 10 minutes after ingestion a temporary frequency decrease is observed, followed by an increase to just above the fasting values ($3.3 \pm 0.17$ cpm) (Fig. 3C). In normal volunteers the ratio between the postprandial and fasting power of the 3-cpm peak in the spectrum is above 2.0.

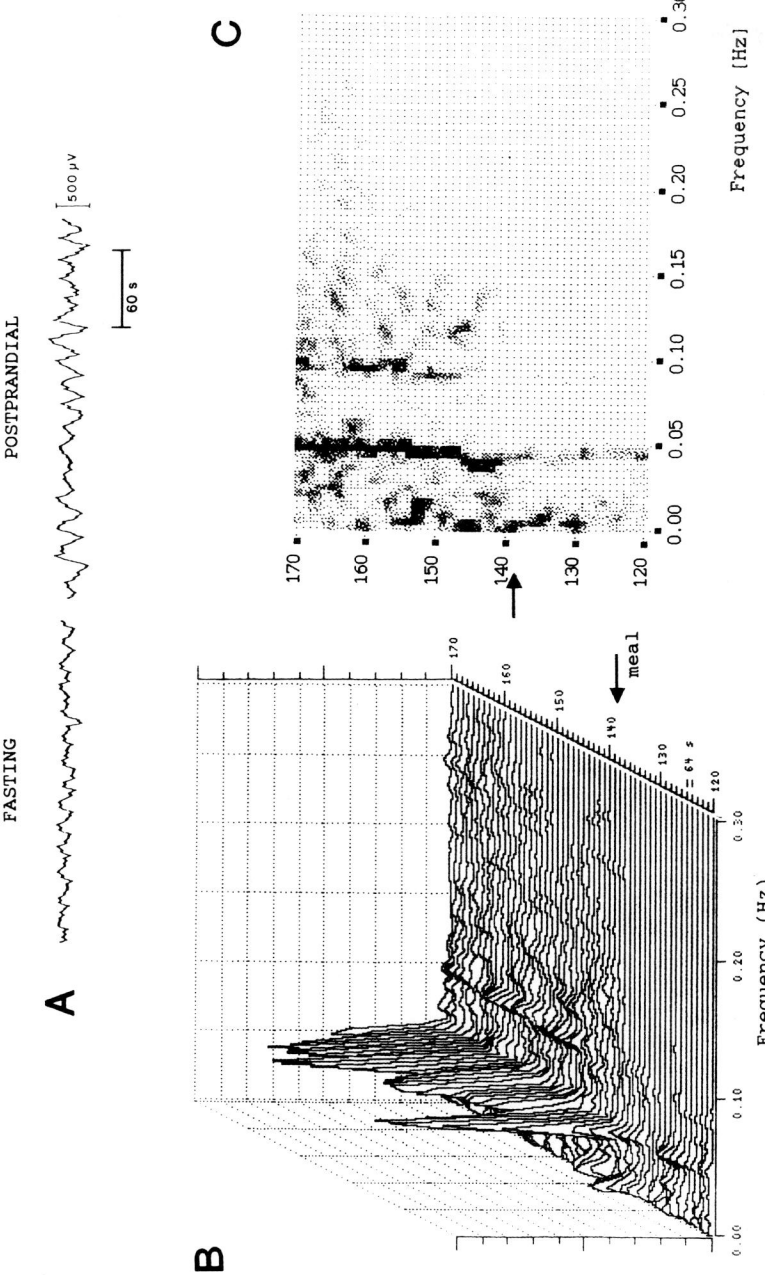

**Figure 3.** **A.** Example of normal electrogastrographic signals, recorded from a healthy human subject, in fasting state (left) and after a meal (right).
**B.** Result of running spectrum analysis of electrogastrographic signals recorded from a healthy human subject, displayed as pseudo-3-dimensional plot. Frequency is on the x-axis, amplitude (power) on the y-axis, and time (in units of 64 sec) on the z-axis. After administration of the test meal (at line 138) an increased amplitude of the 3-cpm (0.05-Hz) component can be seen.
**C.** Running spectra identical to those in figure 3B, displayed as grey-scale plot. The amplitude (power) of each of the spectral components is represented by its blackness.

*A.J.P.M. Smout, H.J.A. Jebbink, P.P.M. Bruijs, D.R. Fone*

**Abnormalities of gastric myoelectrical activity**

Abnormalities of gastric myoelectrical activity can be divided into disturbances of the ECA rhythm (ECA dysrhythmias or arrhythmias), and abnormal (usually diminished) ERA.

**Abnormal ECA**

Arrhythmias of the gastric ECA are of 2 types: ectopic and non-ectopic. In the former, impulses are generated in an ectopic focus in the distal stomach; in the latter the rhythm generated in the normal pacemaker area is irregular.

The simplest type of *ectopic* dysrhythmia is the *ectopic CP*. Ectopic CPs are single CPs or bursts of CPs (shorter than 1 minute) that originate outside the normal pacemaker area, usually in the antrum. In a manner analogous to ventricular premature beats in the heart, single ectopic gastric CPs may be interpolated between two normal Cps, or may be followed by a compensatory pause. An example of this phenomenon is shown in Figure 4. In healthy conscious dogs ectopic CPs occur spontaneously, especially during the quiescent phase (phase I) of the interdigestive migrating motor complex [2, 21]. In anaesthetized dogs, ectopic CPs can be evoked by administration

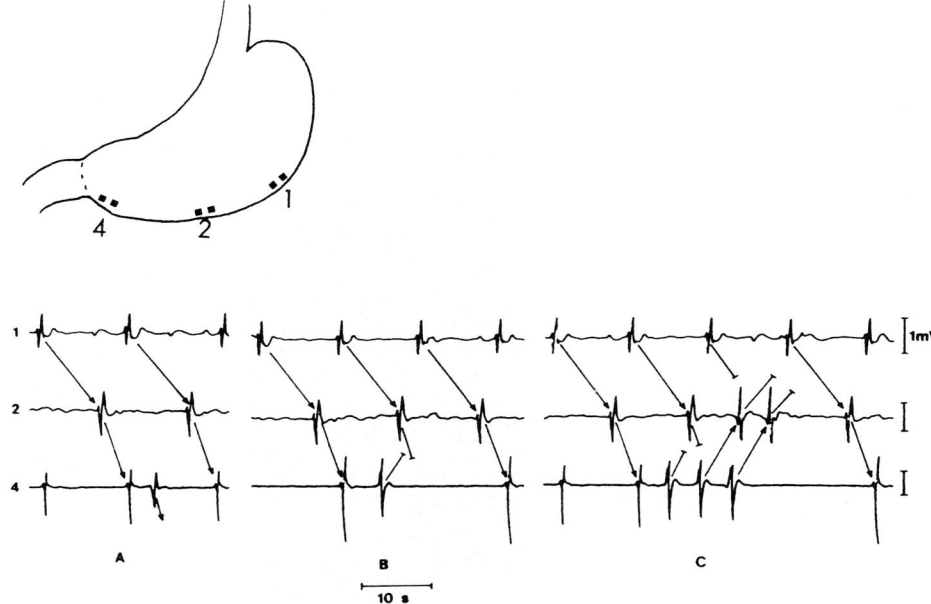

**Figure 4.** Types of ectopic CPs, recorded from the stomach of a healthy conscious dog with implanted serosal electrodes.
A. Single, interpolated CP, not interfering with the normal non-ectopic rhythm.
B. Single CP with compensatory pause.
C. Burst of repetitive CPs, followed by compensatory pause.

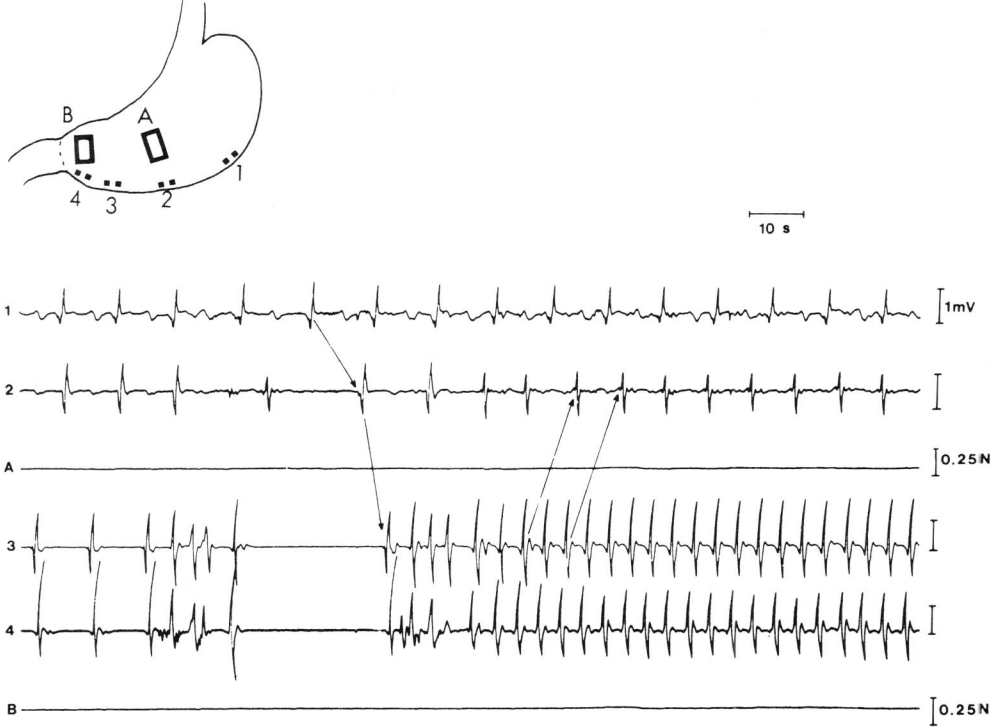

**Figure 5.** Regular tachygastria, recorded with implanted serosal electrodes (1-4) in a conscious dog.
Signals A and B, obtained from strain gauge force transducers, show complete motor quiescence associated with the tachygastria.

of acetylcholine into an artery supplying the stomach [3]. Ectopic CPs can only be recorded with implanted serosal electrodes or with mucosal electrodes; they cannot be detected reliably by surface EGG. Ectopic CPs have previously received little attention in studies of human gastric myoelectrical activity. This probably reflects the assumption that CPs have no effect on gastric motility and emptying, and are unlikely to be associated with symptoms.

Bursts of repetitive ectopic CPs lasting for more than 1 minute are called *tachygastrias* or *gastric tachyarrhythmias*. In the early seventies, episodes of fast ectopic antral activity were found to occur spontaneously in fasting, conscious dogs [22]. The term tachygastria was proposed for regular fast ectopic rhythms (Fig. 5) and tachyarrhythmias for irregular fast ectopic rhythms (Fig. 6). These dysrhythmias were observed most often during phase I of the interdigestive cycle and were also usually abolished by feeding [22].

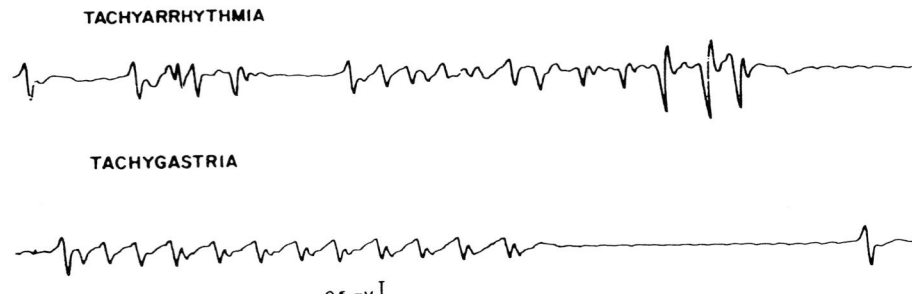

**Figure 6.** Tachyarrhythmia and tachygastria recorded by mucosal electrode in patients with unexplained upper abdominal symptoms. (From ref. [33], with permission).

In anaesthetized dogs, intra-arterial administration of adrenergic substances not only abolishes ERA and contractions, but also induces ectopic CPs and tachyarrhythmias [3, 12]. Since the same changes can be produced by administration of atropine, this was called "the sympathetic dominance pattern" [3]. Our (unpublished) observation in conscious dogs that fear is often associated with the occurrence of antral tachyarrhythmias is in accordance with this concept. Also consistent with this concept is the finding that all types of gastric dysrhythmias are observed more often after vagotomy [6, 8, 23]. The concept of dominance of sympathetic over parasympathetic activity is likely to be oversimplistic, however, since recent studies in dog and man have shown that intra-arterial administration of metenkephalin and prostaglandin $E_2$ [24], and intravenous administration of insulin, secretin, and glucagon [4, 9], also induce episodes of antral dysrhythmia.

The first reports of tachygastria in man date from the fifties. Using intragastric electrodes, abnormally high slow wave frequencies were recorded in some patients with gastric carcinoma [25, 26]. Hinder and Kelly observed tachygastria in a patient with antral carcinoma via peroperative serosal recording [1]. Persistent tachygastria was also reported in an infant with intractable gastric retention, both *in vivo* (peroperative serosal recording), and *in vitro,* after resection of the distal three-quarters of the stomach [10]. Since these early reports, tachygastrias and tachyarrhythmias in humans have been described by several other investigators [2, 4, 5, 7, 11, 14, 16, 23, 27, 30-34]. Antral tachygastria has been successfully recorded by surface EGG (Fig. 7) [4, 16, 20, 29]. It is well established that these dysrhythmias are rare in healthy human subjects. For example in a study of 52 healthy volunteers, Geldof and coworkers found no evidence of tachygastria [16].

There is ample evidence indicating that the presence of a tachygastria or a tachyarrhythmia is always associated with complete absence of motor activity of the distal stomach and that prolonged tachygastria can lead to gastric retention [2-4, 10, 22, 24].

*Non-ectopic dysrhythmias* are those that originate in the pacemaker area, and are subsequently propagated over the distal stomach. An example of this is the unstable

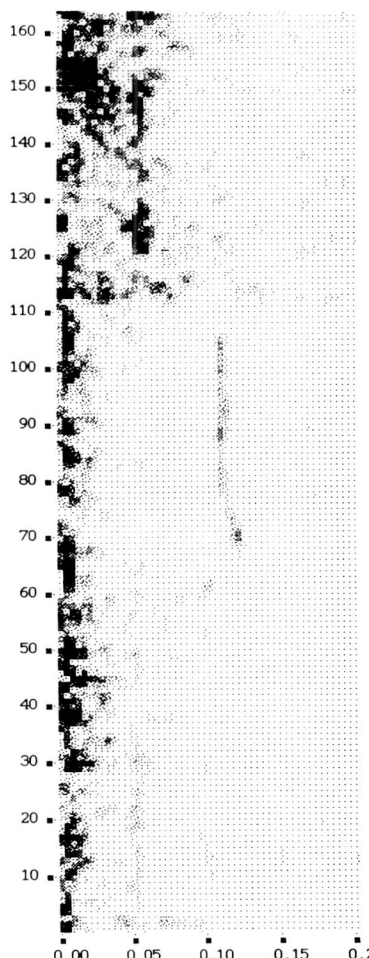

**Figure 7.** Tachygastria recorded electrogastrographically in a patient with non-ulcer dyspepsia, analysed with running spectrum analysis and displayed as grey-scale plot.

rhythm (increased beat-to-beat variability) that is often observed in patients with non-ulcer dyspepsia [16]. Another example is bradygastria, in which the ECA frequency is lower than normal (usually below 2 cpm). Some authors also recognize absence of an electrical rhythm ("asystolia" or "flat-line pattern") as a type of dysrhythmia. Care must be taken, however, not to overdiagnose this latter abnormality, since failure to record a 3-cpm rhythm can also be caused by technical problems, or, in the case of surface recording, by a low signal-to-noise ratio.

**Abnormal ERA**

Abnormal electrical response activity of gastric smooth muscle is, by definition, associated with abnormal phasic contractile activity. Increased ERA has not yet been described. In contrast, one would predict that decreased ERA, associated with impaired motor activity, might occur frequently in patients with a variety of gastric motor disorders. Indeed this appears to be the case. Antral hypomotility after meals has been observed in a significant proportion of patients with non-ulcer dyspepsia [35]. The electrical counterpart of postprandial antral hypomotility is a decreased incidence and amplitude of postprandial ERA. Electrogastrographically this is reflected in a decreased amplitude of the postprandial EGG signal and as a decreased postprandial/fasting power ratio (Fig. 8).

## Relationships between abnormalities of gastric myoelectrical activity and upper abdominal symptoms

One of the first reports suggesting a correlation between antral tachygastria and functional upper abdominal symptoms (non-ulcer dyspepsia) was published in 1980. In their initial study You and coworkers from Rochester, New York, described the electromyographic findings in 14 patients with unexplained nausea, bloating and

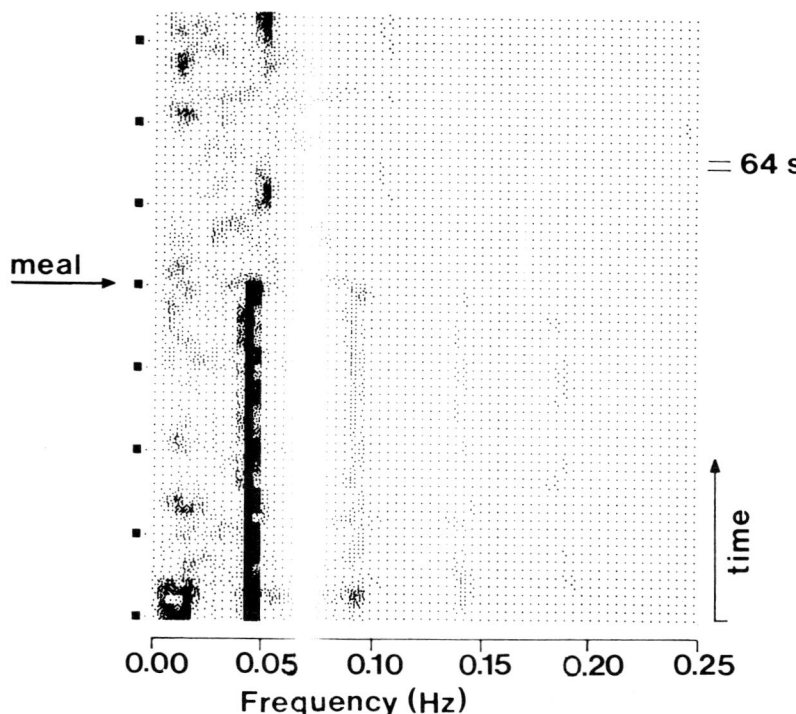

**Figure 8.** Decreased postprandial amplitude (power) of the gastric (3 cpm) peak in the cutaneously recorded EGG in a patient with non-ulcer dyspepsia.

vomiting [11]. These patients were studied in the fasting state, using the peroral mucosal electrode shown in Figure 2. Successful recording (for 1.5 - 3 hours) was achieved in nine out of these 14 patients. In all of these nine patients tachyarrhythmias and tachygastrias were observed. No dysrhythmias were recorded in nine normal subjects. In four of the patients, serosal electrodes were implanted to confirm the existence of arrhythmias. All four subjects were shown to have tachygastria or tachyarrhythmia in the antrum which was propagated either in orad or aborad direction.

One year later, the same group described a 26-year-old woman with persistent nausea, vomiting and upper abdominal pain in whom electromyographic studies with mucosal electrodes revealed antral tachygastria. Radionuclide studies made it clear that gastric emptying in this patient was markedly delayed. Subtotal gastrectomy finally brought relief of her symptoms [14].

In 1983, the Rochester group reported that 35 of 70 patients with unexplained dyspeptic symptoms were found to have antral myoelectrical arrhythmias, whereas no abnormalities were found in 25 healthy volunteers [33].

Perhaps the most convincing evidence comes from the results of a large electrogastrographic study in patients with non-ulcer dyspepsia published in 1986 [16]. EGG was performed in 48 patients with non-ulcer dyspepsia and in 52 control subjects. Abnormal myoelectrical activity of the stomach was found in 23 (48%) of the patients. These abnormalities were of three types: (1) instability of the gastric pacemaker (non-ectopic arrhythmia), (2) tachygastrias (both fasting and postprandial), and (3) absence of the normal postprandial amplitude increase (decreased power ratio) (Fig. 9). These three types of abnormality were present in 25%, 17% and 33% of the patients, respectively. In 30 of the 48 patients, gastric emptying was studied using a radionuclide-labelled solid meal (pancake). Emptying was delayed in 13 patients, all of whom displayed an abnormal electrogastrogram. Thirty-six of the 48 patients were available for follow-up study, and approximately one year after the initial study, 12 of the 36 patients had become free of symptoms. In all of these 12 patients, the EGG was normal, whereas abnormalities had been present a year earlier in seven.

The prevalence of tachygastrias in this study was considerably lower than in the above-cited studies using mucosal electrodes [11, 33]. One explanation for this discrepancy is that the presence of mucosal electrodes may increase the incidence of tachyarrhythmias. Alternatively, it is possible that irregular and short-lived arrhythmias may remain undetected with spectral analysis of EGG signals.

Apart from these observations in non-ulcer dyspepsia, some reports on the association between symptoms and abnormal gastric myoelectrical activity in other diseases and under other experimental conditions should be mentioned.

In the double-blind phase of their study on glucagon-evoked dysrhythmias, Abell and colleagues observed that all four subjects who developed gastric dysrhythmias in response to intravenous glucagon experienced nausea, whereas the other six subjects experienced no symptoms [4]. Hamilton and colleagues described gastric myoelectrical activities in five patients with nausea and vomiting, studied by mucosal and cutaneous recording techniques [7]. Four of these five patients had a history of diabetes mellitus with neuropathy, and the fifth had been diagnosed as having atrophic gastritis. In four of the five patients episodes of tachygastria were seen. The authors reported that each of the patients was symptomatic during the episodes of tachygastria and that the nausea resolved when the abnormally fast rate abated. Geldof and coworkers found that a large proportion of their group of 31 patients with gastric ulcer had abnormal myoelectrical activity of the stomach (dysrhythmia and decreased postprandial amplitude increase). These abnormalities were found to be associated not with the ulcer itself, but with the presence of nausea and vomiting [34]. Koch and colleagues reported that gastric dysrhythmias were present in six out of six insulin-dependent diabetics with nausea and vomiting. After successful treatment with domperidone, leading to a significant reduction in symptom scores, normal 3-cpm activities were recorded from each of the six patients [28]. A significant association between gastric dysrhythmias and nausea was found in an electrogastrographic study of 32 pregnant women [29]. Another recent publication described the relation between tachygastria and motion sickness. Ten of 15 healthy subjects seated in a circular vection drum reported symptoms of motion sickness and showed tachygastria, recorded with EGG,

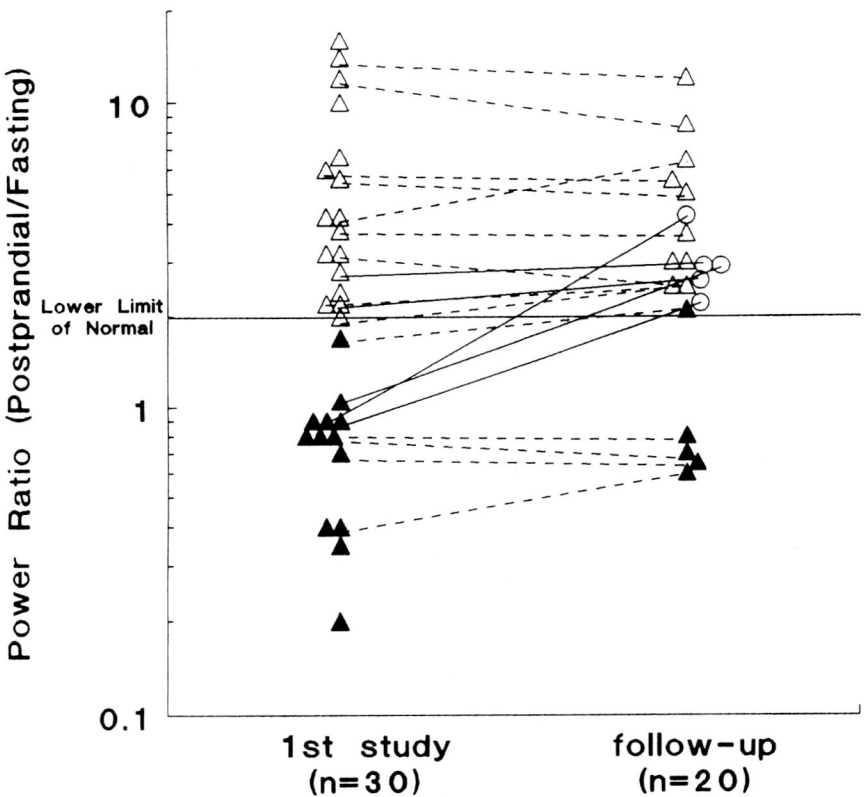

**Figure 9.** Power ratio (postprandial/fasting) in patients with unexplained nausea and vomiting and its relation to symptoms and gastric emptying of a solid meal. Open triangles: symptomatic patients with normal gastric emptying. Closed triangles: symptomatic patients with delayed gastric emptying. Open circles: patients in remission, gastric emptying normalized. Continuous lines in case of remission. Dotted lines with persisting complaints. (From ref. [16], with permission).

five subjects reported no symptoms and showed a continuation of their normal 3-cpm activity [30]. A close correspondence over time between tachygastria and symptoms was observed.

## Conclusions and speculations

Available information strongly suggests a role for myoelectrical abnormalities of the gastric antrum (ECA dysrhythmias and decreased postprandial ERA) in the pathogenesis of non-organic upper abdominal symptoms. These abnormalities can be recorded in a non-invasive manner, using surface recording (EGG). Unequivocal proof that these abnormalities are the cause and not the consequence of the symptoms is difficult to provide, but circumstantial evidence certainly points to a causal role.

Whereas it is easy to understand how postprandial hypomotility (recognized in myoelectrical recordings as decreased ERA) would cause postprandial upper abdominal discomfort, the mechanisms by which short-lived gastric arrhythmias in the fasting state would lead to symptoms need further elucidation. Another goal of future research in this area should be to identify drugs that effectively and safely abolish gastric ECA arrhythmias, without interfering with the normal mechanisms that control gastric motility and emptying.

Studies of gastric myoelectrical activity in patients with non-ulcer dyspepsia are not only of scientific, but also of potential clinical interest. In some symptomatic patients the gastric myoelectrical abnormality is the only demonstrable gastrointestinal abnormality. In these patients, therapeutic efforts should be directed towards (pharmacological) correction of these abnormalities, whereas in dyspeptic patients without any demonstrable dysfunction of the stomach other treatment modalities (for example psychotherapy) should be tried at an earlier stage.

## References

1. Hinder RA, Kelly KA. Human gastric pacesetter potential. Site of origin, spread and response to gastric transection and proximal gastric vagotomy. Am J Surg 1977;133:29-33.
2. Smout AJPM. Myoelectric activity of the stomach. Gastroelectromyography and electrogastrography. Delft University Press, 1980.
3. Daniel EE. The electrical and contractile activity of the pyloric region in dogs and the effects of drugs. Gastroenterology 1965;49:403-18.
4. Abell TL, Malagelada JR. Glucagon-evoked gastric dysrhythmias in humans shown by an improved electrogastrographic technique. Gastroenterology 1985;88:1932-40.
5. Abell TL, Malagelada JR, Lucas AR, Brown ML, Camilleri M, Go VL, Azpiroz F, Callaway CW, Kao PC, Zinsmeister AR, Huse DM. Gastric electromechanical and neurohormonal function in anorexia nervosa. Gastroenterology 1987;93:958-65.
6. Bortolotti M, Labo G, Serantoni C, Ciani P. Effect of highly selective vagotomy on gastric motor activity of duodenal ulcer patients. Digestion 1978;17:108-20.
7. Hamilton JW, Bellahsene BE, Reichelderfer M, Webster JG, Bass P. Human electrogastrograms. Comparison of surface and mucosal recordings. Dig Dis Sci 1986;31:33-9.

8. Stoddard CJ, Smallwood R, Brown BH, Duthie HL. The immediate and delayed effects of different types of vagotomy on human gastric myoelectrical activity. Gut 1975;16:165-70.
9. Stoddard CJ, Smallwood RH, Duthie HL. Electrical arrhythmias in the human stomach. Gut 1981;22:705-12.
10. Telander RL, Morgan RG, Kreulen DL, Schmalz PF, Kelly KA, Szurszewski JH. Human gastric atony with tachygastria and gastric retention. Gastroenterology 1978;75:497-501.
11. You CH, Lee KY, Chey WY, Menguy R. Electrogastrographic study of patients with unexplained nausea, bloating and vomiting. Gastroenterology 1980;79:311-4.
12. You CH, Chey WY. Study of electromechanical activity of the stomach in humans and in dogs with particular attention to tachygastria. Gastroenterology 1984;86:1460-8.
13. Abell TL, Malagelada JR. Electrogastrography. Current assessment and future perspectives. Dig Dis Sci 1988;33: 982-92.
14. You CH, Chey WY, Lee KY, Menguy R, Bortoff A. Gastric and small intestinal myoelectric dysrhythmia associated with chronic intractable nausea and vomiting. Ann Intern Med 1981;95:449-51.
15. Alvarez WC. The electrogastrogram and what it shows. JAMA 1922; 78: 1116-9.
16. Geldof H, Van der Schee EJ, Van Blankenstein M, Grashuis JL. Electrogastrographic study of gastric myoelectrical activity in patients with unexplained nausea and vomiting. Gut 1986;27:799-808.
17. Van der Schee EJ, Grashuis JL. Running spectrum analysis as an aid in the representation and interpretation of electrogastrographic signals. Med Biol Eng Comput 1987; 25:57-62.
18. Chen JD, Vandewalle J, Sansen W, Vantrappen G, Janssens J. Multichannel adaptive enhancement of the electrogastrogram. IEEE Trans Biomed Eng 1990;37:285-94.
19. Geldof H, Van der Schee EJ, Grashuis JL. Electrogastrographic characteristics of interdigestive migrating complex in humans. Am J Physiol 1986;250:G165-71.
20. Smout AJ, Van der Schee EJ, Grashuis JL. What is measured in electrogastrography? Dig Dis Sci 1980;25:179-87.
21. Gullikson GW, Okuda H, Shimizu M, Bass P. Electrical arrhythmias in gastric antrum of the dog. Am J Physiol1980;239:G59-68.
22. Code CF, Marlett JA. Canine tachygastria. Mayo Clin Proc1974;49:325-32.
23. Geldof H, Van der Schee EJ, Van Blankenstein M, Smout AJ, Akkermans LM. Effects of highly selective vagotomy on gastric myoelectrical activity. An electrogastrographic study. Dig Dis Sci 1990;35:969-75.
24. Kim CH, Zinsmeister AR, Malagelada JR. Effect of gastric dysrhythmias on postcibal motor activity of the stomach. Dig Dis Sci 1988;33:193-99.
25. Morton HS. The potentialities of the electrogastrograph. Ann R Coll Surg Engl 1954;15:351-73.
26. Goodman EN, Colcher H, Katz GM, Dangler CL. The clinical significance of the electrogastrogram. Gastroenterology 1955;29:598-608.
27. Reynolds RP, Bardakjian BL, Diamant NE. A case of antral tachygastria: symptomatic and myoelectric improvement with gastroenterostomy and domperidone therapy. Can Med Assoc J 1983;128:826-9.
28. Koch KL, Stern RM, Stewart WR, Vasey MW. Gastric emptying and gastric myoelectrical activity in patients with diabetic gastroparesis: effects of long-term domperidone treatment. Am J Gastroenterolog 1989; 84:1069-75.
29. Koch KL, Stern RM, Vasey M, Botti JJ, Creasy GW, Dwyer A. Gastric dysrhythmias and nausea of pregnancy. Dig Dis Sci 1990;35:961-8.
30. Liberski SM, Koch KL, Atnip RG, Stern RM. Ischemic gastroparesis: resolution after revascularization. Gastroenterology 1990;99:252-7.
31. You CH, Lee KY, Chey WY. Gastric electromyography in normal and abnormal states in humans. In: Chey WY, ed. *Functional Disorders of the Digestive Tract*. New York: Raven Press, 1983:167-74.

32. Stern RM, Koch KL, Stewart WR, Lindblad IM. Spectral analysis of tachygastria recorded during motion sickness. Gastroenterology 1987;92:92-7.
33. Chey WY, You CH, Lee KY, Menguy R. Gastric dysrhythmia: clinical aspects. In: Chey WY, ed. *Functional Disorders of the Digestive Tract.* New York: Raven Press, 1983:175-82.
34. Geldof H, Van der Schee EJ, Smout AJ, Van de Merwe JP, Van Blankenstein M, Grashuis JL. Myoelectrical activity of the stomach in gastric ulcer patients: an electrogastrographic study. J Gastrointest Mot 1989;1:122-30.
35. Camilleri M, Malagelada JR, Kao PC, Zinsmeister AR. Gastric and autonomic responses to stress in functional dyspepsia. Dig Dis Sci 1986;31:1169-77.

# 10

# Disturbances of gastric emptying

S. BRULEY des VARANNES

*Groupe Fonctions Digestives et Nutrition, CHU G et R Laënnec, 44035 Nantes Cedex, France*

**Introduction**

Non-ulcer dyspepsia (NUD) is an ill-defined clinical condition with symptoms referable to the upper alimentary tract in which no organic abnormality can be found. In several of these patients, the symptoms suggest that a digestive motor abnormality might be responsible for the condition. The postprandial occurrence of symptoms suggests an abnormality of motor gastric response to food.

Several digestive motor abnormalities have been described in patients with NUD, both during fasting and in the postprandial period [1-5]. Disorders of gastric emptying are frequently evoked and sometimes documented. However the frequency and the precise characteristics of those abnormalities are not well-known. Indeed, there is neither a clear definition of this syndrome nor any objective characteristics which enable the diagnosis to be made with certainty. As a result, the studies frequently concern few patients and are difficult to compare because the criteria chosen for the selection of patients are too varied. In addition, there is not a good correlation between the symptoms and objectively demonstrable functional abnormalities, also making evaluation difficult [6, 7].

In this paper an attempt is made to review the incidence of abnormalities of gastric emptying in NUD, and to identify some motor characteristics and some aetiopathogenic hypotheses attached to these abnormalities. Patients with organic causes of delayed gastric emptying (diabetic gastroparesis, hypertrophic pyloric stenosis, post-surgical gastroparesis) are not considered as having NUD in this chapter. Except when stated otherwise, NUD is considered to be idiopathic functional or essential dyspepsia.

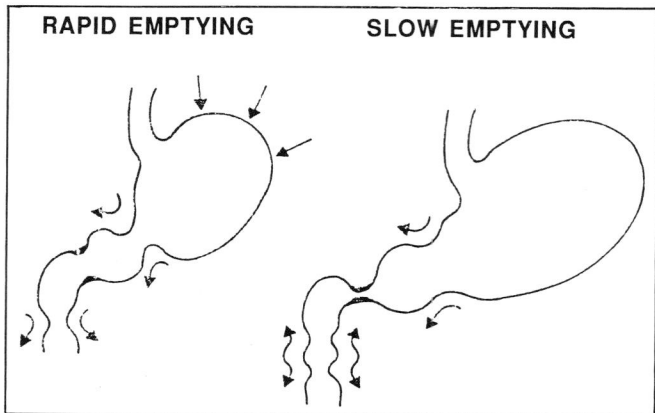

**Figure 1.** Schematic illustration of the integrated gastroduodenal motor activities that take place during rapid gastric emptying of bland liquids (on the left) and slow gastric emptying of nutrient-rich liquids. Arrows represent the main events. Rapid emptying is associated with an increase in fundal tone, strong phasic contractions of the antrum, a wide open pylorus and coordinated duodenal contractions. Slow emptying is associated with fundal relaxation, shallow phasic contractions of the antrum, an increase in phasic and tonic activity of the pylorus, and uncoordinated or random duodenal contractions. (Figure and legend reproduced from Read and Houghton [9], with permission).

## Mechanical events in gastric emptying in normal individuals

Contrasting with its relatively elementary anatomical structure, the functional capacities of the stomach are complex. To assume its role of provider of qualitatively and quantitatively adapted nutrients to the small intestine, the functions of the stomach are controlled by highly sophisticated neurohumoral regulating mechanisms. For an exhaustive review the reader is invited to consult two recent publications [8, 9]. However some functional characteristics of the organ have to be recalled.

The swallowing and the ingestion of a meal induce a vagally-mediated relaxation of the fundus. This relaxation allows volume to be accommodated to content with no concomitant increase in fundic pressure. Thereafter, the pressure in the fundus gently increases, inducing a tonic contraction. This low but sustained fundal pressure, by generating a pressure gradient between stomach and duodenum, is the primary mechanism for emptying liquids out of the stomach. The gastric antrum is characterized by tonic and contractile activity, and this mechanical activity is responsible for mixing and grinding. The mechanical electrically-controlled activity is made by waves of pressure descending from the corpus towards the pylorus. These waves propel the gastric contents forwards and gradually squeeze them by narrowing the antral walls. As the wave approaches the pylorus, the lumen shuts down, allowing only fluid and the smallest particles through into the duodenum. Other particles and solid components are retropropelled into the antrum for further mixing and grinding in order to reduce their size. In the analysis of gastric emptying results, the "lag" period is the time taken for solids to move from fundus to antrum and to be ground by antral contractions to a size (about 1-2 mm) that allows them to pass through the pylorus.

Some recent work completes this classical description of the events of gastric emptying (Fig. 1). The fundal pressure gradient does not appear to be the only mechanism for the ejection of liquids from the stomach [10-12]. Liquids empty in gushes associated with coordinated contractions of the antrum, pylorus and duodenum. While the role of antral motility in the emptying of solids has been clearly demonstrated [13], the role of the antro-pyloro-duodenal coordination has also been recently highlighted. Indeed Houghton *et al.* [14] showed in healthy subjects that the half time for solid emptying was inversely correlated with the rate of coordinated contractions involving the antrum. In this study it was also found that the rate emptying of solids was dependent on the rate of emptying of liquids, and finally that isolated pyloric pressure waves may serve as an intermittent resistance. Finally, it has been shown that non-disruptible solids are emptied from the stomach as boluses at around the same time that phase III of the interdigestive migrating motor complex occurs in the stomach and in the duodenum.

Ideally one should be able with the above functions to determine the causes of functional gastric motor disorders and to explain which abnormal functions, either alone or in combination, explain the symptoms. In theory, to explain abnormalities of gastric emptying one can suggest three main levels of disturbance, which are summarized in Table I. Unfortunately, though some results are presently available, we are still a long way from achieving this approach because only a few studies have investigated systematically the possible pathogenic mechanisms involved in patients with NUD.

## Symptoms of gastric emptying dysfunction

In patients with NUD, are there any symptoms which point to gastric emptying disorders? Patients usually complain about epigastric pain, nausea, and an inability to finish a meal. They may also describe an impression of slow digestion, sometimes accompanied by epigastric fullness and bloating. Symptoms may vary from almost none to rather dramatic symptoms such as postprandial vomiting and even loss of weight [15]. Recently a working party differentiated subgroups of patients with NUD or essential dyspepsia on specific symptoms related to different causative factor patterns. The above mentioned symptoms would probably be included under "dysmotility-like dyspepsia" [16].

Symptoms of patients with NUD are chronic and very close to the symptoms caused by mechanical obstruction, at least in "dysmotility like-dyspepsia". As a result, it will be essential in clinical practice to make certain that morphological evidence of disease is excluded, especially if symptoms are of recent onset. While all these symptoms and their relation with food ingestion suggest a digestive origin, and in particular a motor disorder, there is no evidence of a clear relationship between such symptoms and an abnormality of gastric emptying. On the contrary, several studies have failed to demonstrate any relation between dyspeptic symptoms and delayed emptying [7, 17].

**Table I.** Frequency of delayed gastric emptying of digestible and non-digestible solids (S) and liquids (L) in non-ulcer dyspepsia.

| Authors [ref] | patients (n) | women (n) | S* (%) | L* (%) | calories (kcal) | method | remarks |
|---|---|---|---|---|---|---|---|
| Talley et al. [17] | 32 | 23 | D | Unk | Unk | IM,PD,SI | Delay only in women |
| Bertrand et al. [30] | 46 | 26 | D | Unk | 650 | RM | No relationship between symptoms and emptying rate. Indigestible solids ingested with a digestible meal. |
| Jian et al. [22] | 27 | Unk | 26 | 41 | 440 | IM,DD,DI | Meal content: F: 36%; CH:38%; P: 26% |
| Bolondi et al. [26] | 36 | 18 | | 64 | 800 | EM | Standard italian meal |
| Urbain et al. [23] | 8 | 5 | D | D | 390 | IM,DD,DI | Meal content: F: 56%; CH: 28%; P: 16% |
| Mc Callum et al. [31] | 16 | 16 | 31 | Unk | 0 | IM,AD | Abstract. Indigestible solids (4 diabetics, 2 sclerodermias) All those patients had a delay of digestible solids emptying |
| Corinaldesi et al. [24] | 118 | 77 | D | Unk | 688 | IM | 30 patients had also gastro-oesophageal symptoms. |
| Fisher et al. [34] | 191 | Unk | 41 | 8 | Unk | IM,DI | Emptying was delayed regardless of gastro-oesophageal symptoms 91% of patients with delayed emptying were women. |
| Jian et al. [7] | 27 | 18 | 30 | 30 | 440 | IM,DD,DI | Meal content: F: 36%; CH: 38%; P: 26% |
| Geldof et al. [35] | 30 | Unk | 43 | Unk | Unk | IM | Electrogastrographic study |
| Wegener et al. [18] | 43 | 30 | Unk | 30 | 440 | IM,AD[a],SI | Concomitant mouth-to-caecum transit and whole gut transit Delay predominantly in women (12 of 13) |

IM: Isotopic measurement. AD or PD: Anterior or posterior detection; DD: Double detection; SI or DI: Simple or double isotope.
EM: Echographic measurement. RM: Radiologic method. Unk: Unknown.
*: Results for solid and liquid gastric emptying are indicated either using D when there is a significant delay in the group of patients or by a number in % when the proportion of patients with delayed emptying was indicated.
[a]: lateral acquisition to correct for attenuation.

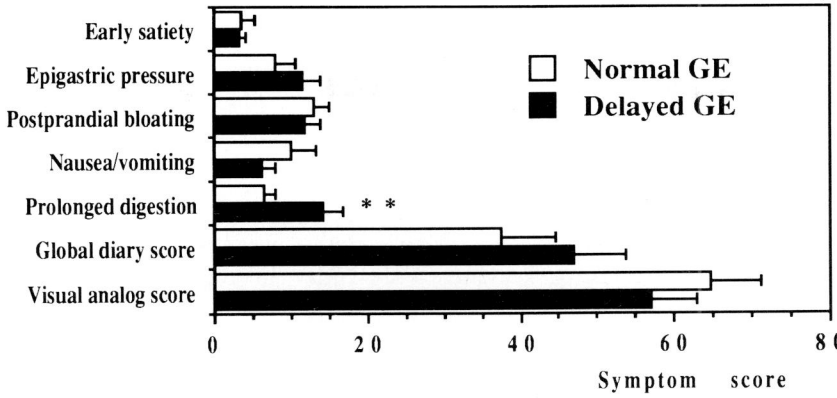

**Figure 2.** Severity of symptoms measured using scores calculated from diary records by patients with non-ulcer dyspepsia. Open boxes represent patients without objective gastric stasis (n=11), and black boxes represent patients with objective delayed gastric emptying (GE) of solids or liquids (n=16). **:P<0.01. (Adapted from Jian et al. [7]).

Jian et al. (Fig. 2) observed that one of the seven variables examined (i.e., the symptom score "prolonged digestion") was significantly higher in patients with objectively delayed emptying than in those with normal emptying. In fact, there was a major overlap and these workers concluded that no clinical feature was able to distinguish between patients with normal and abnormal gastric emptying [7]. Likewise, in a study conducted in 43 well-defined patients with NUD, Wegener et al. [18] did not observe any significant difference in the frequency and in the intensity of symptoms between dyspeptic patients with normal and delayed gastric emptying of liquids. On this point, some additional information can be obtained by examining the results of therapeutic studies conducted in patients with NUD. Information is usually included in such studies as to whether the above mentioned symptoms were or were not associated with documented delayed gastric emptying. Several studies have been able to demonstrate a beneficial effect on symptoms and on gastric emptying with the use of prokinetic drugs. However, in most cases, the improvement in symptoms is not, or only marginally, correlated with gastric emptying results [6, 19]. This apparent discrepancy between objective delay in gastric emptying and the severity of symptoms reflects the difficulty in determining the mechanism of symptoms occurring in patients with upper gut disturbances. Hopefully, a better understanding of symptoms in these patients will be obtained by increasing knowledge on sensory perception and adaptation to distension. A recent study showed that dyspepsia patients had a lower pain threshold to gastric distension with or without delayed gastric emptying [20].

We can conclude from all of these studies that neither the occurrence nor the characteristics of symptoms in the clinical presentation of patients with NUD allow us to make the diagnosis of a gastric emptying abnormality with sufficient predictive value [7]. As a result, it is necessary to make an objective measurement of gastric emptying to establish whether there is a disturbance of gastric emptying in these patients. Proof of delayed gastric emptying could be of therapeutic interest because patients with NUD having this abnormality do seem to get more benefit with gastrokinetic drugs than patients with normal emptying [7].

## Gastric emptying in NUD

Gastric emptying has been examined using several different techniques under a variety of different technical conditions and of patients. These technical differences, and the different inclusion criteria for patients with NUD in the studies, make some comparisons difficult. But all of these studies are consistent in finding that gastric emptying is delayed in a proportion of the patients [7, 21-24]. In this paper we shall focus on the results of the main studies of gastric emptying conducted in patients with NUD. In relation to the technical aspects of gastric emptying measurements, the interested reader should refer to a recent and exhaustive review by Scarpignato [25]. The results of some gastric emptying studies in symptomatic patients with NUD are given in Table I.

### Global measurement of gastric emptying

Recently, Bolondi *et al.* [26], using a non-invasive ultrasonographic method, measured gastric emptying in 36 patients with NUD and in 18 controls. The ultrasonographic method is based on repeated measurements of the width of the gastric antrum before and after a meal of standardized energy content (800 kcal). Final emptying time, defined as the time when the cross-sectional area and the volume of the antrum returned to basal values and remained unchanged for a least 30 min, was significantly increased in NUD patients (359±64 *vs* 248±39 min, m±SD). Interestingly, this method allows one to evaluate the degree of dilatation of the gastric antrum by calculating the ratio between gastric antral area and the baseline value at different times. In both patients and controls, the maximal cross-sectional areas of the antrum were reached about 60 min after the beginning of the meal, but the antral cross-sectional area was significantly larger in patients than in controls (Fig. 3). This result suggests that, as observed in manometrically performed recordings, tonic and/or phasic antral motility is reduced in fed patients with NUD. Moreover the same group showed that a drug-induced acceleration of gastric emptying in patients with NUD was accompanied by a reduction in maximal antral volume [27]. Using the same methodology other studies have also found this increased distension in NUD patients [28], and in one of these studies the authors were able to note a good relation between symptoms and an increase of antral distension [29].

Gastric emptying of indigestible solids is also delayed in patients with NUD [30, 31]. This delay is likely to result from disturbances of the regular motor activity of the motor migrating complex [2, 25].

### Emptying of solids and liquids

The radionuclide technique is of particular interest in determining the characteristics of gastric emptying for the two components of the meal in NUD patients (Fig. 4).

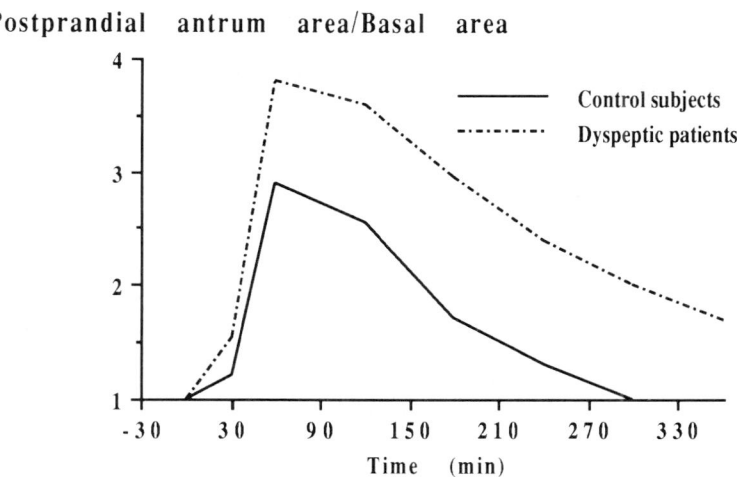

**Figure 3.** Degree of dilatation of the gastric antrum measured using ultrasonographic method following the ingestion of a meal in healthy subjects and in patients with non-ulcer dyspepsia. This measurement is calculated as the ratio between gastric antrum area at different times and basal values. Note that in both groups the maximum rate is observed at about 60 min, but in dyspeptic patients, the degree of dilatation remains significantly higher than in controls. (Reproduced from Bolondi et al. [26] with permission).

Several studies have been conducted using this technique. However, in addition to the previously mentioned problem of defining the patients with NUD, these studies also differ in technique and in the meals used.

Some studies have found a delay only for the solid component of the meal (Table I). In one documented observation of a patient with severe and gradually increasing NUD symptoms, Rees et al. [32] observed marked gastric stasis of solids associated with a weak antral pressure response, whereas gastric emptying of fluids was normal. In a small series of eight patients, Urbain et al. [23] did not find any significant difference for emptying of liquids, but showed a significantly delayed emptying of the solid component 100 min after the completion of a small meal (390 kcal) with a high fat content (56%). Together with the increased ultrasonographic antral volume in these patients [26] and the fundamental role of antral motility in emptying of solids, all these observations suggest that the delayed emptying of solids is likely to be related to disturbances of antral motility [2, 13, 14]. However, Jian et al. [7], in a group of 27 patients with NUD, found a delayed emptying of solids in 30%, but in this study, the $\beta$ coefficient of patients, considered either globally or only in patients with prolonged emptying, was not different from that of the controls. Likewise, Talley et al., measuring emptying of solids, failed to find any significant difference in the $\beta$ coefficient between patients (only women had delayed emptying) and controls [17]. The $\beta$ parameter is the coefficient of the power exponential function that characterizes the early emptying of solids and is closely related to antral motility [13]. The lack of

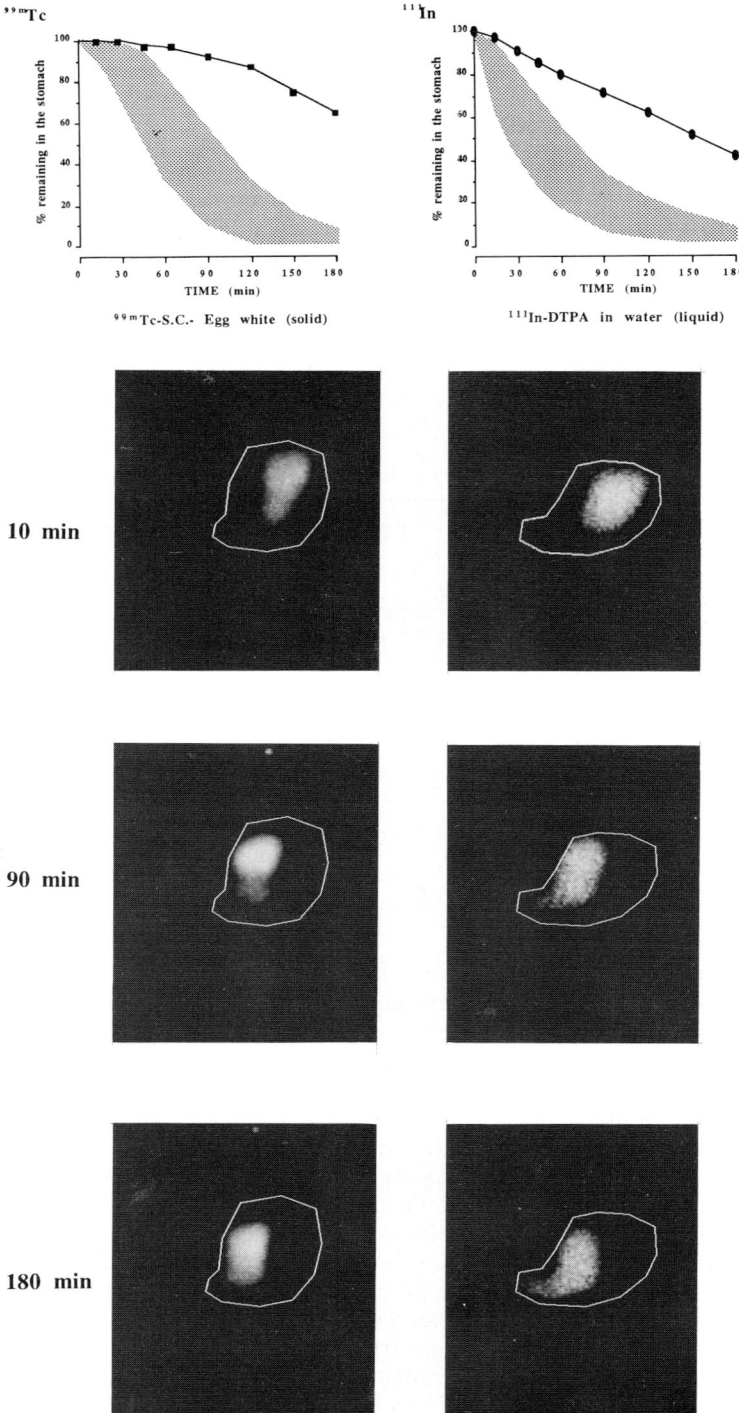

**Figure 4.** Serial gastric emptying scans for solids ($^{99m}$Tc window) and liquids ($^{111}$In window) in a patient with symptoms of non-ulcer dyspepsia. Close line is the gastric region of interest. Scintiscans were obtained during 180 min after meal ingestion (440 kcal). On the top are the curves of emptying showing the percentage remaining in the stomach for each isotope. Shaded areas indicate range (m±2SD) of normal values calculated in 16 healthy asymptomatic subjects. In this patient, emptying is delayed both for solids and liquids. Note the increase of lag phase for solids, and the low slope.

a significant difference in this parameter between patients and controls suggests that, even if antral motility is an important parameter, other factors should be involved.

In fact, emptying of liquids has frequently been found to be slow, and some workers have even found a predominant delay in liquid emptying [3, 22]. Measuring the emptying of liquids included in a caloric solid-liquid meal, Wegener et al. [18] observed that 30% of the patients with NUD had delayed emptying. Labelling the liquid phase is readily done, but the stability and specificity of this labelling is not very high [33]; so $^{99m}$Tc incorporated in the liquid phase becomes partially adsorbed to the solid food, and the measurement is likely to reflect an unknown proportion of the gastric emptying of solids. In Jian et al.'s study a delayed gastric emptying of liquids and/or solids (defined by the T1/2>m+2SD of controls) was observed in 44% of the patients [22]. The rate is much higher in postvagotomy (90%) or in secondary dyspepsia (83%) groups [22]. Recently, Fisher et al. [34] measured emptying using $^{99m}$Tc egg white and $^{111}$In water in a large group of patients suffering from NUD symptoms. Among the 362 patients investigated, 191 could be classified as NUD patients as defined at the beginning of this chapter (essential dyspepsia). 41% had delayed emptying of solids. Although those results have only been published in abstract form, it appears that delayed emptying of liquids was less frequent, representing 20% of patients with delayed emptying of solids. In this last study, a selective delay for liquids (with emptying of solids normal) was never observed.

Acceleration of gastric emptying has not been often reported in patients with NUD. This situation is probably more frequent in postsurgical situations or in peculiar pharmacological conditions, and essentially concerns the emptying of liquids. It might be related to a failure of fundic relaxation.

Put together, these results show that between 40 and 70% of patients with NUD have delayed gastric emptying. This delay seems to be related more often to the solid component of the meal, but in some groups of patients, the delay is predominantly for liquids. These sometimes conflicting results again illustrate the heterogeneous characteristics of patients with NUD, and suggest that various motor abnormalities may be involved (Table II). Other points remain unexplained, especially the frequent female predominance not only in symptomatic patients but also in patients with delayed emptying [17]. The natural history of gastric emptying disturbances is almost

**Table II.** Potential gastroduodenal motor anomalies that can alter gastric emptying in patients with non-ulcer dyspepsia.

*Proximal stomach*
Decrease in the postprandial fundic tone
Excessive accommodation to fundic distension

*Distal stomach*
Weakness of antral contractions
(decrease in frequency and/or amplitude)

*Gastroduodenal junction*
Perturbation of antro-pyloro-duodenal coordination
Increase of isolated pyloric pressure waves
Alteration in duodenojejunal motor activity

unknown. In one study re-examining patients with initial delayed emptying, it was found that the majority of patients did not have essential changes in their emptying rate one year later [35].

## Motor abnormalities and gastric emptying disorders

Several gastrointestinal motor abnormalities have been described in various groups of patients with NUD, both fasting and fed [2, 3, 36]. Malagelada and Stanghellini [2], in a large group of patients including idiopathic and secondary dyspepsia, observed that approximately half of them had antral fasting or postprandial hypomotility. Though no measure of gastric emptying was performed in these patients, it is highly likely, considering the relationships between antral motor activity and gastric emptying [10, 13, 14], that most patients with antral hypomotility have delayed emptying. This high proportion of cases with antral hypomotility is about the same that has been found in some studies measuring gastric emptying in patients with NUD.

In a subset of symptomatic patients with delayed gastric emptying, Labò et al. [1] found that a dysfunction in the fasting interdigestive motor activity was frequent. This absence of phase 3 activity cannot, however, directly explain the delayed emptying and is only a reflection of a fasting motility disturbance. On the other hand it could slow down the emptying of the gastric contents in the late postprandial period, and principally the emptying of indigestible particles.

In fact, manometric recordings of the upper digestive tract in fasting and fed subjects yield two main types of abnormalities in patients with delayed gastric emptying. As previously stated, antral hypomotility is frequently observed during the postprandial period [3] but also during fasting [4]. The second abnormality is a disturbance of intestinal pressure activity in the fasting or fed state with bursts of non-propagated or retrograde phasic pressure activity, incoordinated activity or even inability of the ingested meal to change fasting intestinal activity to a fed pattern [3, 4, 37]. In some of these studies, the two types of abnormalities were not present in the same subject.

Camilleri et al. [3] found delayed gastric emptying of liquids in patients with severe symptoms of gut dysmotility, either with objected antral hypomotility alone or with intestinal dysmotility alone. In the same study, only the patients with antral hypomotility had delayed emptying of solids (Fig. 5) whereas patients with intestinal dysmotility did not, as it was also observed in another recent study [36]. Consequently, gastric stasis of solids does seem to be predominantly associated with postcibal antral hypomotility. These results suggest that delayed emptying of liquids is likely to be connected with a more diffuse disturbance of the digestive motility.

When measured, neither the mouth to caecum transit time nor the whole gut transit time was found prolonged in patients with NUD. Surprisingly, even in the subgroup of patients with prolonged gastric emptying times, the mouth-to-caecum transit time was not prolonged [18]. These similar mouth-to-caecum transit times, independent of gastric emptying rates, suggest that the transit time in the small intestine might be faster when there is a prolonged gastric emptying time.

In the digestive tract, the mechanical activity is electrically controlled. Gastric electrical activity has frequently been found to be abnormal in patients with NUD. In patients with delayed emptying, whether proven or not, a large variety of dysrhythmias can be recorded, which may be related to an ectopic antral pacemaker. A decrease in

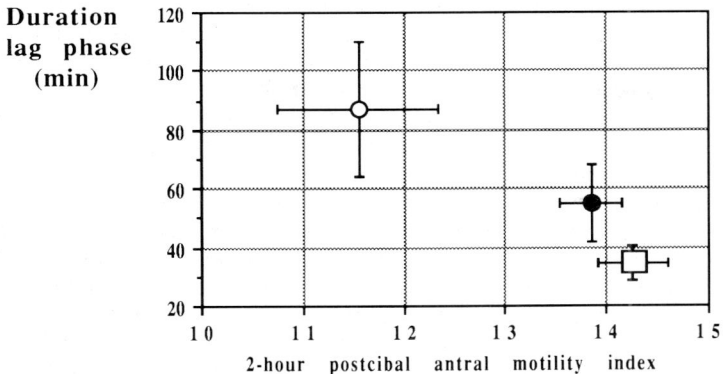

**Figure 5.** Relationship between 2-h postcibal antral motility index and the duration of lag phase for solids in healthy controls (□) and in patients with non-ulcer dyspepsia and antral hypomotility (○) or intestinal dysmotility (●). Each point shows the mean and standard error bar. Note the visual inverse relation between antral motility index and duration of the lag phase. (Adapted from Camilleri et al. [3] with permission).

the fasting and postcibal amplitude of electrical power has also been observed [15, 33, 38, 39]. In patients with NUD, Geldof et al. [35] demonstrated that, compared to patients with a normal emptying rate, those with delayed gastric emptying of solids had absence of the normal postprandial power increase, or even a power decrease after the test meal. Some of these electrical aspects are also observed in pregnant women with nausea and in subjects with motion sickness [40].

## Aetiopathogenic hypothesis for delayed emptying in NUD

An excessive response to stress has been evoked in the disturbances in these patients. The decrease in antral motility during stress is a physiological phenomenon observed in control subjects, which induces a delay in gastric emptying [41, 42]. Patients with NUD but with normal antral postcibal motility may change to hypomotility under stress. On the other hand in the patients with postprandial antral hypomotility, the motility pattern does not change during stress [41]. Patients with NUD seem to have intact afferent and efferent neural pathways and to exhibit normal autonomic and humoral response to stress when applied with transcutaneous electrical nerve stimulation [41]. This last study did not find any relation between the antral motor response and the autonomic humoral variables or the personality or the clinical presentation of these patients. In fact the role of stress in the symptoms and in the motor disorders in these patients has not yet been elucidated, and the studies have almost always involved acute stress, and not a chronic one comparable to a real-life situation.

However, in some patients, the role of endogenous opiate-like substances, the enkephalins, could be involved in the delayed gastric emptying. Naloxone, a specific opioid antagonist, can induce a significant acceleration of gastric emptying in patients with NUD [4]. This effect was only observed in a subgroup of patients with duodenal dyskinesia, and there was no effect in patients with antral hypomotility (Fig. 6). This selective effect on patients with duodenal dyskinesia links with the absence of change in the β-endorphin level found by Camilleri *et al.* in patients with antral hypomotility [41]. Moreover, the alterations in gastric motility and gastric emptying resulting from numerous noxious stimuli increasing plasma β-endorphin level suggest that endogenous opiates could play a role in the mediation of these events [42, 43].

Some interesting data have emerged from studies on anorexia nervosa. Patients with anorexia nervosa complain of early satiety and bloating after meals [44]. Several studies have shown slow gastric emptying for solids and/or liquids [45-48]. As previously shown in animals submitted to prolonged food starvation, food restriction seems to be a major determinant of delayed gastric emptying in anorexia nervosa [44, 48]. However this mechanism is unlikely to be involved very often in patients with NUD, who usually do not have such peculiar alimentary behaviour.

A possible infectious aetiology of dyspepsia has been suggested because in some patients the onset of symptoms could be related in time to a bout of gastroenteritis. However, there has been no study in patients with NUD that allows a precise link to be made between delayed gastric emptying and an infective agent. A recent study did not observe any relation between delayed gastric emptying of a mixed solid-liquid meal and *Helicobacter pylori* antral gastritis in patients with NUD [49].

Gastric acid secretion does not seem to be altered in patients with NUD [21] and cannot be considered responsible for delayed emptying in these patients. Moreover symptoms are not improved by antisecretory agents [50]. Some hormonal abnormalities have also been shown but deserve further studies. In Labò *et al.*'s study, the absence of phase 3 activity in the gastroduodenal area was associated with the

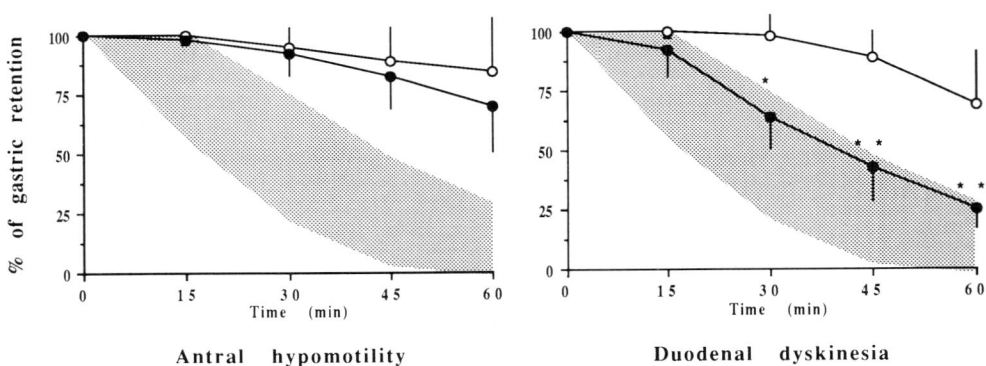

**Figure 6.** Percentage of marker $^{99m}$Tc-SC egg white remaining in the stomach in two groups of patients with non-ulcer dyspepsia compared to healthy controls (shadowed areas). Treatment with naloxone (black dots) did not change the gastric emptying rate of patients with antral hypomotility (left), whereas naloxone restored normal emptying in patients with duodenal dyskinesia (right). (Reproduced from Narducci *et al.* [4], with permission).

absence or diminution of motilin fluctuations [1]. Recently, a study using a specific antagonist of CCK receptors has shown a beneficial effect, suggesting a possible involvement of CCK in the delayed emptying [27, 51].

## Summary and conclusions

Patients with NUD are a heterogeneous group [16]. Even inside the individualized group of "dysmotility-like" dyspepsia, patients appear to be different. Approximately half of the patients have a delayed emptying. Among these patients, there are several different possible causes of this functional abnormality. In fact the pathophysiological significance of a selective delay in gastric emptying of liquids is likely to be different from a delayed emptying for both liquids and solids. The lack of correlation between symptoms and gastric emptying abnormalities makes the following question unsolved: how do the gastric motor abnormalities recorded in dyspeptic patients give rise to the specific sensations of which the patient complains? A sense of fullness and epigastric bloating symptoms, such as the inability to finish a normal sized meal, might relate to failure of fundic receptive relaxation, since these symptoms are also observed in patients following gastric surgery and vagotomy. The large preponderance of female patients observed in numerous studies has not yet been explained.

Progress will come from extensive clinical studies in which the characteristics of symptoms are very precisely defined. Longitudinal studies should help in elucidating the natural history of this group of patients. Finally some additional information could be gained by using non-invasive techniques such as electrogastrography or impedance measurements allowing determinations to be repeated in the same patients; and by using more invasive new techniques such as barostat to explain especially the abnormalities of fundic relaxation and/or of sensory perception [20] which may occur during the emptying of a meal.

## References

1. Labò G, Bortolotti M, Vezzadini P, Bonora G, Bersani G. Interdigestive gastroduodenal motility and serum motilin levels in patients with idiopathic delay in gastric emptying. Gastroenterology 1986;90:20-6.
2. Malagelada JR, Stanghellini V. Manometric evaluation of functional upper gut symptoms. Gastroenterology 1985;88:1223-31.
3. Camilleri M, Brown ML, Malagelada JR. Relationship between impaired gastric emptying and abnormal gastrointestinal motility. Gastroenterology 1986;91:94-9.
4. Narducci F, Bassotti G, Granata MT, Gaburri M, Farroni F, Palumbo R, Morelli A. Functional dyspepsia and chronic idiopathic gastric stasis. Role of endogenous opiates. Arch Intern Med 1986;146:716-20.
5. Malagelada JR. Functional disorders of gastrointestinal motility. In: Szurszewski JH, ed. *Cellular Physiology and Clinical Studies of Gastrointestinal Smooth Muscle*. New York: Elsevier, 1987:339-61.
6. Corinaldesi R, Stanghellini V, Raiti C, Rea E, Salgemini R, Barbara L. Effect of chronic administration of cisapride on gastric emptying of a solid meal and on dyspeptic symptoms in patients with idiopathic gastroparesis. Gut 1987;28:300-5.

7. Jian R, Ducrot F, Ruskoné A, Chaussade S, Rambaud JC, Modigliani R, Rain JD, Bernier JJ. Symptomatic, radionuclide and therapeutic assessment of chronic idiopathic dyspepsia. A double-blind controlled evaluation of cisapride. Dig Dis Sci 1989;34:657-64.
8. Meyer JH. Motility of the stomach and gastroduodenal junction. In: Johnson LR, ed. *Physiology of the Gastrointestinal Tract*. 2nd ed. New York: Raven press, 1987:613-30.
9. Read NW, Houghton LA. Physiology of gastric emptying and pathophysiology of gastroparesis. Gastroenterol Clin North Am 1989;18:359-73.
10. Houghton LA, Read NW, Heddle R, Maddern GJ, Downton J, Toouli J, Dent J. Motor activity of the gastric antrum, pylorus, and duodenum under fasted conditions and after a liquid meal. Gastroenterology 1988;94:1276-84.
11. Dooley CP, Valenzuela JE. Antropyloroduodenal activity during gastric emptying of liquid meals in humans. Am J Physiol 1988;255:G93-8.
12. Paraskevopoulos JA, Houghton LA, Eyre-Brooke I, Johnson AG, Read NW. Effect of composition of gastric contents on resistance to emptying of liquids from stomach in humans. Dig Dis Sci 1988,33:914-8.
13. Camilleri M, Malagelada JR, Brown ML, Becker G, Zinsmeister AR. Relation between antral motility and gastric emptying of solids and liquids in humans. Am J Physiol 1985;249:G580-5.
14. Houghton LA, Read NW, Heddle R, Horowitz M, Collins PJ, Chatterton B, Dent J. Relationship of the motor activity of the antrum, pylorus, and duodenum to gastric emptying of a solid-liquid mixed meal. Gastroenterology 1988;94:1285-91.
15. You CH, Chey WY, Lee KY, Menguy R, Bortoff A. Gastric and small intestinal myoelectric dysrhythmia associated with chronic intractable nausea and vomiting. Ann Intern Med 1981;95:449-51.
16. Colin-Jones DG, Bloom B, Bodemar G, Crean GP, Freston J, Gugler R, Malagelada J, Nyrén O, Petersen H, Piper D. Management of dyspepsia: report of a working party. Lancet 1988;1:576-9.
17. Talley NJ, Shuter B, McCrudden G, Jones M, Hoschl R, Piper DW. Lack of association between gastric emptying of solids and symptoms in non-ulcer dyspepsia. J Clin Gastroenterol 1989;11:625-30.
18. Wegener M, Borsch G, Schaffstein J, Reuter C, Leverkus F. Frequency of idiopathic gastric stasis and intestinal transit disorders in essential dyspepsia. J Clin Gastroenterol 1989;11:163-8.
19. Davis RH, Clench MH, Mathias JR. Effects of domperidone in patients with chronic unexplained upper gastrointestinal symptoms: a double-blind, placebo-controlled study. Dig Dis Sci 1988;33:1505-11.
20. Dederding JP, Lemann M, Jian R, Rambaud JC. Study of sensory perceptor and adaptation to distension of proximal stomach in chronic idiopathic dyspepsia (CID). Gastroenterology 1988;94:A91(abstr).
21. Corinaldesi R, Stanghellini V, Raiti C, Rea E, Salgemini R, Paternico A, Paparo GF, Barbara L. Gastric acid secretion and gastric emptying (GE) of solids in patients with chronic idiopathic dyspepsia (CID). Dig Dis Sci 1986;31(suppl 10):343S(abstr).
22. Jian R, Ducrot F, Piedeloup C, Mary JY, Najean Y, Bernier JJ. Measurement of gastric emptying in dyspeptic patients: effect of a new gastrokinetic agent (cisapride). Gut 1985;26:352-8.
23. Urbain JL, Siegel JA, Debie NC, Pauwels SP. Effect of cisapride on gastric emptying in dyspeptic patients. Dig Dis Sci 1988;33:779-83.
24. Corinaldesi R, Tosetti C, Stanghellini V, Ricci Maccarini M, Ghidini C, Levorato L, Monetti N, Barbara L. Gastric emptying of solids in dyspeptic patients with and without symptoms suggestive of gastroesophageal reflux disease. Gastroenterology 1990;98:A339(abstr).
25. Scarpignato C. Gastric emptying measurement in man. In Scarpignato C, Bianchi-Porro G, eds. *Clinical Investigation of Gastric Function*. Basel: Karger, 1990:198-246.

26. Bolondi L, Bortolotti M, Santi V, Calleti T, Gaiani S, Labò G. Measurement of gastric emptying time by real-time ultrasonography. Gastroenterology 1985;89:752-9.
27. Li Bassi S, Rovati LC, Giacovelli G, Bolondi L, Barbara L. Effects of loxiglumide, a cholecystokinin antagonist, in non-ulcer dyspepsia. Gastroenterology 1990;98:A77(abstr).
28. Savarino V, Percario G, Neumaier CE, Fera G, Isotta A, Scalabrini P, De Paolis M, Celle G. Clinical evaluation of real-time ultrasonic scanning in the measurement of gastric emptying in normal subjects and dyspeptic patients. Ital J Gastroenterol 1987;19:317-20.
29. Ricci R, Bontempo I, La Bella A, De Tschudy A, Corazziari E. Dyspeptic symptoms and gastric antrum distension. An ultrasonographic study. Ital J Gastroenterol 1987;19:215-7.
30. Bertrand J, Metman EH, Dorval ED, Rouleau P, d'Hueppe A, Itti R, Philippe L. Etude du temps d'évacuation gastrique de repas normaux au moyen de granules radio-opaques. Applications cliniques et validation. Gastroentérol Clin Biol 1980;4:770-6.
31. McCallum RW, Valenzuela G, Polepalle S, Stubbs J. Gastric emptying of indigestible solids in normals and patients with gastroparesis. A new radionuclide study. Gastroenterology 1990;98:A374(abstr).
32. Rees WD, Miller LJ, Malagelada JR. Dyspepsia, antral motor dysfunction, and gastric stasis of solids. Gastroenterology 1980;78:360-5.
33. Jobin G, Jian R. Isotope studies in gastric emptying. Dig Dis Sci 1982;27:571-2.
34. Fisher RS, Lockerman Z, Maurer A, Krevsky B, Miller L, Vitti R. Gastroparesis (GP) as a cause of non-ulcer dyspepsia (NUD): new insights into a common disorder. Gastroenterology 1990;98:A350(abstr).
35. Geldof H, Van Der Schee EJ, Van Blankenstein M, Grashuis JL. Electrogastrographic study of gastric myoelectrical activity in patients with unexplained nausea and vomiting. Gut 1986;27:799-808.
36. Bassotti G, Pelli MA, Morelli A. Duodenojejunal motor activity in patients with chronic dyspeptic symptoms. J Clin Gastroenterol 1990;12:17-21.
37. Pandolfo N. Duodenal motility: emphasis on some physiological, pathophysiological and therapeutic aspects. In: Bertaccini G *et al.*, eds. *The Duodenum: Selected Topics*. New York: Raven Press 1988:57-66.
38. Bortolotti M, Sarti P, Barbara L, Brunelli F. Gastric myoelectric activity in patients with chronic idiopathic gastroparesis. J Gastrointest Mot 1990;2:104-8.
39. You CH, Lee KY, Chey WY, Menguy R. Electrogastrographic study of patients with unexplained nausea, bloating, and vomiting. Gastroenterology 1980;79:311-4.
40. Koch KL, Stern RM, Vasey M, Botti JJ, Creasy GW, Dwyer A. Gastric dysrhythmias and nausea of pregnancy. Dig Dis Sci 1990;35:961-8.
41. Camilleri M, Malagelada JR, Kao PC, Zinsmeister AR. Gastric and autonomic responses to stress in functional dyspepsia. Dig Dis Sci 1986;31:1169-77.
42. Fone DR, Horowitz M, Maddox A, Akkermans LM, Read NW, Dent J. Gastroduodenal motility during the delayed gastric emptying induced by cold stress. Gastroenterology 1990;98:1155-61.
43. Stanghellini V, Malagelada JR, Zinsmeister AR, Go VLW, Kao PC. Stress-induced gastroduodenal motor disturbances in humans: possible humoral mechanisms. Gastroenterology 1983;85:83-91.
44. Robinson PH. Gastric function in eating disorders. Ann NY Acad Sci 1989;575:456-65.
45. Dubois A, Gross HA, Ebert MH, Castell DO. Altered gastric emptying and secretion in primary anorexia nervosa. Gastroenterology 1979;77:319-23.
46. McCallum RW, Grill BB, Lange R, Planky M, Glass EE, Greenfeld DG. Definition of a gastric emptying abnormality in patients with anorexia nervosa. Dig Dis Sci 1985;30:713-22.
47. Stacher G, Bergmann H, Wiesnagrotzki S, Kiss A, Schneider C, Mittelbach G, Gaupmann G, Hobart J. Intravenous cisapride accelerates delayed gastric emptying and increases antral contraction amplitude in patients with primary anorexia nervosa. Gastroenterology 1987:92:1000-6.

48. Robinson PH, Clarke M, Barrett J. Determinants of delayed gastric emptying in anorexia nervosa and bulimia nervosa. Gut 1988;29:458-64.
49. Wegener M, Borsch G, Schaffstein J, Schulz-Flake C, Mai U, Leverkus F. Are dyspeptic symptoms in patients with *Campylobacter pylori*-associated type B gastritis linked to delayed gastric emptying? Am J Gastroenterol 1988;83:737-40.
50. Nyrén O, Adami HO, Bates S, Bergstrom R, Gustavsson S, Loof L, Nyberg A. Absence of therapeutic benefit from antacids or cimetidine in non-ulcer dyspepsia. N Engl J Med 1986;314:339-43.
51. Brunelli F, Bortolotti M, Sarti P, Barbara L. Effect of CCK on gastric electric and manometric activities in normal subjects and in patients with idiopathic dyspepsia. Proceedings of the World Congress of Gastroenterology. Sydney, 1990: 143.

# 11

# Role of acid and pepsin

H. PETERSEN

*Section of Gastroenterology, Department of Medicine, Trondheim Regional and University Hospital, Trondheim, Norway*

The relationship between peptic ulcer disease and gastric acid secretion is well-known and not subject to much dispute. Furthermore, patients with duodenal ulcer on average secrete nearly twice as much acid and pepsin as normal. Non-ulcer dyspepsia (NUD) is a poorly defined and heterogeneous condition (Fig. 1). The term "non-ulcer", however, tends to make one think that this is a condition similar to peptic ulcer disease with regard to acid dependency, only lacking the defect in the duodenal or gastric mucosa. Because of the often burning character of the pain, the acid-tasting regurgitations and the frequent relief by antacids, the patients themselves also tend to regard their complaints as a consequence of "too much acid". Previously such a belief was strongly supported by the frequent use of unpleasant gastric secretory tests. In this chapter the evidence favouring a relationship between NUD and gastric acid will be discussed.

## Hypersecretion of acid in NUD

The belief in the existence of an "acid hypersecretory non-ulcer dyspepsia syndrome" was supported by Rhodes *et al.* in 1968 [1] when they reported on acid hypersecretion in patients with ulcer-like dyspepsia and coarse duodenal mucosal folds but no ulcer. The patients were not studied endoscopically, however, and probably suffered from peptic ulcer disease or severe duodenitis. Subsequent studies have failed to confirm that hypersecretion of acid is a characteristic feature of NUD [2]. In 1971 Bonnevie *et al.* [3] even reported a negative correlation between peak acid output and the degree of symptoms in such patients. Novis *et al.* in 1973 [4] found no relationship between gastric acid secretion and subsequent development of significant or minor dyspepsia.

Quite recently Collen *et al.* [5] again failed to show any abnormality of basal acid secretion in patients with NUD.

In good agreement with the above studies we found that the basal gastric secretion of acid and pepsin, as well as in response to modified sham-feeding or pentagastrin was normal in 72 patients with NUD and definitely lower than in patients with duodenal ulcer disease [6]. We also failed to discover any relationship between acid and pepsin secretion and symptom profiles or endoscopic features of gastritis. Patients with endoscopic duodenitis, however, tended to secrete more acid than those without such features. This finding is in good accordance with those of Rhodes *et al.* [1] and others [7, 8], but some studies have found that the acid secretion is normal in patients with duodenitis [5, 9]. It has been suggested that duodenitis is a part of the pathophysiological spectrum of duodenal ulcer disease and that in many patients with duodenitis a duodenal ulcer later develops [10, 11]. In good accordance with this we have found that the symptoms in patients with NUD and endoscopic duodenitis are similar to those of patients with duodenal ulcer (unpublished results).

When excluding a few patients with duodenitis, one can safely conclude that there is no evidence for the existence of a condition deserving the label "acid hypersecretory non-ulcer dyspepsia syndrome".

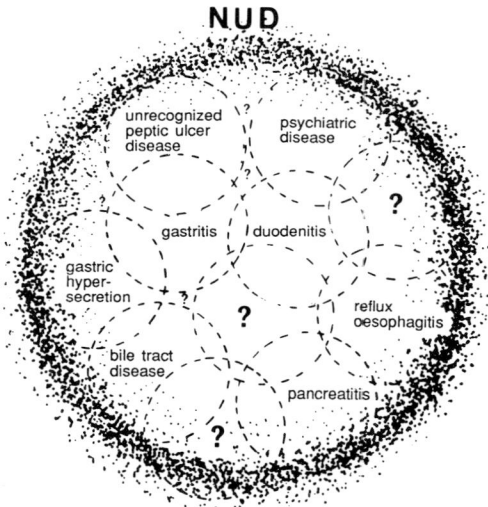

**Figure 1.** Non-ulcer dyspepsia (NUD).

## Acid as a cause of NUD

The fact that acid secretion tends to be normal in patients with NUD does not at all preclude the possibility that gastric acid plays a part in the creation of symptoms in these patients. In patients with true "acid-induced NUD" attempts to remove acid from the upper gastrointestinal tract would be expected to give symptomatic relief.

In 1973, Christiansen *et al.* [12] reported on a highly selected group of patients with NUD and hypersecretion of acid who were operated on with truncal vagotomy and drainage. The effect on acid secretion was good, but in most patients the clinical course was poor.

According to our study [13] about one third of the patients with NUD reports relief from antacids. The proportion of patients with peptic ulcers or oesophagitis who report relief from antacids is considerably greater [13]. A controlled study has failed to confirm a better effect of antacids than of placebo in patients with NUD [2, 14]. According to Graham *et al.* [15] heavy users of antacids tend to suffer from symptoms compatible with gastro-oesophageal reflux.

The effect of $H_2$-receptor antagonists in NUD is still judged as uncertain. Some have found a small effect [16, 17], but most studies have failed to show a beneficial effect of such drugs in patients with NUD [18-20]. Differences in patient selection may explain the different results.

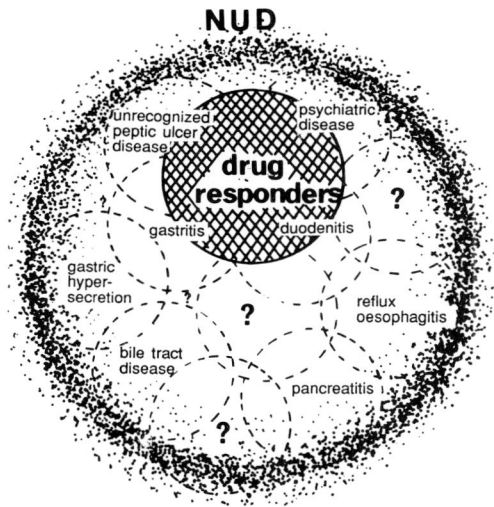

**Figure 2.** Drug responders in non-ulcer dyspepsia (NUD).

Because the term NUD includes such a heterogeneous group of patients it's highly unlikely that more than a subgroup may benefit from one type of treatment (Fig. 2). Such a subgroup may easily be missed when performing conventional randomized parallel group studies with a limited number of patients. In Trondheim we have therefore designed single case study models based on multiple cross-overs between cimetidine and placebo (Table I) [21-26]. We have used six or twelve treatment periods of 1, 2 or 4 days' duration and the symptoms have been measured daily on a visual analogue scale. Initially we used a model randomized only with regard to the treatment given first [21, 22], but because of statistical criticism [27] we subsequently changed to a model with pairwise randomization of the treatment periods (Table I) [23]. With

**Table I.** Multi cross-over models.

| Regular interchanges | AP | AP | AP | AP | AP | AP |
|---|---|---|---|---|---|---|
|  | PA | PA | PA | PA | PA | PA |
| Interchanges randomized in blocks: | PA | AP | PA | AP | AP | PA |
|  | AP | AP | PA | PA | AP | AP |
|  | AP | PA | AP | PA | PA | AP |
|  | ...... | | | | | |

A = active drug
P = placebo

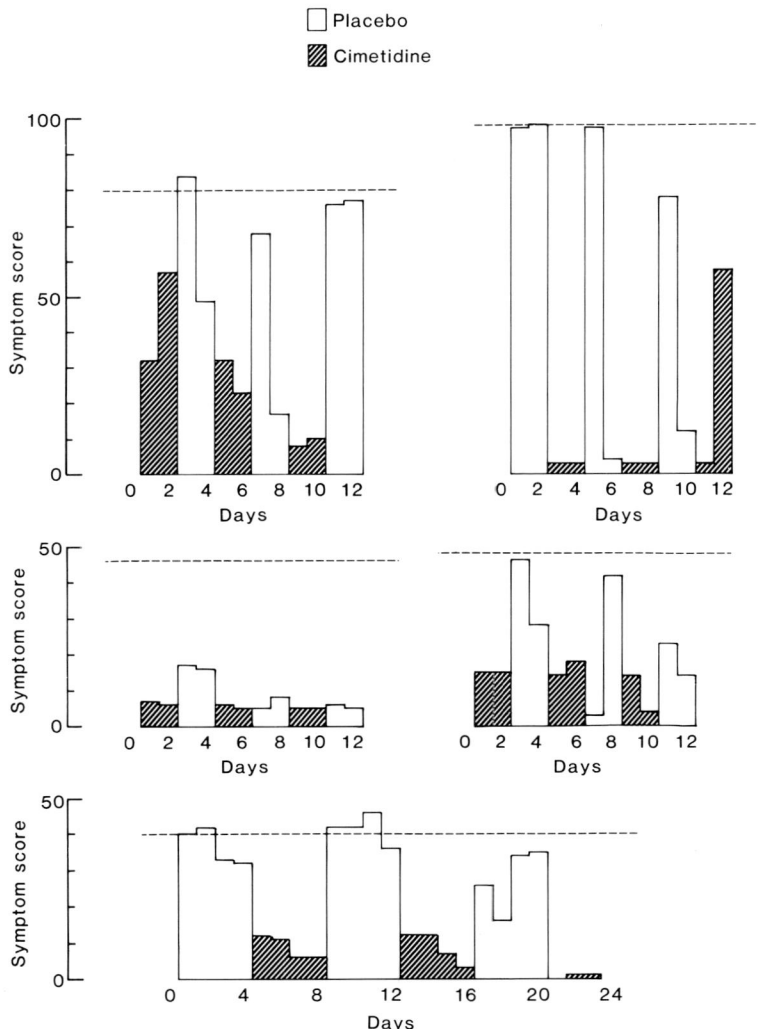

**Figure 3.** Examples of individual responders to cimetidine in non-ulcer dyspepsia (NUD) [21].

the use of such models we have been able to make statements about the effect of cimetidine compared to that of placebo in individual patients (Fig. 3) with a defined degree of certainty. When using such randomized models even individual p-values may be given [23, 26].

Altogether using the single case study approach we have compared the symptom-relieving effect of cimetidine with that of placebo in more than 500 patients with NUD. When evaluated as group studies cimetidine has been convincingly shown to be associated with a reduction in symptoms compared with placebo indicating that the groups studied include true individual responders to cimetidine, and thus patients with "acid-induced NUD". The proportion of patients identified as responders will depend very much on the demand for certainty included in the definition of responders. Taken together our studies indicate that responders to $H_2$-blockers among patients with NUD are characterized by peptic-ulcer-like or gastro-oesophageal-reflux-like symptoms, endoscopic hiatus hernia or endoscopic duodenitis. Patients with "acid-induced NUD" therefore probably suffer from gastro-oesophageal reflux disease without oesophagitis or from peptic ulcer disease with duodenitis as the actual organic manifestation.

Surprisingly we could not find any difference between responders and non-responders to cimetidine with regard to acid and pepsin secretion, either during basal or stimulated conditions (Fig. 4) [22]. Also no relationship was found between the response to cimetidine and the sensitivity of the oesophagus to acid or endoscopic features of gastritis.

Quite recently we have compared the symptom-relieving effect of single doses of cimetidine and placebo taken on demand because of actual gastro-oesophageal-reflux-like or peptic-ulcer-like NUD, using a pairwise randomized single case study model

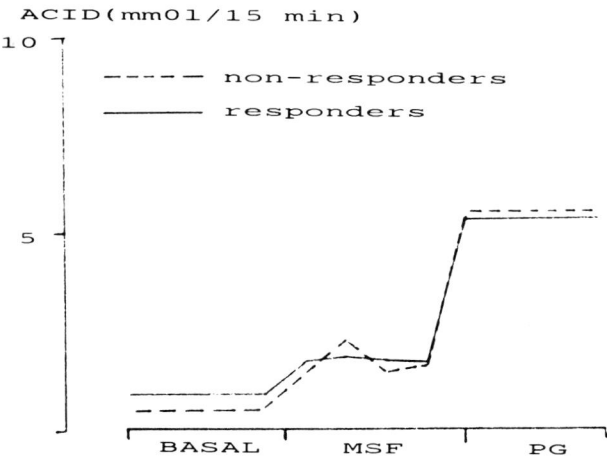

**Figure 4.** Gastric acid secretion basally, in response to modified sham feeding (MSF), and in response to pentagastrin (PG) in responders and non-responders to cimetidine among patients with non-ulcer dyspepsia (NUD).

[28]. This approach circumvents the disturbing spontaneous day to day variations in dyspeptic symptoms [29]. The preliminary results are very promising, fully confirming the beneficial effect of cimetidine in these subgroups of patients with NUD and showing that the effect is already present 30 minutes after drug intake. This model obviously may identify individual responders to $H_2$-blockers with a better sensitivity than similar models based on fixed treatment periods. The model may turn out to be useful for identification of individual $H_2$-blockers responders in clinical practice.

## Conclusions

In general patients with NUD have normal gastric secretion and there is no relationship between gastric secretion and symptom profile or endoscopic gastritis. Patients with endoscopic duodenitis, however, tend to secrete more acid than those without.

In a subgroup of patients with NUD, symptoms are relieved by $H_2$-blockers [30, 31]. These patients most probably suffer from gastro-oesophageal reflux disease without oesophagitis or from peptic ulcer disease with duodenitis as the actual organic manifestation.

Patients with NUD responding to $H_2$-blockers are not characterized by hypersecretion of acid and measurement of gastric secretion is of little value in the evaluation of patients with NUD.

## References

1. Rhodes J, Evans KT, Lawrie JH, Forrest AP. Coarse mucosal folds in the duodenum. Q J Med 1968;37:151-69.
2. Petersen H. Antacids in non-ulcer dyspepsia. Scand J Gastroenterol 1982;17(suppl 75): 77-8.
3. Bonnevie O, Kallehauge HE, Wulff HR, Wulff MR. Prognostic value of the augmented histamine test in ulcer disease and x-ray negative dyspepsia. Scand J Gastroenterol 1971;6:723-9.
4. Novis BH, Marks IN, Bank S, Sloan AW. The relation between gastric acid secretion and body habitus, blood groups, smoking, and the subsequent development of dyspepsia and duodenal ulcer. Gut 1973;14:107-12.
5. Collen MJ, Loebenberg MJ. Basal gastric acid secretion in non-ulcer dyspepsia with or without duodenitis. Dig Dis Sci 1989;34:246-50.
6. Petersen H, Johannessen T, Fjøsne U, Kleveland PM, Halvorsen T, Kristensen P, Sandbakken P, Hafstad PE, Løge I. Gastric secretion in non-ulcer dyspepsia. Scand J Gastroenterol 1989;24(suppl 159):71.
7. Myren J. Gastric secretion in duodenitis. Scand J Gastroenterol 1982;17(suppl 79):98-101.
8. Joffe SN. Relevance of duodenitis to non-ulcer dyspepsia and peptic ulceration. Scand J Gastroenterol 1982;17(suppl 79):88-97.
9. Beck IT, Kahn DS, Lacerte M, Solymar J, Callegarini U, Geokas MC. "Chronic duodenitis": a clinical pathological entity? Gut 1965;6:376-83.
10. Venables C. Duodenitis. Scand J Gastroenterol 1988;23(suppl 155):61-7.
11. Thomson WO, Joffe SN, Roberston AG, Lee FD, Imrie CW, Blumgart LH. Is duodenitis a dyspeptic myth? Lancet 1977;1:1197-8.
12. Christiansen J, Aagaard P, Koudahl G. Truncal vagotomy and drainage in the treatment of ulcer-like dyspepsia without ulcer. Acta Chir Scand 1973;139:173-5.

13. Johannessen T, Petersen H, Kleveland PM, Dybdahl JH, Sandvik AK, Brenna E, Waldum H. The predictive value of history in dyspepsia. Scand J Gastroenterol 1990;25:689-97.
14. Norrelund N, Helles A, Schmiegelow M. Uncharacteristic dyspepsia in general practice. A controlled trial with an antacid (Alminox). Ugeskr Laeger 1980;142:1750-3.
15. Graham DY, Smith JL, Patterson DJ. Why do apparently healthy people use antacid tablets? Am J Gastroenterol 1983;78:257-60.
16. Delattre M, Malesky M, Prinzie A. Symptomatic treatment of non-ulcer dyspepsia with cimetidine. Curr Ther Res 1985;37:980-91.
17. Talley NJ, Mc Neil D, Hayden A, Piper DW. Randomized, double-blind, placebo-controlled cross-over trial of cimetidine and pirenzepine in non-ulcer dyspepsia. Gastroenterology 1986;91:149-56.
18. Kelbæk H, Linde J, Eriksen J, Mungaard S, Moesgaard F, Bonnevie O. Controlled clinical trial of treatment with cimetidine for non-ulcer dyspepsia. Acta Med Scand 1985;217:281-7.
19. Nyrén O, Adami HO, Bates S, Bergstrom R, Gustavsson S, Loof L, Nyberg A. Absence of therapeutic benefit from antacids of cimetidine in non-ulcer dyspepsia. N Engl J Med 1986;314:339-43.
20. Dobrilla G, Comberlato M, Steele A, Vallaperta P. Drug treatment of functional dyspepsia. A meta-analysis of randomized controlled clinical trials. J Clin Gastroenterol 1989;11:169-77.
21. Kleveland PM, Larsen S, Sandvik L, Kristensen P, Johannessen T, Hafstad PE, Sandbakken P, Løge I, Fjøsne U, Petersen H. The effect of cimetidine in non-ulcer dyspepsia. Experience with a multi cross-over model. Scand J Gastroenterol 1985;20:19-24.
22. Johannessen T, Fjøsne U, Kleveland PM, Halvorsen T, Kristensen P, Løge I, Hafstad PE, Sandbakken P, Petersen H. Cimetidine responders in non-ulcer dyspepsia. Scand J Gastroenterol 1988;23:327-36.
23. Johannessen T, Kristensen P, Petersen H, Fosstvedt D, Løge I, Kleveland PM, Dybdahl J. The symptomatic effect of one-day treatment periods with cimetidine in dyspepsia. (Submitted for publication).
24. Petersen H, Løge I, Johannessen T, Fjøsne U, Kleveland PM, Kristensen P, Sandbakken P, Hafstad PE, Halvorsen T. Dyspepsia: therapeutic response as a diagnostic tool. Scand J Gastroenterol 1987;22(suppl 128):108-13.
25. Johannessen T, Fosstvedt D, Petersen H. Experience with a multi cross-over model in dyspepsia. Scand J Gastroenterol 1988;23(suppl 147):33-7.
26. Johannessen T, Fosstvedt D, Petersen H. Statistical aspects of controlled single subject trials. Fam Pract 1990;7:325-8.
27. Spiedgelhalter DJ. Statistical issues in studies of individual response. Scand J Gastroenterol 1988;23(suppl 147):40-5.
28. Johannessen T, Petersen H, Kristensen P, Fosstvedt D, Kleveland PM, Dybdahl J, Løge I. Cimetidine on-demand in dyspepsia. Preliminary experience with a randomized controlled single subject trial (N of 1 RCT) (Submitted for publication).
29. Johannessen T, Petersen H, Kristensen P, Kleveland PM, Dybdahl J, Sandvik A, Brenna E, Waldum H. The intensity and variability of symptoms in dyspepsia (Submitted for publication).
30. Farup PG, Hofstad B, Wetterhus S, Nerdrum T, Stray N, Breckan R, Tholfsen J, Ulshagen K, Larsen S. Ranitidine (Ran) for non-ulcer dyspepsia (NUD). Scand J Gastroenterol 1990;25(suppl 176):85(abstr).
31. Saunders JHB, Oliver RJ, Higson DL. Dyspepsia incidence of non-ulcer disease in a controlled trial of ranitidine in general practice. Br Med J 1986;292:645-8.

# 12

# Duodenogastric reflux

S.A. MÜLLER-LISSNER

*Department of Gastroenterology, Medizinische Klinik, Klinikum Innenstadt, University of München, Germany*

## Introduction

Duodenogastric reflux is defined as the flow of duodenal contents into the stomach [1]. It occurs intermittently and is a normal event both in the fasted state and after eating. Increased duodenogastric reflux has been claimed to be pathogenic for a couple of diseases which may cause dyspepsia. The role of duodenogastric reflux for classic causes of dyspepsia such as gastric ulcer is beyond the scope of this chapter and has been discussed elsewhere [2]. In the following, the possible role of duodenogastric reflux for functional dyspepsia of different causes will be discussed after a short note on the measurement of duodenogastric reflux.

## Duodenogastric reflux

Since the composition of the duodenal contents is variable due to factors such as feeding, bile flow, and pancreatic secretion, the reflux rates of the different constituents of duodenal contents do not necessarily parallel each other [3]. In most studies, duodenogastric bile reflux has been measured. Due to gastric secretion and emptying the reflux rate in terms of amount refluxed per unit time is not the only determinant of gastric concentrations of bile. This concentration, however, is likely to be the main determinant of mucosal damage, beside factors of mucosal resistance.

Duodenogastric reflux occurs intermittently as short pulses [4]. Therefore mean values over a couple of seconds or minutes do not properly reflect the time pattern of reflux. But even if mean values over several minutes are obtained, reflux may vary by a factor of more than 100 from one experimental period to another both in the fasting state and after a meal [5].

Attempts have been made to overcome partly the shortcomings of continuous gastric aspiration (removal of gastric contents applicable only while fasting, invasiveness) by scintigraphic and pH-metric techniques. The appearance in the stomach of radiopharmaceutics used for hepatobiliary scintigraphy may be used to semiquantify duodenogastric reflux [6, 7]. Due to technical problems such as overlap between liver, small intestine and stomach, complicated corrections are necessary which render the quantitation unreliable.

The alkalinity of the refluxate has been used to monitor reflux by means of long term gastric pH monitoring [8]. Though it is clear that a gush of duodenal juice into the stomach leads to temporary increase in gastric pH, the opposite conclusion is not necessarily true, namely that each temporary increase in gastric pH is caused by duodenogastric reflux. In addition, short alkaline spikes during pH monitoring provide no information about the gastric concentrations of noxious material such as bile salts and their duration. Thus, gastric pH monitoring is unreliable in diagnosing duodenogastric reflux.

## Gastro-oesophageal reflux disease

Increased acid exposure of the distal oesophagus can be demonstrated in most but not all patients with erosive oesophagitis and/or typical reflux symptoms (heartburn and acid regurgitation). Reflux disease in the absence of apparently increased acid reflux could either be due to an increased mucosa susceptibility to damage or to reflux constituents other than acid, e.g. bile salts.

In one study [9] using oesophageal aspiration, trace amounts of bile acids ($\leq$ 40 µmol/l) could be detected in two of 10 controls, but in 39 of 45 patients with oesophageal erosions. Eleven of the patients had concentrations in excess of 200 µmol/l in the supine position, but only one patient had no demonstrable acid reflux. In another study oesophageal bile salts could neither be found in controls nor in reflux patients, either fasting or postprandially [10]. In acute experiments, the minimum damaging concentrations of bile salts are in the millimolar range [11].

It is therefore unlikely that duodeno-gastro-oesophageal reflux by itself plays a role in gastro-oesophageal reflux disease in the unoperated stomach. A contributing role in the presence of acid gastro-oesophageal reflux is possible.

## Duodenogastric reflux and gastroparesis

Slowed gastric emptying can be found in a proportion of patients with functional dyspepsia. It is hence of interest whether duodenogastric reflux may slow gastric emptying.

No correlation has been observed between gastric liquid emptying and reflux of duodenal markers in volunteers [5]. Similar results were obtained in fasting volunteers [12]. In contrast, progressive destruction of the pylorus by surgical measures increases gastric liquid emptying and duodenogastric marker reflux in parallel [13].

Parr *et al.* examined whether intragastric bile would modify gastric emptying [14]. Bile was administered intragastrically, resulting in gastric concentrations of bile acids similar to those found in Billroth II resected patients, but no alteration of gastric emptying could be demonstrated.

Increased duodenogastric reflux therefore does not produce functional dyspepsia via slowing of gastric emptying.

## The duodenogastric reflux syndrome

Destruction of the gastroduodenal junction by pyloroplasty or distal gastric resection with gastroenterostomy leads to an enormous increase in duodenogastric reflux as long as no Roux-en-Y loop is constructed [15, 16]. In some patients after refluxogenic operations a syndrome occurs which is characterized by epigastric pain, nausea and in particular vomiting of large amounts of bilious fluid. This is called the duodenogastric reflux syndrome [1]. The precise pathogenesis is not known. Since the symptoms are not specific, other causes have to be excluded, e.g. anastomotic ulceration and gastroparesis. The diagnosis is probable if a fasting bile reflux of more than 120 µmol/h can be shown [15] and if the symptoms can be reproduced when the patients own small intestinal contents or alkali are infused intragastrically [17, 18]. However, the overall results of remedial operations are not convincing [19]. Therefore, extreme caution should be applied before Roux-en-Y reconstruction is advocated.

## Reflux gastritis

Chronic duodenogastric reflux produces a characteristic histological appearance of the gastric mucosa with hyperplastic changes (Table I), but a paucity of both acute and chronic inflammatory cells [20]. These characteristics have been derived from patients after refluxogenic gastric surgery in comparison with unoperated stomachs with and without peptic ulcers. They have been validated in patients in whom reflux was eliminated by Roux-en-Y anastomosis [21]: whereas the macroscopic changes and the microscopic hyperplastic changes improved, gastritis in terms of inflammation remained unchanged. It is, however, unclear whether these characteristics are specific for the diagnosis of significant duodenogastric reflux in patients without the duodenogastric reflux syndrome.

Table I. Microscopic characteristics of the gastric mucosa in patients with high duodenogastric reflux [20].

Hyperplasia
Oedema
Smooth muscle fibers in the lamina propria
Vasodilation and congestion of superficial mucosal capillaries
Paucity of both acute and chronic inflammatory cells

## Postcholecystectomy syndrome

Fractional reflux of duodenal contents is similar in the fasted state and after fatty, protein, and mixed meals [5]. In contrast, bile acid reflux following a meal is higher than in the fasted state [22]. This is due to an increased amount of bile delivered to the duodenum by gallbladder contraction. (During emptying of a solid-liquid meal from the stomach the gallbladder empties progressively over approximately two hours by about 50% [23].)

Elimination of variations in bile flow due to gallbladder contraction should reverse the relation between fed and fasted bile reflux. Fasting bile salt concentrations in the range of those after Billroth II resection could in fact be shown in patients after cholecystectomy [22, 24]. In such patients the occurrence of the duodenogastric reflux syndrome seems therefore possible, but no clear correlation between high gastric bile salt concentrations and dyspeptic symptoms could be demonstrated [22, 25].

## Duodenogastric reflux and functional dyspepsia

If all known causes of dyspepsia, either classic causes such as peptic ulcer or motility disorders such as gastro-oesophageal reflux disease and gastroparesis, have been excluded, the dyspepsia is called functional, idiopathic, or essential. A shortcoming of all studies dealing with dyspepsia which is possibly due to duodenogastric reflux is that not all other known causes of dyspepsia had been excluded.

In several studies, no difference in bile reflux between controls and dyspeptic patients has been found, whether prepyloric erosive changes were present or not [24, 26, 27]. In contrast, three other groups have claimed that duodenogastric reflux is associated with an increase in functional dyspepsia on the basis of scintigraphy [7] or gastric pH monitoring [8, 28]. One of the latter groups even performed biliary diversion surgery (duodenal switch operation) in five such patients [6]. The success of this operation does not, however, prove that duodenogastric reflux was really responsible for the dyspepsia, since this is not the only phenomenon to be affected (e.g. CCK release, which acts on upper GI motility, is certainly modified by the procedure). In one of the studies an association was observed between acid gastro-oesophageal reflux and typical gastro-oesophageal reflux symptoms (acid regurgitation and heartburn) on the one hand, and antral alkalinization and non-specific epigastric dyspeptic symptoms on the other [28]. It is, however, unclear whether the duodenogastric reflux events suspected to cause the antral alkalinization are the cause of the symptoms or not; for example, could nausea of whatever cause lead to increased duodenogastric reflux? These results therefore deserve further investigation.

Cisapride, which is able to reduce high reflux rates [29, 30], has improved dyspeptic symptoms in many studies [31, 32], but this could also be due to its effects on gastro-oesophageal reflux and/or gastric emptying. A role of duodenogastric reflux in the pathogenesis of dyspepsia of unknown cause has in my view therefore not been proven.

## Duodenogastric reflux and *Helicobacter pylori*

*Helicobacter pylori*-induced gastritis has been implicated in the pathogenesis of otherwise unexplained dyspepsia [33]. Patients with high gastric bile salt concentrations after distal gastric resection were less likely to be *H. pylori* positive than unoperated controls [34] but this could be due to different sites of biopsies: near the pylorus in unoperated patients (who have low reflux) but in the mid-corpus in operated patients (who have high reflux). In addition, no relation between *H. pylori* status and degree of duodenogastric reflux could be found in unoperated patients [35]. However, it could be shown that *H. pylori* was cleared from the stomach of about half of the patients who underwent gastric resection with Billroth II anastomosis, but in no patient who underwent gastric resection with Roux-en-Y anastomosis [36]. It seems therefore that *H. pylori* tolerates poorly high duodenogastric reflux.

## Conclusions

Increased duodenogastric reflux in the absence of refluxogenic gastric surgery is still a condition looking for its responsibility in the pathophysiology of a disease. As long as no methodology is available to quantify reflux, taking into account its temporal and spatial distribution, the role of duodenogastric reflux in dyspepsia will remain unclear.

## References

1. Blum AL, Heading R, Müller-Lissner S, Olbe L. Is duodenogastric reflux clinically relevant? Gastroenterol Int 1989;2:3-8.
2. Müller-Lissner SA. Does duodenogastric reflux cause diseases? Z Gastroenterol 1988;26:637-42.
3. Müller-Lissner SA, Fraass C. Dissociation of duodenogastric marker reflux and bile salt reflux. Dig Dis Sci 1985;30:733-8.
4. King PM, Adam RD, Pryde A, McDicken WN, Heading RC. Relationships of human antroduodenal motility and transpyloric fluid movement: non-invasive observations with real-time ultrasound. Gut 1984;25:1384-91.
5. Sonnenberg A, Müller-Lissner SA, Weiser HF, Müller-Duysing W, Heinzel F, Blum AL. Effect of liquid meals on duodenogastric reflux in humans. Am J Physiol 1982;243:G42-7.
6. DeMeester TR, Fuchs KH, Ball CS, Albertucci M, Smyrk TC, Marcus JN. Experimental and clinical results with proximal end-to-end duodenojejunostomy for pathologic duodenogastric reflux. Ann Surg 1987;206:414-26.
7. Dufresne F, Carrier L, Gagnon M, Picard D, Chartrand R, Dumont A. Scintigraphic study of duodenal-gastric reflux in cases of primary gastropathy, chronic ulcer of the duodenal bulb, and Moynihan's disease. J Nucl Med 1988;29:17-22.
8. Stein HJ, Hinder RA, DeMeester TR, Lloyd BA, Fuchs KH, Attwood SE, Gupta NC. Clinical use of 24-hour gastric pH monitoring vs O-diisopropyl iminodiacetic acid (DISIDA) scanning in the diagnosis of pathological duodenogastric reflux. Arch Surg 1990;125:966-71.
9. Gotley DC, Morgan AP, Cooper MJ. Bile acid concentrations in the refluxate of patients with reflux oesophagitis. Br J Surg 1988;75:587-90.

10. Mittal RK, Reuben A, Whitney JO, McCallum RW. Do bile acids reflux into the esophagus? A study in normal subjects and patients with gastroesophageal reflux disease. Gastroenterology 1987;92:371-5.
11. Harmon JW, Johnson LF, Maydonovitch CL. Effects of acid and bile salts on the rabbit esophageal mucosa. Dig Dis Sci 1981;26:65-72.
12. Schindlbeck NE, Heinrich C, Müller-Lissner SA. Relation between fasting antroduodenal motility and transpyloric fluid movements. Am J Physiol 1989; 257:G198-G201.
13. Müller-Lissner SA, Blum AL. To-and-fro movements across the canine pylorus. Scand J Gastroenterol 1984;19(suppl 92):1-3.
14. Parr NJ, Baker PR, Grime JS, Mackie CR. Intragastric bile does not perturb gastric emptying of liquids in humans. Dig Dis Sci 1988, 33:289-92.
15. Hoare AM, McLeish A, Thompson H, Alexander-Williams J. Selection of patients for bile diversion surgery: use of bile acid measurement in fasting gastric aspirates. Gut 1978;19:163-5.
16. Keighley MR, Asquith P, Alexander-Williams J. Duodenogastric reflux: a cause of gastric mucosal hyperaemia and symptoms after operations for peptic ulceration. Gut 1975;16:28-32.
17. Meshkinpour H, Marks JW, Schoenfield LJ, Bonnoris GG, Carter S. Reflux gastritis syndrome: mechanisms of symptoms. Gastroenterology 1980;79:1283-7.
18. Warshaw AL. Intragastric alkali infusion. A simple, accurate provocative test for diagnosis of symptomatic alkaline reflux gastritis. Ann Surg 1981;194:297-304.
19. Malagelada JR, Phillips SF, Shorter RG, Higgins JA, Magrina C, Van Heerden JA, Adson MA. Postoperative reflux gastritis: pathophysiology and longterm outcome after Roux-en-Y diversion. Ann Intern Med 1985; 103:178-83.
20. Dixon MF, O'Connor HJ, Axon AT, King RF, Johnston D. Reflux gastritis: distinct histopathological entity? J Clin Pathol 1986;39:524-30.
21. Bechi P, Amorosi A, Mazzanti R, Buccarelli A, Pantalone D, Cortesini C. Short-term effects of bile diversion on postgastrectomy gastric histology. Dig Dis Sci 1988;33:1288-96.
22. Müller-Lissner SA, Schindlebeck NE, Heinrich C. Bile salt reflux after cholecystectomy. Scand J Gastroent 1987;22(suppl 139):20-4.
23. Lawson M, Everson GT, Klingensmith W, Kern F. Coordination of gastric and gallbladder emptying after ingestion of a regular meal. Gastroenterology 1983;85:866-70.
24. Watson RG, Love AH. Intragastric bile acid concentrations are unrelated to symptoms of flatulent dyspepsia in patients with and without gallbladder disease and postcholecystectomy. Gut 1987;28:131-6.
25. Warshaw AL. Bile gastritis without prior gastric surgery: contributing role of cholecystectomy. Am J Surg 1979;137:527-31.
26. Bost R, Hostein J, Valenti M, Bonaz B, Payen N, Faure H, Fournet J. Is there an abnormal fasting duodenogastric reflux in non-ulcer dyspepsia? Dig Dis Sci 1990;35:193-9.
27. Nesland AA, Rydning A, Berstad A. Intragastric bile acid concentrations in patients with erosive prepyloric changes. Scand J Gastroenterol 1987;22:505-8.
28. Mattioli S, Pilotti V, Felice V, Lazzari A, Zannoli R, Bacchi ML, Loria P, Tripodi A, Gozzetti G. Ambulatory 24-hr pH monitoring of esophagus, fundus, and antrum. A new technique for simultaneous study of gastroesophageal and duodenogastric reflux. Dig Dis Sci 1990;35:929-38.
29. Müller-Lissner SA, Fraass C. Chronic oral treatment with cisapride decreases high bile salt reflux rates. Am J Gastroenterol 1986;81:354-7.
30. Rezende-Filho J, di Lorenzo C, Dooley CP, Valenzuela JE. Cisapride stimulates antral motility and decreases biliary reflux in patients with severe dyspepsia. Dig Dis Sci 1989;34:1057-62.
31. Dobrilla G, Comberlato M, Steele A, Vallaperta P. Drug treatment of functional dyspepsia. A meta-analysis of randomized controlled clinical trials. J Clin Gastroenterol 1989;11:169-77.

32. Müller-Lissner SA, Klauser AG. The treatment of gastrointestinal diseases with motility-stimulating drugs. Internist 1989;30:797-804.
33. Rokkas T, Pursey C, Uzoechina E, Dorrington L, Simmons NA, Filipe MI, Sladen GE. Non-ulcer dyspepsia and short term DeNol therapy; a placebo-controlled trial with particular reference to the role of *Campylobacter pylori*. Gut 1988;29:1386-91.
34. O'Connor HJ, Dixon MF, Wyatt JI, Axon AT, Ward DC, Dewar EP, Johnston D. Effect of duodenal ulcer surgery and enterogastric reflux on *Campylobacter pyloridis*. Lancet 1986;2:1178-81.
35. Karttunen T, Niemelä S. *Campylobacter pylori* and duodenogastric reflux in peptic ulcer disease and gastritis. Lancet 1988;1:118.
36. Offerhaus GJ, Rieu PN, Janssen JB, Joosten HJ, Lamers CB. Prospective comparative study of the influence of post-operative bile reflux on gastric mucosal histology and *Campylobacter pylori* infection. Gut 1989;30:1552-7.

# SESSION III
# Pathophysiology (continued)

Chairman: J. FREXINOS

# 13

# Gastric mucosal barrier and non-steroidal anti-inflammatory drugs

F. HALTER

*Gastrointestinal Unit, University Hospital, Inselspital, Bern, Switzerland*

The stomach and duodenum are protected from endogenous damaging luminal contents — particularly acid and pepsin — by several mechanisms. The underlying principle also represents the first line of defence against ingested damaging agents, e.g. ethanol or non-steroidal anti-inflammatory agents (NSAIDs). The precise mechanisms whereby NSAIDs produce gastroduodenal damage are unknown, although depletion of mucosal prostaglandins with a corresponding reduction in the competence of mucosal defence mechanisms is widely thought to be important [1-3]. The defence line appears to be multifactorial (Table I). It includes the mucus gel layer, bicarbonate secretion by epithelial cells, surface active phospholipids, the apical membrane itself, and the process of restitution and healing. In addition mucosal blood flow plays a vital role in the prevention of injury to the surface epithelium by delivering oxygen, nutrients, and bicarbonate and by removing $H^+$ ions which have penetrated the mucus-bicarbonate barrier. Among these the "mucus bicarbonate barrier" acts as the first line of defence, with bicarbonate secretion by the surface epithelial cells in the mucus gel

Table I. Proposed mechanisms for mucosal protection: possible role of prostaglandins.

- Stimulation of bicarbonate and mucus secretion
- Stimulation of surface-active phospholipids
- Maintenance or enhancement of gastric mucosal blood flow
- Stimulation of cellular transport processes
- Liberation of cAMP and polyamines
- Stabilization of tissue lysosomes
- Preservation of basal membrane

layer setting up a pH gradient and maintaining juxtamucosal neutrality in the environment of low luminal pH. Such a gradient has been demonstrated *in vitro* and *in vivo* in many animals models as well as in man [4-9]. NSAIDs have been shown in animal models to reduce both epithelial bicarbonate secretion [10] and mucus synthesis and secretion. The mucus gel layer is thus diminished, exposing the epithelial cells to a more acidic environment [6, 7].

Intragastric acidity can enhance the mucosal toxicity of aspirin by changing its solubility. Aspirin (pK 3.5) is mostly ionized at pH 3.5 or higher. These charged particles do not cross cell membranes, and only physical injury of surface epithelium occurs from unsolubilized crystal particles. In an acidic environment (i.e. below pH 3.5) aspirin remains unionized and as a lipid-soluble molecule it can easily cross the lipid-protein layer in the cell membrane. Although several mechanisms of intracellular toxicity of aspirin have been suggested, the most likely pathway involves a decrease in mitochondrial oxidative phosphorylation with a resultant depletion of ATP. The increased membrane permeability and intracellular accumulation of sodium and water leads to epithelial cell death and exfoliation, similar to those described for ethanol, except that the mucosal penetration of aspirin and the erosions are not as extensive as those after ethanol [11].

## Role of eicosanoids in defence, damage and repair of gastric mucosal barrier

Local synthesis of eicosanoids has been suggested to be involved in resistance against noxious agents and in injury and repair processes. Eicosanoids are derived from arachidonic acid with various enzymatic pathways (Fig. 1). The cyclo-oxygenase pathway with its formation of prostaglandins protects the gastric mucosa against a wide variety of damaging agents. Indeed, this protective activity of prostaglandins and synthetic analogues has resulted in a surge of popularity for investigating gastric mucosal injury and has initiated the concept of "cytoprotection". Gastric "cytoprotection" can be defined as prevention of haemorrhagic gastric mucosal injury without inhibition of acid secretion [11, 12]. Despite obvious protection superficial epithelial layers are not initially preserved, so the term "mucosal protection" is therefore preferred by many. Of particular importance in this still not fully understood phenomenon appears to be the integrity of mucosal blood flow and the preservation of the basal lamina, which can be achieved by prostaglandins [11]. This allows rapid replacement of necrotic superficial cell layers by migrating adjacent surviving cells [13]. The concept that prostaglandins are causatively involved in mucosal protection is strengthened by two important observations: arachidonic acid can induce mucosal protection by itself, most likely by enhanced local synthesis of prostaglandins [14]; while in experimental animals inhibition of prostaglandin formation by NSAIDs weakens the resistance of the gastric mucosa against naturally occurring noxious agents and results in the development of mucosal erosions within 3-5 hours [11].

Other metabolites of arachidonic acid include cyclo-oxygenase-derived thromboxane $(TX)A_2$, and the 5-lipoxygenase-derived cysteinyl leukotrienes (LT) $C_4$ and $D_4$ [3,4]. $(TX)A_2$ and the cysteinyl leukotrienes are potent vasoconstrictors in the stomach and cause flow disturbances in the gastric mucosal/submucosal microcirculation [15-17]. These metabolites of arachidonic acid have been shown to be pro-ulcerogenic (Fig. 1). The initially widely accepted concept that an intact balance between protective mucosal prostaglandins and pro-ulcerogenic leukotrienes represents the basis of understanding the principle of mucosal protection has recently been challenged. It was soon realized that prostaglandins are not the only agents with mucosal protective properties. Gastric mucosal resistance can also be strengthened by a series of other substances, such as sulphydryls, hormones, polyamines, metal ions, mild irritants, and several drugs such as conventional antacids, sucralfate and colloidal bismuth [11, see Table II]. Increasing evidence is accumulating that cytoprotection can be maintained even when tissue prostaglandin synthesis is partially or fully

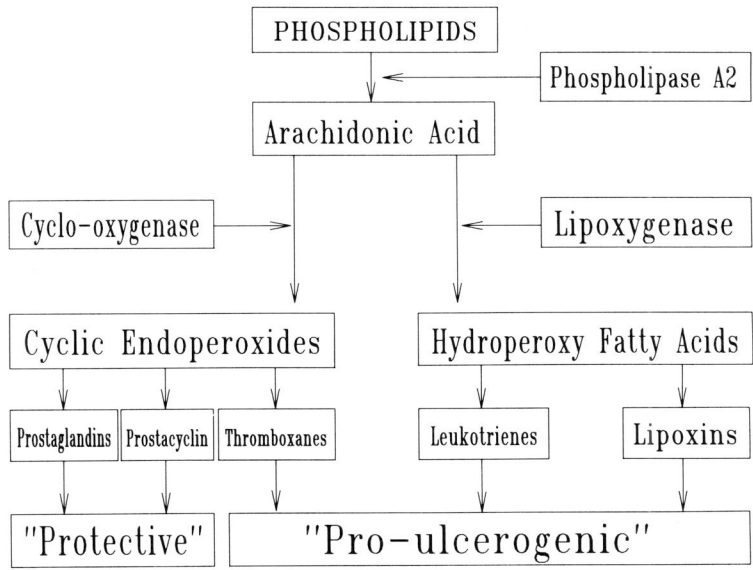

**Figure 1.** Arachidonic acid cycle with cyclo-oxygenase and lipoxygenase pathways and conventional separation into "protective" and pro-ulcerogenic actions of the various derivatives.

**Table II.** Cytoprotective agents.

|  | Endogenous | Exogenous |
|---|---|---|
|  | Prostaglandins | Mild stress |
|  | Sulphydryls | Non-specific irritants |
|  | N-Acetylcysteine | and stimulants |
|  | Penicillamine | Several drugs: |
|  | Dimercaprol | — sucralfate |
|  | BAL | — colloidal bismuth |
|  | Hormones | — antacids |
|  | EGF |  |
|  | Gastrin |  |
|  | Polyamines |  |

suppressed by cyclo-oxygenase blockers such as indomethacin [18]. Moreover it was shown that suppression of leukotrienes by potent and specific inhibitors does not necessarily enhance protection of gastro-duodenal mucosa.

## Eicosanoids and repair of experimental mucosal damage and healing of experimental ulcers

The concept of mucosal protection coupled with the clinical experience that NSAIDs are an established risk factor in peptic ulcer disease led to a widespread, almost missionary belief, that "cytoprotection" would implicitly enhance ulcer healing.

Prostaglandins did not however fulfil this promise [19]. It was soon realized that prostaglandins only enhance ulcer healing with high acid inhibitory doses while healing was uninfluenced by small "cytoprotective" doses. It has since been firmly established that drugs modulating the endogenous gastric mucosal prostaglandin and leukotriene system differ in protective and healing processes. Prostaglandins are apparently unable to accelerate repair of superficial mucosal defects [20], this despite their established trophic properties [21]. This comes as no surprise since the trophic effects of prostaglandins are mainly based on a delayed senescence of gastric mucosal tissue [22] and since the phenomenon of gastric reconstitution occurs within minutes to hours [13], before trophic effects based on cell reproduction could theoretically occur. As an example, gastrin-induced enhancement of DNA synthesis has a minimum lag time of 8-14 hours [23]. Similarly, suppression of prostaglandin synthesis does not necessarily result in delayed restitution of superficial mucosal defects. It is of interest that in one recent study both proquazone and indomethacin, when given at doses that substantially diminish tissue prostaglandin levels, enhanced the healing of superficial mucosal defects [18].

Conversely, prostaglandins did not enhance healing of ulcers in most experimental models [24, 25]. Several studies, including one from our own laboratories, have, however, shown that indomethacin can delay healing of experimental ulcers, in conjunction with diminished cell reproduction in the ulcer margin [25, 26]. Some preliminary evidence points, however, towards the possibility that such a delay can be overcome by a particularly profound decrease in prostaglandin synthesis. This observation was made when indomethacin treatment was combined with fish oil diet, which *per se* reduces prostaglandin synthesis [27]. Indomethacin, 1.5 mg b.d. subcutaneously, did not delay but rather accelerated healing of gastric cryo-ulcers in rats given a fish oil diet [28]. Even if the reason for the failure of indomethacin to delay ulcer healing in the above mentioned study is not fully established, the acceleration of repair and healing by high dose indomethacin therapy is not fully unexpected. It is indeed well-established that both high doses of aspirin or indomethacin can enhance cell reproduction in gastric corpus mucosa, possibly as an overcompensation for the increase in cell loss which is well-known to occur with cyclo-oxygenase inhibitors [29, 31]. Growth regulation of gastric mucosa indeed depends on the equilibrium between cell death and cell renewal [31]. Both prostaglandins and indomethacin can thus, albeit through different pathways, challenge this equilibrium in favour of an overall increase in gastric mucosal cell mass [31, Fig. 2]. In this context, it is of particular interest that the prostanoid enprostil, which

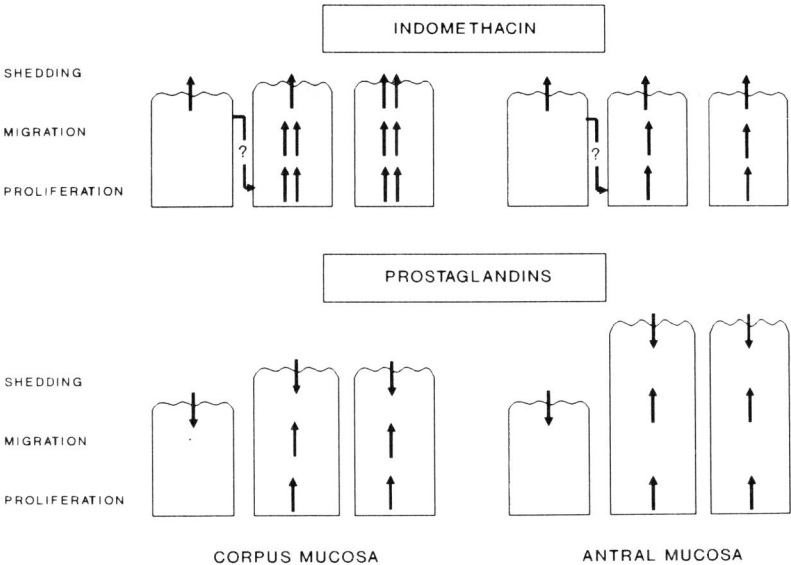

**Figure 2.** Possible mechanisms responsible for the differences in the mucosal mass of the gastric corpus and antrum after prostaglandin or indomethacin treatment. ↑ = increase, ↓ = decrease in shedding, migration and proliferation.

has been shown to exert protection in the gastric mucosa [32], can nevertheless induce mucosal damage by itself or potentiate ethanol-induced damage in man [33, 34].

## The phenomenon of adaptive mucosal protection

Soon after the discovery was made that prostaglandins can enhance the resistance of mucosal protection, it was realized that mucosal protection can also be induced by short and long term application of mild irritants such as 10-20% ethanol [35]. This phenomenon was subsequently named "adaptive cytoprotection". It was initially postulated that "adaptive cytoprotection" was the consequence of enhanced tissue prostaglandin synthesis. In more recent studies it was however shown that suppression of tissue prostaglandin synthesis does not abolish "adaptive cytoprotection". Several studies performed in experimental animals and man have indeed shown that adaptive mucosal protection can occur during prolonged treatment with NSAIDs [36-38]. This phenomenon may be of major clinical importance since the prevalence of peptic ulcer formation during prolonged NSAID therapy is relatively low if one considers that during acute intake most patients develop multiple gastric erosions [39].

## Conclusion

The so-called gastric mucosal barrier is an important, albeit incompletely understood, protective measure against the well-established potential damage of NSAID therapy. Even though it is established beyond doubt that prostaglandins can partly protect the stomach against this risk factor, it is now well-established that they share this protective role with many other substances, including sulphydryl agents and metal ions. The role of prostaglandins in mucosal protection even appears to be optional and it has been shown that at least one prostanoid used in ulcer therapy can *per se* induce superficial gastro-duodenal mucosal damage. Similarly, some preliminary evidence points towards a dual effect of cyclo-oxygenase inhibitors on healing of superficial and deep mucosal gastro-duodenal defects.

## References

1. Vane JR. Inhibition of prostaglandin synthesis as a mechanism of action for aspirin-like drugs. Nature New Biol 1971;231:232-5.
2. Whittle BJ, Higgs GA, Eakins KE, Moncada S, Vane JR. Selective inhibition of prostaglandin production in inflammatory exudates and gastric mucosa. Nature 1980;284:271-3.
3. Whittle BJR. Prostaglandin cyclo-oxygenase inhibition and its relationship to gastric damage. In: Harmon JW, ed. *Basic Mechanisms of Gastrointestinal Mucosal Cell Injury and Protection*. Baltimore, London: Williams and Wilkins, 1981:197-210.
4. Takeushi K, Magee D, Critchlow J, Matthews J, Silen W. Studies of the pH gradient and thickness of frog gastric mucus gel. Gastroenterology 1983;84:331-40.
5. Williams SE, Turnberg LA. Demonstration of a pH gradient across mucus adherent to rabbit gastric mucosa: evidence for a mucus-bicarbonate barrier. Gut 1981;22:94-6.
6. Flemstrom G, Kivilaakso E. Demonstration of a pH gradient at the luminal surface of rat duodenum *in vivo* and its dependence on mucosal alkaline secretion. Gastroenterology 1983;84:787-94.
7. Ross IN, Bahari HM, Turnberg LA. The pH gradient across mucus adherent to rat fundic mucosa *in vivo* and the effect of potential damaging agents. Gastroenterology 1981;81:713-8.
8. Bahari HM, Ross IN, Turnberg LA. Demonstration of a pH gradient across the mucus layer on the surface of human gastric mucosa *in vitro*. Gut 1982;23:513-6.
9. Quigley EM, Turnberg LA. pH of the microclimate lining human gastric and duodenal mucosa *in vivo*. Studies in control subjects and in duodenal ulcer patients. Gastroenterology 1987;92:1876-84.
10. Rees WD, Gibbons LC, Turnberg LA. Effects of non-steroidal anti-inflammatory drugs and prostaglandins on alkali secretion by rabbit gastric fundus *in vitro*. Gut 1983;24:784-9.
11. Szabo S. Mechanisms of mucosal injury in the stomach and duodenum: time-sequence analysis of morphological, functional, biochemical and histochemical studies. Scand J Gastroenterol 1987;22(suppl 127):21-8.
12. Robert A, Nezamis JE, Lancaster C, Hanchar AJ. Cytoprotection by prostaglandins in rats. Prevention of gastric necrosis produced by alcohol, HCl, NaOH, hypertonic NaCl, and thermal injury. Gastroenterology 1979;77:433-43.
13. Lacy ER, Ito S. Ethanol-induced insult to the superficial rat gastric epithelium. A study of damage and rapid repair. In: Allen A *et al.*, eds. *Mechanisms of Mucosal Protection in the Upper Gastrointestinal Tract*. New York: Raven Press, 1984:49-56.

14. Hollander D, Tarnawski A. The role of dietary essential fatty acids and fish oils in gastroduodenal mucosal protection against injury. Proceedings Falk Symposium 59, 1990 (in press).
15. Whittle BJ, Kauffman GL, Moncada S. Vasoconstriction with thromboxane A2 induces ulceration of the gastric mucosa. Nature 1981;292:472-4.
16. Pihan G, Rogers C, Szabo S. Vascular injury in acute gastric mucosal damage. Mediatory role of leukotrienes. Dig Dis Sci 1988;33:625-32.
17. Konturek SJ, Brzozowski T, Drozdowicz D, Beck G. Role of leukotrienes in acute gastric lesions induced by ethanol, taurocholate, aspirin, platelet-activating factor and stress in rats. Dig Dis Sci 1988;33:806-13.
18. Peskar BM, Trautmann M, Pallapies D, Respondek M, Müller KM. Actions of eicosanoids. Proceedings Falk Symposium 59, 1990 (in press).
19. Hawkey CJ, Walt RP. Prostaglandins for peptic ulcers: a promise unfulfilled. Lancet 1986;2:1084-7.
20. Schmidt KL, Bellard RL, Smith GS, Henagan JM, Miller TA. Influence of prostaglandin on repair of rat stomach damaged by absolute ethanol. J Surg Res 1986;41:367-77.
21. Reinhart WH, Müller O, Halter F. Influence of long-term 16,16-dimethyl prostaglandin $E_2$ treatment on the rat gastrointestinal mucosa. Gastroenterology 1983;85:1003-10.
22. Uribe A, Rubio C, Johansson C. Cell kinetics of rat gastrointestinal mucosa. Autoradiographic study after treatment with 15(R)15-methyl-prostaglandin $E_2$. Scand J Gastroenterol 1986;21:246-52.
23. Willems G, Vansteenkiste Y, Limbosch JM. Stimulating effect of gastrin on cell proliferation kinetics in canine fundic mucosa. Gastroenterology 1972;62:583-9.
24. Konturek SJ, Stachura J, Radeki T, Drozdowicz D, Brzozowski T. Cytoprotective and ulcer healing properties of prostaglandin $E_2$, colloidal bismuth sucralfate in rats. Digestion 1987;38:103-13.
25. Inauen W, Wyss PA, Kayser S, Baumgartner A, Schürer-Maly CC, Koelz HR, Halter F. Influence of prostaglandins, omeprazole, and indomethacin on healing of experimental gastric ulcers in the rat. Gastroenterology 1988;95:636-41.
26. Levi S, Goodlad RA, Lee CY, Stamp G, Walport MJ, Wright NA, Hodgson JH. Inhibitory effect of non-steroidal anti-inflammatory drugs on mucosal cell proliferation associated with gastric ulcer healing. Lancet 1990;336:840-3.
27. Hansen HS, Fjalland B, Jensen B. Extremely decreased release of prostaglandin $E_2$-like activity from chopped lung of ethyl linolenate-supplemented rats. Lipids 1983;18:691-5.
28. Schürer-Maly CC, Hoeflin F, Lauterburg B, Flogerzi B, Halter F. Fish oil: role in development and healing of experimental gastric ulcers in the rat. Gastroenterology 1990;98:A121(abstr).
29. Eastwood GL, Quimby GF. Effect of chronic aspirin ingestion on epithelial proliferation in rat fundus, antrum and duodenum. Gastroenterology 1982;82:852-6.
30. Kuwayama H, Eastwood GL. Effects of water immersion, restraint stress and chronic indomethacin ingestion on gastric antral and fundic epithelial proliferation. Gastroenterology 1985;88:362-5.
31. Baumgartner A, Koelz HR, Halter F. Indomethacin and turnover of gastric mucosal cells in the rat. Am J Physiol 1986;250:G830-5.
32. Cohen MM, McCready DR, Clark L, Sevelius H. Protection against aspirin-induced antral and duodenal damage with enprostil. A double-blind endoscopic study. Gastroenterology 1985;88:382-6.
33. Lanza FL, Robinson MG, Isenberg JI, Basuk PM, Karlin DA. Effect of enprostil on the gastroduodenal mucosa of healthy volunteers. Aliment Pharmacol Ther 1990;4:601-13.
34. Cohen MM, Yeung R, Wang HR, Clark L. Human antral damage induced by alcohol is potentiated by enprostil. Gastroenterology 1990;99:45-50.
35. Robert A. Cytoprotection by prostaglandins. Gastroenterology 1979;77;761-7.

36. Hawkey CJ, Kemp RT, Walt RP, Bhaskar NK, Davies J, Filipowicz B. Evidence that adaptive cytoprotection in rats is not mediated by prostaglandins. Gastroenterology 1988;94:948-54.
37. Graham DY, Smith JL, Spjut HJ, Torres E. Gastric adaptation. Studies in humans during continuous aspirin administration. Gastroenterology 1988;95:327-33.
38. Shorrock CJ, Prescott RJ, Rees WD. The effects of indomethacin on gastroduodenal morphology and mucosal pH gradient in the healthy human stomach. Gastroenterology 1990;99:334-9.
39. Langman MJS. Epidemiologic evidence of the association between peptic ulceration and anti-inflammatory drug use. Gastroenterology 1989;96:640-6.

# 14

# Weakness of gastric mucosal barrier: myth or reality?

CH. FLORENT, B. FLOURIÉ(**), B. DESAINT, C. LEGENDRE(*)

*Service de Gastroentérologie, (*) Service d'Anatomie Pathologique, Hôpital Saint-Antoine, 184 rue du Faubourg Saint-Antoine, 75012 Paris, France (**) INSERM U. 290, Hôpital Saint-Lazare, 107 bis rue du Faubourg Saint-Denis, 75010 Paris, France*

## The gastric mucosal barrier

The gastric mucosa is permanently exposed to various noxious agents, either endogenous (mainly acid, pepsin and duodeno-gastric reflux) or exogenous (e.g. food, hypertonic drinks, drugs such as aspirin and non-steroidal anti-inflammatory drugs [NSAIDs]). The gastric mucosa withstands aggressions remarkably well, due to protective mechanisms referred to, since Davenport's studies, as the so-called "gastric mucosal barrier". This barrier consists in several more or less interdependent components:

— Secretion of mucus and bicarbonate, creating a non-acid medium between gastric juice and the apical membranes of the epithelial cells [1-2].

— Gastric mucosal blood flow, which supplies gastric cells with oxygen and nutrients, and also allows clearance of noxious agents. The latter (aspirin, NSAIDs, back-diffusion of $H^+$, other reactive chemicals) may indeed accumulate on the basal side of the epithelium via cellular or paracellular routes, and induce cell death [3-7].

— Cell renewal and migration, which are of major importance for the rapid repair of epithelial disruption [8]. Cell migration allows lamina propria to be covered before "cell renewal" (to be understood as "cell production") starts. The restitution of the gastric mucosa depends on the depth of lesions. It starts a few minutes after an aggression and the lamina propria is covered by cells growing in from the margins of the ulceration within 30 minutes. Such a mechanism, however, has not been demonstrated in chronic ulceration in man, even in experimental conditions.

— Gastric epithelial trophic factors: growth factors, gastrin, eicosanoids (prostaglandins E) [9-10].

The equilibrium of this barrier is permanently challenged by numerous endogenous, exogenous and iatrogenic factors. NSAIDs and aspirin decrease gastric mucosal protection by inhibiting the synthesis of endogenous prostaglandins. This results in epigastric pain without any detectable endoscopic lesion in many patients (30 to 50%, according to the series) and sometimes in lesions of the gastric mucosa, either diffuse (erosions and haemorrhage) or focal (erosions, ulcers), with or without digestive symptoms.

## Assessment of functional digestive disease

Functional digestive disease has been considered for a long time to be a psychosomatic disorder, without any demonstrable anatomical support. This was due to the lack of accurate means of investigation, and does not now hold true since new techniques have shown undisputed abnormalities in so-called "psychofunctional disorders". In some cases, a clear relation has been established between normalization of a measured parameter (mainly a motor disturbance) and improvement in patient's clinical status, thus establishing the causative nature of the motor dysfunction:

— delayed gastric emptying in patients with postprandial discomfort and sensations of slow digestion (non-ulcer dyspepsia, diabetic gastroparesis, post-vagotomy syndrome);

— decrease in small bowel transit time in patients with the irritable bowel syndrome (evidenced by scintigraphic studies and hydrogen breath-test with non-absorbable sugars);

— Oddi's sphincter dysfunction, evidenced by manometry, during biliary pain without gallstones ("functional Odditis").

All these well-described functional disorders are related to a motor disturbance. Whether mucosal anomalies without any detectable endoscopic lesions are responsible for the symptoms remains an open question. In other words, is endoscopy appropriate to visualize any gastric, duodenal and even colonic lesions? Does the absence of gross macroscopic lesion, mainly erosions or ulcers, allow confirmation of mucosal integrity?

One may of course answer negatively. Improvements in endoscopic techniques (electronic video-endoscopes with opto-electronic zoom lens) permits visualization of ulceration less than 0.1 mm in diameter. Moreover, gastric epithelium cannot be assessed directly with endoscopy; scanning electron microscopy is able to show normal or disrupted apical cell membranes.

Impairment of mucosal protection, leading to mucosal lesions, has been demonstrated in man but in particular conditions, mainly in critically-ill patients or during NSAID consumption. In order to establish a causal relationship between symptoms and impaired mucosal protection in a subset of patients, one should require: (a) clear-cut digestive complaints; (b) absence of endoscopic lesions; (c) the existence of a simple, reliable and reproducible technique already validated, demonstrating the mucosal abnormality.

We described six years ago [11-14] a subset of dyspeptic patients, referred to as "hypersthenic dyspeptic patients", presenting with anomalies in gastric transepithelial potential difference (PD). Our findings have been confirmed by A. Pfeiffer et al. in Müncken (personal communication), but not by others [15]. Such discrepancies are not surprizing since our results were preliminary. PD measurement meets the above mentioned criteria and a dramatic decrease in PD value is observed during gastric mucosal aggression in animal and in man, whatever the aggressive agent is:

concentrated ethanol, acidified aspirin, biliary salts. A relation between basal PD values and mucosal surface integrity (as observed by scanning electron microscopy) has been clearly established in the animal. We drew the same conclusion in patients with weakness of gastric mucosal barrier syndrome, according to our criteria [Fig. 1-5].

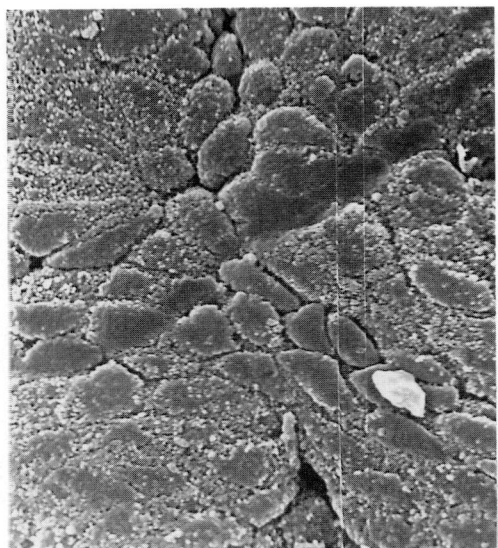

**Figure 1.** Normal gastric mucosa observed with scanning electron microscopy (x 800). Note the cell density, the close vicinity of cells and the dense apical microvilli.

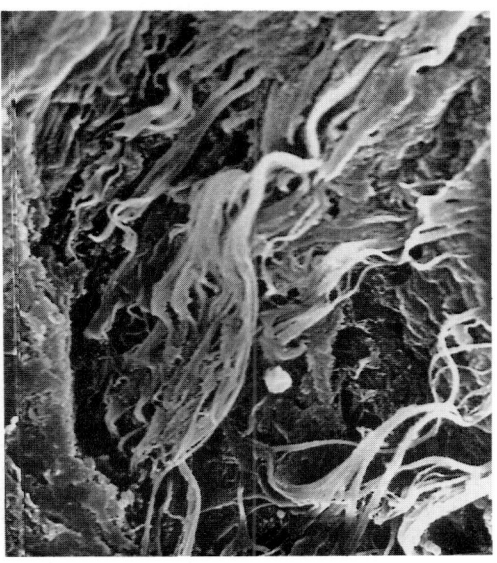

**Figure 2.** Slight aggression against the gastric mucosa. Note the hypersecretion of a filamentous mucus insufficient to cover surface cells (x 800).

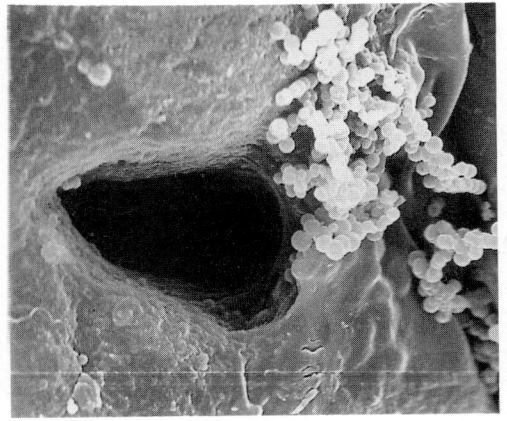

**Figure 3.** Scanning electron microscopy aspect of the opening of an oxyntic crypt (x 600). Note the mucus thickness and the extravasation of platelets on a cellular defect.

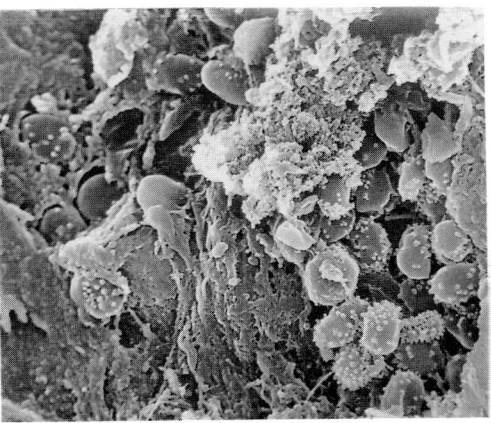

**Figure 4.** Inflamed mucosa with mucus concretions making a discontinuous network. Activated lymphocytes are present at the surface (x 800).

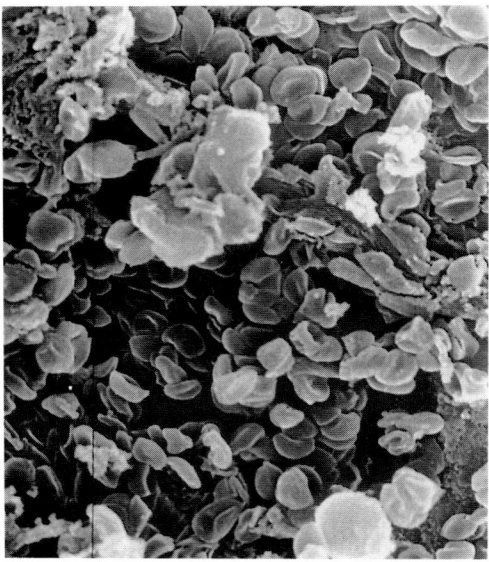

**Figure 5.** Gastric microbleeding from an antral micro-ulceration (x 800).

### The concept of gastric transepithelial potential difference: a reappraisal

In order to assess the importance of PD abnormalities in non-ulcer dyspepsia, we studied several groups of subjects:
— 200 healthy subjects;
— 20 patients with the irritable bowel syndrome;
— 25 patients with active peptic ulcer disease, confirmed by endoscopy;
these three groups serving as controls;
— 25 patients with "hypersthenic dyspepsia", defined by early postprandial, food-related epigastric pain, without clinical evidence of irritable bowel syndrome and with normal upper GI endoscopy and biopsies, and normal abdominal ultrasonography.

Symptoms were recorded with a questionnaire by two independent observers whose quotations were compared. Upper GI endoscopy was performed in all subjects, with fundic and antral biopsies in order to assess chronic atrophic gastritis. *Helicobacter pylori* was not searched for at that time; however, scanning electron microscopy was often performed and allowed us to exclude its presence in most cases.

PD was measured using the intragastric catheter technique, infused with sodium chloride 154 mM, forming an intragastric electrode. The reference electrode was constituted by a second catheter filled with agar-agar potassium chloride 3 M, set in an epicranian needle subcutaneously implanted in the forearm. PD was measured in the basal state, i.e. after manual emptying of the stomach and infusion of 100 ml of sodium chloride 154 mM, during 30 minutes, and after infusion of 500 mg aspirin in 100 ml hydrochloric acid 0.1 M (pH 1). The following parameters were assessed: (a) intragastric pH during the test period (initially by gastric juice sampling at fixed intervals; thereafter by continuous intragastric pH recording, using a combined probe and an analogue recorder); (b) maximum drop in PD absolute value (PDmax), expressed in millivolts; (c) time for PDmax (in minutes); (d) time to recover PD baseline (in minutes); (e) area under the curve of falling PD (AUC); (f) irritation index (RI), defined as AUC x PDmax/100.

We showed that basal PD was significantly lower in dyspeptic patients (i.e. with epigastric pain without endoscopic lesions) than in healthy subjects, patients with duodenal ulcer or irritable bowel syndrome. Aspirin infusion (not performed in ulcer patients) resulted in the same drop in PD (absolute values), occurring at the same time in all subjects tested. Dyspeptic patients, however, exhibited a longer time for basal PD recovery. Ten per cent ethanol induced a slight drop in PD in healthy subjects, and in patients with peptic ulcer or irritable bowel syndrome. This was at variance with dyspeptic patients, in whom ten per cent ethanol induced a marked and sustained drop in PD (Tables I and II).

**Table I.** Effects of aspirin 500 mg on gastric PD.

|  | Healthy subjects | Dyspeptic patients | Irritable bowel patients |
|---|---|---|---|
| Basal PD (mv) | 39.4 ± 3.3 | 26.6** ± 6.4 | 37.7 ± 4.0 |
| Maximum drop in PD (mv) | 10.5 ± 4.5 | 10.2 ± 4.0 | 8.7 ± 1.6 |
| Area under the curve (mv.min) | 99.5 ± 22.7 | 79 ± 8.5 | 87.5 ± 11.7 |
| Time to recover PD baseline (min) | 18.2 ± 3.5 | 52** ± 8 | 27.5 ± 3.5 |
| Irritation index (mv$^2$.min) | 1.04 ± 0.33 | 0.93 ± 0.15 | 0.98 ± 0.48 |

** $p<0.001$ vs healthy subjects and other groups.

**Table II.** Effects of ten per cent ethanol on gastric PD.

|  | Healthy subjects | Dyspeptic patients | Peptic ulcer patients | Irritable bowel patients |
|---|---|---|---|---|
| Maximum drop in PD (mv) | 4.0 ± 0.2 | 9.8** ± 1.3 | 3.6 ± 0.5 | 4.0 ± 1.6 |
| Area under the curve (mv.min) | 12.3 ± 0.8 | 72 ± 15 | 10.0 ± 4.3 | 16.4 ± 5.5 |
| Time to recover PD baseline (min) | 11.0 ± 0.7 | 52** ± 7 | 14.5 ± 1.0 | 17.6 ± 3.7 |
| Irritation index (mv$^2$.min) | 0.049 ± 0.0024 | 1.03 ± 0.36 | 0.038 ± 0.34 | 0.086 ± 0.03 |

** $p<0.001$ vs healthy subjects and other groups.

As compared with controls, superficial gastric mucosal abnormalities disclosed by scanning electron microscopy were more frequent in dyspeptic patients. Pfeiffer et al. in München observed the same variations in PD after aspirin and ethanol intake. Gignoux et al. [15], however, did not confirm these results in a small group of dyspeptic patients apparently presenting with the same characteristics. These authors performed acid infusion of the stomach instead of using sodium chloride 154 mM and used a different technique for PD measurement. These differences make comparisons difficult. Weakness of mucosal barrier assessed by several parameters including PD measurement has been demonstrated in other circumstances, such as congestive gastropathy during portal hypertension, in animal and in man [16]. Studies are currently in progress in cirrhotic patients, in order to determine whether a relation exists between decrease in portal pressure, restitution of normal PD and reduced bleeding risk from hypertensive gastropathy.

Available data provide conflicting results about the value of PD measurements characterizing a subset of dyspeptic patients. This is at least in part due to a lack of standardization of experimental procedures. The main unresolved problem is still to know whether some groups of dyspeptic patients, characterized by specific symptoms and easily identified by simple investigations, can be included in homogeneous therapeutic trials. We have shown in two previously published studies [12, 13] that mucosal protective drugs with or without antacid activity were able to modify the gastric mucosal barrier and to induce activity partially protective against aspirin injury.

**Conclusion**

These results suggest that drug-induced changes in the mucosal barrier can oppose exogenous and perhaps endogenous aggressions. Studies with prostaglandins (used at non-antisecretory doses) have confirmed that mucosal protection can be improved by drugs. It is not yet possible to determine with certainty one or more subgroups of dyspeptic patients. More studies are necessary; they should be multicentre and be based upon clinical data as well as functional tests. The latter are of course not restricted to PD measurement. Moreover, PD determination is not actually accepted as a routine procedure, while detection of gross mucosal lesions by upper GI endoscopy is still considered as the gold standard. Others, mainly in Japan, have shown anomalies in mucosal blood flow using laser-Doppler in non-ulcer dyspepsia. Such disturbances have also been found during stress (extensive burns) with endoscopic laser-Doppler or reflectance spectrometry. Sato et al. [7] found that a decrease in mucosal blood flow in patients with extensive burns correlated with the risk of subsequent gastric bleeding (ischaemia/reperfusion syndrome). These simple techniques have not been widely evaluated so far and should be part of therapeutic studies, in order to be correlated with symptoms (personal communication), and to determine their respective outcomes under treatment. We are personally convinced that weakness of the gastric and/or duodenal mucosal barrier is an undisputable concept, supported by numerous experimental data, in animals as well as in man.

## References

1. Allen A, Leonard AJ, Sellers LA. The mucus barrier. Its role in gastroduodenal mucosal protection. J Clin Gastroenterol 1988;10 (suppl 1):S93-8.
2. Allen A, Garner A. Mucus and bicarbonate secretion in the stomach and their possible role in mucosal protection. Gut 1980;21:249-62.
3. Guth PH. Gastric blood flow in restraint stress. Am J Dig Dis 1972;17:807-13.
4. Holm L. Gastric mucosal blood flow and mucosal protection. J Clin Gastroenterol 1988;10(suppl 1):S114-9.
5. Kitajima M, Otsuka S, Shimizu A, Nakajima M, Kiuchi T, Ikeda Y, Oshima A. Impairment of gastric microcirculation in stress. J Clin Gastroenterol 1988;10(suppl 1):S120-8.
6. Mac Greevy JM, Moody FG. Protection of gastric mucosa against aspirin-induced erosions by enhanced blood flow. Surg Forum 1977;28:357-9.
7. Sato N, Kawano S, Tsuji S, Kamada T. Micro-vascular basis of gastric mucosal protection. J Clin Gastroenterol 1988;10(suppl 1):S13-8.
8. Lacy ER. Epithelial restitution in the gastrointestinal tract. J Clin Gastroenterol 1988;10(suppl 1):S72-7.
9. Ogino K, Oka S, Okazaki Y, Takemoto T. Gastric mucosal protection and superoxide dismutase. J Clin Gastroenterol 1988;10(suppl 1):S129-32.
10. Takeuchi K, Johnson LR. Pentagastrin protects against stress ulcerations in rats. Gastroenterology 1979;76:327-34.
11. Bernier JJ, Florent C. La faiblesse de la barrière muqueuse gastrique et la dyspepsie hypersthénique. Ann Gastroentérol Hépatol 1986;22:33-5.
12. Florent C, Flourié B, Bernier JJ. Effets d'un pansement anti-acide sur les modifications de la différence de potentiel gastrique induites par l'aspirine chez l'homme. Gastroentérol Clin Biol 1984;8:359-63.
13. Florent C, Flourié B, Pfeiffer A, Bernier JJ. Mesure de la différence de potentiel transépithéliale gastrique. Effets des agents agressifs (aspirine, alcool ) et des pansements gastriques. Gastroentérol Clin Biol 1985;9(suppl):58-64.
14. Florent C, Pfeiffer A. Bernier JJ. La faiblesse de la barrière muqueuse gastrique: un nouveau concept. Gastroentérol Clin Biol 1985; 9(suppl):65-71.
15. Gignoux C, Fricamps C, Bonaz B, Hostein J, Fournet J. Le syndrome de faiblesse de la barrière muqueuse gastrique définit-il un sous-groupe de malades dyspeptiques? Gastroentérol Clin Biol 1990;14:604-5.
16. Pienkowski P, Payen JL, Calès P, Monin JL, Gerin P, Pascal JP, Frexinos J. Etude fonctionnelle, chez l'homme, de la gastropathie congestive au cours de la cirrhose par la mesure de la différence de potentiel. Gastroentérol Clin Biol 1989;13:763-8.

# 15

# *Helicobacter pylori,* gastritis and non-ulcer dyspepsia

P. MAINGUET, J.-C. DEBONGNIE

*Cliniques Universitaires Saint-Luc, Université Catholique de Louvain, Avenue Hippocrate 10, 1200 Brussels, Belgium*

There is accumulating evidence that *Helicobacter pylori (H. pylori)* plays a significant role in chronic antral gastritis (type B), that it could be a predisposing factor to duodenal ulcer, and that it may contribute to its chronic evolution.

*H. pylori* colonizes the human gastric mucosa without any competition from other micro-organisms. The urease activity, spiral shape and gas requirements seem to be factors enabling *H. pylori* to survive in a viscous, poorly-oxygenated environment. When *H. pylori* is associated with antral gastritis (type B), the mucus-bicarbonate barrier is compromised. The micro-organism does not penetrate through the mucosal epithelium, but the inflammatory response seen in type B chronic gastritis seems to be directed at least in part at *H. pylori* antigens.

Thus the relationship between *H. pylori* infection and "non-ulcer dyspepsia" (NUD) is strictly linked to the presence of a chronic type B gastritis, or more rarely to an acute gastritis, as in human ingestion studies.

The link between *H. pylori* and NUD remains unclear. The present review will consider the pathogenicity of *H. pylori* with regard to gastritis, the criteria to histological and endoscopic diagnosis of *H. pylori* gastritis, and the relationship of *H. pylori* gastritis with NUD (Fig. 1).

## *Helicobacter pylori* as a cause of gastritis (Table I)

In microbiology, Koch's postulates are basic requirements for a causal relationship. Extended causal postulates have been proposed [1], not specifically for micro-organisms, and have been applied for the relationship between *H. pylori* and peptic ulcer [2].

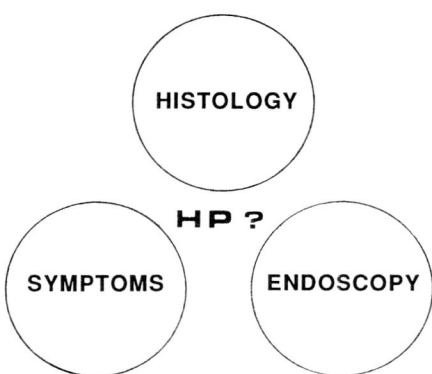

**Figure 1.** What is gastritis?
HP: *Helicobacter pylori*

**Table I.** Is *Helicobacter pylori* a cause of gastritis?

| Proposal | Answer |
|---|---|
| Koch's postulates | |
| 1. The germ should always be found in the animals having the disease and in that disease only | Yes |
| 2. The germ should be obtained from the diseased animal and grown outside the body | Yes |
| 3. The inoculation of these germs should produce the same disease in a susceptible animal | Yes |
| 4. The germs should be found in the diseased areas so produced in the animal | Yes |
| Extended postulates | |
| 1. Time-order: colonization should precede effect | Unclear |
| 2. Specificity | Unclear |
| 3. Dose-response relationship | Unclear |
| 4. Plausibility | Yes |

### First postulate

"The germ should always be found microscopically in the bodies of animals having the disease and in that disease only; it should occur in such a manner as to explain the lesion of the disease."

a — *H. pylori* is always found in the gastric mucosa of patients with chronic active antral gastritis, the lesion caused by the micro-organism. The bacteria were found in 88% of 1393 patients with chronic active gastritis and the negative cases may be due to the limited number of samples or the limited sensitivity of diagnostic methods. The same relationship does not hold for body and fundic mucosa: in studies covering antral and fundic mucosa [3-9], *H. pylori* is frequently associated with antral gastritis but the infected fundic mucosa is normal in 18-66% of cases [3-6, 10], the frequency being higher [6] in duodenal ulcer patients (84%) than in gastritis patients (39%).

b — *H. pylori* is not found in normal stomachs. *H. pylori* was present in 5% of 1049 patients with normal mucosa on biopsy. This incidence could represent either histological false positives in which some curved bacterial structures were incorrectly taken to be *H. pylori,* or to a false negative diagnosis of gastritis, the mucosa sampled being in the neighbourhood of, but not actually involving, inflamed gastric mucosa. Until now, no case of cultured *H. pylori* has been described from histologically completely normal stomachs [3, 6, 11].

c — Location of *H. pylori* explains the lesion. The target of *H. pylori* is the gastric mucus surface cell [12] and *H. pylori* is thus also found in Barrett's mucosa [13] and in gastric metaplasia in the duodenal bulb [14, 15], but not in intestinal metaplasia in the antrum. When numerous bacteria seen on electron-microscopy (EM) sections are adherent to the epithelium, mainly by abutting but also by pedestals of indentation, signs of epithelial degeneration are always present [16]. A close spatial relationship is found between the juxtamucosal bacteria and the granulocytic infiltrate [17]. Gastric mucosa from patients with *H. pylori* produces specific immunoglobulin *in vitro* and this antibody production correlates with the plasma cell infiltrate seen in these patients [18], reflecting the local humoral immune reaction. Lymphoid follicles in gastric mucosa, implying local antigenic stimulation, are a specific feature of *Helicobacter*-associated gastritis [18] and are associated with the highest levels of systemic antibodies to *H. pylori* [19]. In addition, an increase in epithelial and lamina propria T-lymphocytes is present, reflecting the local immune cellular reaction [2].

In contrast to type B gastritis, in a new entity — lymphocytic gastritis — characterized by a dense intra-epithelial infiltration with T-lymphocytes [20, 21] the prevalence of *H. pylori* is low, only 8% of 102 cases of lymphocytic gastritis being positive [22]. Furthermore, Fléjou *et al.* [23] found on follow-up of *H. pylori*-positive patients that two among those who became negative revealed a histological picture of lymphocytic gastritis. The relationship between these features remains unclear.

## Second postulate

"The germ should be obtained from the diseased animal and grown outside the body."

Although, gastric bacteria were described as long ago as the last century [24] and rediscovered recently on gastric sections [25], only modern bacteriological methods have enabled this fragile micro-organism to be cultured [26], and it has recently been renamed *Helicobacter,* a new family [27]. *H. pylori* obtained from gastric biopsies with chronic active gastritis can thus be cultured.

## Third postulate

"The inoculation of these germs, in pure cultures freed by successive transplantations from the smallest particle of matter taken from the original animal, should produce the same disease in a susceptible animal."

Two scientific investigators with a normal gastric mucosa ingested pure cultures of *H. pylori* but additional pharmacological inhibition of acid production was needed to produce acute symptoms and inflammation. Antibiotic treatment normalized the mucosa in one [26] but persistence of the infection resulted in chronic gastritis in the other [10]. The same sequence from a normal mucosa to acute and later chronic gastritis was observed in a patient participating in an endoscopic and secretory study of aspirin adaptation [28].

Experimental infection of germ-free pigs resulted in chronic gastritis (35 of 47 experimental models). Naturally occurring *Helicobacter pylori* in monkeys is associated with gastritis [29].

**Fourth postulate**

"The germs should be found in the diseased areas so produced in the animal."

In the human and animal inoculations resulting in gastritis, culture of gastric biopsies confirmed the presence of *H. pylori* [10, 26, 30-35].

Extended postulates of causality have been proposed [1] such as plausibility, time-order, specificity, and dose-response relationship (Table I). A causal relationship is plausible, as *H. pylori* alters mucosal defence mechanisms [39] and as eradication of *H. pylori* is associated with clearance of gastritis. The time-order relationship (colonization preceding gastritis), the specificity and the dose-response relationship (quantitative relation between inflammation and gastritis) are suggestive but provide insufficient support at the present time.

Having fulfilled Koch's four postulates [36], *H. pylori* hit the stage of the "Infectious Disease Theatre" to play the role of the causative agent of gastritis.


## Diagnosis of gastritis

**Histological diagnosis**

A new classification of gastritis — the so-called "Sydney System" — was proposed at the last World Congress of Gastroenterology (1990) [37]. Its advantage is the attempt to correlate more strictly the histological and endoscopic features, stimulating a direct collaboration between the endoscopist and the pathologist.

Both must take into account the topographical distribution of abnormalities located to the antrum alone, to the corpus alone, or to the whole gastric mucosa (pangastritis).

With regard to *H. pylori* gastritis, the "Sydney System" adds grading of morphological appearances and density of *H. pylori* mucosal colonization. The main morphological changes of inflammation, atrophy, "activity" (density of neutrophil polymorphs), metaplasia, and density of *H. pylori*, are graded into four grades: none; mild; moderate; severe. Other variables, such as cell mucin content, epithelial degeneration, foveolar hyperplasia, oedema, fibrosis or vascularity are documented, but not graded. The key elements of this histological division are deriving from the classification of Whitehead [38], which is purely morphological, gives no statement about aetiology, and was largely used in previous studies devoted to the *H. pylori* gastritis.

A correct histo-endoscopic approach is mandatory [37]:
— a minimum of two biopsies for histology (preferably one from the anterior and one from the posterior wall) have to be taken from both the antrum and the corpus (antral biopsies 2 cm proximal to the pylorus). The 7 French gauge biopsy forceps should be used in preference to the other types;
— any specific lesions are biopsied separately;
— biopsies for culture (n = 2) are sampled in the antrum, and ideally also in the body.

**Endoscopic diagnosis**

*H. pylori* might be a tool for a renewed analysis of the macroscopic aspects of chronic gastritis. At the present time, the low sensitivity of endoscopy in the diagnosis of gastritis reflects the imprecision of the description using a mixture of variations of colour and surface. Some abnormalities might better predict *H. pylori* gastritis than others: in our experience, nodules are more often associated with *H. pylori*. This may be an extension of the specificity of lymphoid follicles as predictors of *H. pylori* [39] manifested in children as micronodules.

Antral nodularity is a peculiar endoscopic picture reported in children. Although one third of infected children have a normal appearing stomach at endoscopy, in about half to two thirds of them nodularity of the antral mucosa is found [40-43]. Nodules have various diameters so that the mucosa may appear pseudopolypoid or micronodular, but this endoscopic picture is quite specific for *H. pylori* infection, the micro-organism being found in up to 90% of cases of nodular antritis. Histological examination in nodular antritis reveals a high degree of inflammatory cell infiltration consisting mainly of mononuclear cells, neutrophils and eosinophils and an increased number of lymphoid follicles, closely resembling benign lymphoid hyperplasia, which is frequently seen in small and large bowel mucosa of children. In the paediatric age, gastritis is usually more severe when the antral mucosa is colonized by *H. pylori* [36, 44]. This is a superficial chronic gastritis (SCG) without mucosal atrophy. In about one third of patients, SCG is active (defined as the presence of polymorphonuclear cell infiltration), which seems to be an early stage of the disease. Indeed analysing the relationship between histological findings and clinical manifestations, a significantly shorter duration of symptoms was found in children with active SCG [45].

This suggests that SCG, starting as an active process, progresses over time to quiescent SCG.

**Helicobacter pylori and non-ulcer dyspepsia**

Recently an international working group has defined non-ulcer dyspepsia (NUD) [46] as "upper or retrosternal pain, discomfort, heartburn, nausea, vomiting, or other symptoms considered to be referable to the proximal alimentary tract, lasting for more than 4 weeks, unrelated to exercise, and for which no focal lesion or systemic disease can be found responsible".

Such a definition raises two problems:

1. It may cover a wide range of pathology; in a study of Talley and Piper [47], the main diagnoses found in a series of 327 patients were irritable bowel syndrome, gastro-oesophageal reflux, aerophagy and gallstones.

The term "essential dyspepsia" was suggested for the undiagnosed group, and one can presume that as more information comes to light with an expanding number of tests the importance of this group is likely to diminish.

2. It excludes patients bearing macroscopic lesions, i.e. those with endoscopic features due to *H. pylori* gastritis.

Two questions can be asked about the possible link between *H. pylori* and NUD:

1. Are there specific symptoms, or a symptom profile, that typify NUD in patients with *H. Pylori* gastritis?

2. Does eradication of *H. pylori* lead to a significant resolution of, or reduction in the dyspeptic symptoms?

## Symptomatic profiles in patients with *Helicobacter pylori* gastritis

The ingestion studies of Marshall [26] and Morris [10] have shown that *H. pylori* acute gastritis is accompanied by symptoms that are more severe than expected from a review of published reports. Marshall [26] experienced epigastric fullness, hunger, headache, halitosis and one episode of vomiting. In Morris's case the symptoms were worse [10]: the epigastric pain came in waves, he could not sleep and walked the floor for hours attempting to get relief. The vomitus contained fluid and food ingested up to 8 hours before, and an intestinal obstruction was suspected.

In childhood, *H. pylori* infection occurs mainly in children 8-16 years old, but has been found in children as young as 2 years [48].

The younger the patients, the more severe are the symptoms; this suggests that with increasing age, a sort of clinical tolerance to *H. pylori* gastritis develops.

Recurrent abdominal pain has been the main presenting feature in children with *H. pylori* on gastric endoscopic biopsies [49]. The pain is usually epigastric and suggestive of peptic ulcer disease, but can also be peri-umbilical [42] and is frequently associated with recurrent vomiting, headache and more exceptionally with lethargy [50].

Chronic diarrhoea with malnutrition [51] and protein losing enteropathy [52] have been attributed to acute *H. pylori* gastritis, but further data will be needed to confirm the relationship between these symptoms and the presence of *H. pylori*.

In adults, there are a few endoscopic reports suggesting some association between chronic *H. pylori* infection and "dyspepsia" using a broad definition, but these do not answer more specific questions about NUD, nor define clearly a symptom profile. Rokkas *et al.* [53] studied 55 patients with dyspepsia of at least 6 months duration, excluding those who where taking NSAIDs; 15 normal controls were also studied. Postprandial bloating was the only symptom significantly associated with the presence of *H. pylori*. Moreover, the frequency of *H. pylori* in the NUD group was significantly greater than in the control group (45.5% vs 13.3%). Andersen *et al.* [54] showed a significant difference in only two symptoms between *H. pylori* positive and negative groups in 33 patients with NUD. Conversely Borsch *et al.* [55], in a study of 149 consecutive patients undergoing upper G.I. endoscopy, found no significant differences in symptoms between those with or without *H. pylori*. There were, in this study, differences in the use of ulcer healing drugs, smoking habits, and antibiotic treatment between the two groups.

Perhaps, for methodological reasons, no clear profile emerges from these studies, and up to now they strongly suggest that, except in human ingestion studies and in young children, *H. pylori* does not cause specific symptoms.

**Therapeutic studies**

The therapeutic studies have also been disappointing in not providing a clear-cut symptomatic response to eradication of *H. pylori* and healing of gastritis. McNulty *et al.* [56], in a series of 50 patients evaluated after being randomized to receive bismuth salicylate, observed a greater, but not significant, symptomatic improvement in the group of patients cleared of *H. pylori*.

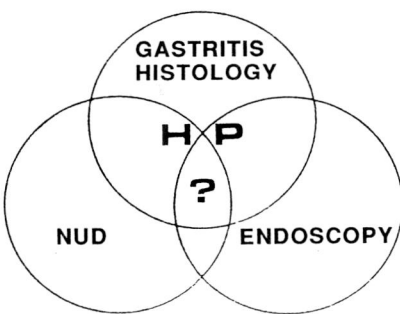

**Figure 2.** *Helicobacter pylori* gastritis.

Rokkas *et al.* [57, 58] reported a significantly better symptomatic response to bismuth compared with placebo in a double-blind study of 40 patients with NUD, but gave no details about *H. pylori* clearance. A better methodological approach has been provided by the study of Glupczinski *et al.* [59]: in 45 patients with NUD and *H. pylori*, randomized treatment with amoxycillin suspension (1 g twice daily for 8 days) *versus* placebo resulted in clearance of *H. pylori* in 91% of the patients in the treated group and resolution of active antral gastritis in 68%; in the cleared group, the improvement in the overall symptom score was higher, but not statistically significant, when compared to the placebo group.

The difficulty in linking *H. pylori* and NUD in therapeutic studies is mostly due to lack of correct diagnostic criteria for NUD and poor attention to the comparability of the control group. A clear-cut response to efficient, eradicating therapeutic agents against *H. pylori* would certainly contribute to demonstrating a significant effect on NUD symptoms, provided that a more reliable scoring system is used for their evaluation. Nevertheless, such studies will remain difficult even with an increased number of patients. A large number of people carry *H. pylori* without dyspepsia, while around 50% of patients with dyspeptic symptoms have no *H. pylori*.

We can conclude (Fig. 2) that, for these reasons, there is presently no place for systematic treatment of *H. pylori* associated with NUD, except within the limits of clinical trials. It is open to the individual clinician to treat, on the basis of his personal experience, any patient whose symptoms of NUD associated with *H. pylori* gastritis are quite evident, as they may be in paediatric practice, and this may justify a double or triple therapy regimen.

## References

1. Spilker B. Concept of cause and effect. In: Spilker B, ed. *Guide to Clinical Interpretation of Data*. New York: Raven Press, 1986:19-26.
2. Wormsley KG. *Campylobacter pylori* and ulcer disease — A causal connection? Scand J Gastroenterol 1989;24(suppl 160):53-8.
3. Dooley CP, Cohen H, Fitzgibbons PL, Bauer M, Appleman MD, Perez-Perez GI, Blaser MH. Prevalence of *Helicobacter pylori* infection and histologic gastritis in asymptomatic persons. N Engl J Med 1989;321:1562-6.
4. Johnston BJ, Reed PI, Ali MH. Prevalence of *Campylobacter pylori* in duodenal and gastric mucosa — Relationship to inflammation. Scand J Gastroenterol 1988;23(suppl 142):69-75.
5. Musgrove C, Bolton FJ, Krypczyk AM, Temperley JM, Cairns SA, Owen WG, Hutchinson DN. *Campylobacter pylori*: clinical, histological and serological studies. J Clin Pathol 1988;41:1316-21.
6. Queiroz DM, Barbosa AJ, Mendes EN, Rocha GA, Cisalpino EO, Lima GF, Oliveira CA. Distribution of *Campylobacter pylori* and gastritis in the stomach of patients with and without duodenal ulcer. Am J Gastroenterol 1988;83:1368-70.
7. Kang JY, Tay HH, Wee A, Guan R, Math MV, Yap I. Effect of colloidal bismuth subcitrate on symptoms and gastric histology in non-ulcer dyspepsia. A double-blind placebo-controlled study. Gut 1990;31:476-80.
8. Marcheggiano A, Iannoni C, Agnello M, Paoluzi P, Pallone F. *Campylobacter*-like organisms in the human gastric mucosa. Relation to type and extent of gastritis in different clinical groups. Gastroenterol Clin Biol 1987;11:376-81.
9. Morvan J, Teyssou R, Botton A, Vialette G, Megraud F. *Campylobacter pylori* et gastrites: résultats à propos de 95 biopsies gastriques. Med Mal Infect 1987;17:543-8.
10. Morris A, Nicholson G. Ingestion of *Campylobacter pyloridis* causes gastritis and raised fasting gastric pH. Am J Gastroenterol 1987;82:192-9.
11. Hazell SL, Hennessy WB, Borody TH, Carrick J, Ralston M, Brady L, Lee A. *Campylobacter pyloridis* gastritis II: distribution of bacteria and associated inflammation in the gastroduodenal environment. Am J Gastroenterol 1987;82:297-301.
12. Bode G, Malfertheiner P, Ditschuneit H. Pathogenetic implications of ultrastructural findings in *Campylobacter pylori* related gastroduodenal disease. Scand J Gastroenterol 1988;23(suppl 142):25-39.
13. Paull G, Yardley JH. Gastric and oesophageal *Campylobacter pylori* in patients with Barrett's esophagus. Gastroenterology 1988; 95:216-8.
14. Carrick J, Lee A, Hazell S, Ralston M, Daskalopoulos G. *Campylobacter pylori*, duodenal ulcer and gastric metaplasia: possible role of functional heterotopic tissue in ulcerogenesis. Gut 1989;30:790-7.
15. Wyatt JI, Rathbone BJ, Dixon MF, Heatley RV. *Campylobacter pyloridis* and acid induced gastric metaplasia in the pathogenesis of duodenitis. J Clin Pathol 1987;40:841-8.
16. Hessey SJ, Spencer J, Wyatt JI, Sobala G, Rathbone BJ, Axon AT, Dixon MF. Bacterial adhesion and disease activity in *Helicobacter* associated chronic gastritis. Gut 1990;31:134-8.

17. Andersen LP, Holck S, Povlsen CO, Elsborg L, Justesen T. *Campylobacter pyloridis* in peptic ulcer disease. I. Gastric and duodenal infection caused by *C. pyloridis*: histopathologic and microbiologic findings. Scand J Gastroenterol 1987;22:219-24.
18. Wyatt JI, Rathbone BJ. Immune response of the gastric mucosa to *Campylobacter pylori*. Scand J Gastroenterol 1988;23(suppl 142):44-9.
19. Fox JG, Correa P, Taylor NS, Zavala D, Fontham E, Janney F, Rodriguez E, Hunter F, Diavolitsis S. *Campylobacter pylori*-associated gastritis and immune response in a population at increased risk of gastric carcinoma. Am J Gastroenterol 1989;84:775-81.
20. Haot J, Hamichi L, Wallez L, Mainguet P. Lymphocytic gastritis: a newly described entity: a retrospective endoscopic and histological study. Gut 1988;29:1258-64.
21. Haot J, Jouret A, Willette M, Gossuin A, Mainguet P. Lymphocytic gastritis — prospective study of its relationship with varioliform gastritis. Gut 1990;31:282-5.
22. Wallez L, Weynand B, Haot J. Evaluation histologique de la présence d'organismes de type *Campylobacter* dans les gastrites lymphocytaires. Acta Endosc 1987;17:283-92.
23. Fléjou JF, Price AB, Smith AC. A natural history of *Campylobacter pylori* in the stomach: a follow-up biopsy study. Gastroenterol Int 1988;1(suppl 1)1085A.
24. Bizzozero G. Uber die schlauchformigen drusen des magendarmkanals und die beziehungen ihres epithels zu dem oberflachenepithel der schleihaut. Arch Mikrobiol Anat 1893;42: 82-152.
25. Marshall BJ. Unidentified curved bacilli on gastric epithelium in active chronic gastritis. Lancet 1983; 1:1273-5.
26. Marshall BJ, Armstrong JA, McGechie DB, Glancy RJ. Attempt to fulfill Koch's postulates for pyloric *Campylobacter* Med J Aust 1985;142:436-9.
27. Goodwin CS, Armstrong JA, Chilvers T, Peters M, Collins MD, Sly L, Mc Connell W, Harper WES. Transfer of *Campylobacter pylori* and *Campylobacter mustelae* to *Helicobacter* new-genus as *Helicobacter pylori* and *Helicobacter mustelae* new combination respectively. Int J Syst Bacteriol 1989;39:397-405.
28. Graham DY, Alpert LC, Smith JL Yoshimura HH. Iatrogenic *Campylobacter pylori* infection is a cause of epidemic achlorhydria. Am J Gastroenterol 1988; 83;974-80.
29. Baskervile A, Newell DG. Naturally occurring chronic gastritis and *C. pylori* infection in the rhesus monkey: a potential model for gastritis in man. Gut 1988;29:465-72.
30. Marshall BJ, Warren JR, Francis GJ, Langton SR, Goodwin CS, Blinow ED. Rapid urease test in the management of *Campylobacter pyloridis*-associated gastritis. Am J Gastroenterol 1987;82:200-10.
31. Marshall BJ. Etude *in vivo* de *Campylobacter pylori* — Modèles expérimentaux. Gastroenterol Clin Biol 1989; 13:50B-2B.
32. Marshall BJ, Goodwin CS, Warren JR, Murray R, Blincow ED, Blackbourn SJ, Phillips M, Waters TE, Sanderson CR. Prospective double-blind trial of duodenal ulcer relapse after eradication of *Campylobacter pylori*. Lancet 1988;2:1439-42.
33. McNulty CA, Dent JC, Uff JS, Gear MW, Wilkinson SP. Detection of *Campylobacter pylori* by the biopsy urease test: an assessment in 1445 patients. Gut 1989;30:1058-62.
34. Miller NM, Naran A, Simjee AE, Spitaels JM, Pettengell KE, Van Den Ende J, Manion G. Incidence of *Campylobacter pylori* in patients with upper gastro-intestinal symptoms. S Afr Med J 1988;74:563-6.
35. Mitchell HM, Lee A, Berkowicz J, Borody T. The use of serology to diagnose active *Campylobacter pylori* infection. Med J Aust 1988;149:604-9.
36. Oderda G, Vaira D, Dell'Olio D, Holton J, Forni M, Altare F, Ansaldi N. Serum pepsinogen I and gastrin concentrations in children positive for *Helicobacter pylori*. J Clin Pathol 1990;43:762-5.
37. Misiewicz JJ, Tytgat GNJ, Goodwin CS, Price AB, Sipponen P, Strickland RG, Cheli R. The Sydney System: a new classification of gastritis. Proceedings of the 9th World Congress of Gastroenterology — Sydney — Australia, 1990;1-10.
38. Whitehead R, Truelobe SC, Gear MW. The histological diagnosis of chronic gastritis in fibreoptic gastroscope biopsy specimens. J Clin Pathol 1972;25:1-11.

39. Droy-Lefaix MT. Mécanismes de défense de l'estomac et *Campylobacter pylori*. Gastroenterol Clin Biol 1989; 13:13B-7B.
40. Bujanover Y, Konikoff F, Baratz M. Nodular gastritis and *Helicobacter pylori*. J Pediatr Gastroenterol Nutr 1990;11:41-4.
41. Cadranel S, Goosens H, De Boeck M, Malengreau A, Rodesch P, Butzler JP. *Campylobacter pyloridis* in children. Lancet 1986;1:735-6.
42. Czinn SJ, Dahms BB, Jacobs GH, Kaplan B, Rothstein FC. *Campylobacter*-like organisms in association with symptomatic gastritis in children. J Pediatr 1986; 109:80-3.
43. Oderda G, Lerro P, Poli E, Tavassoli K, Ansaldi N. Childhood nodular gastritis and *Campylobacter pylori*. Endoscopy 1988;20(suppl II):86.
44. Kilbridge PM, Dahms BB, Czinn SJ. *Campylobacter pylori*-associated gastritis and peptic ulcer disease in children. Am J Dis Child 1988; 142:1149-52.
45. Oderda G, Forni M, Poli E *et al*. *Helicobacter pylori* gastritis in children: wide spectrum of symptoms.Eur J Gastroenterol Hepatol 1990;2(suppl):S75.
46. Colin-Jones DG, Bloom B, Bodemar G, Crean G, Freston J, Gugler R, Malagelada JR, Nyrén O, Petersen H, Piper D. Management of dyspepsia: report of a working party. Lancet 1988;1:576-9.
47. Talley NJ, Piper DW. The association between non-ulcer dyspepsia and other gastrointestinal disorders Scand J Gastroenterol 1985;20:896-900.
48. Cadranel S, Glupczynski Y, Labbé M, Deprez C. *Campylobacter pylori* in children. In: Meuge H, Gregor M, Tytgat GNT, Marshall BJ, eds. *Campylobacter pylori*. Berlin Heidelberg: Springer Verlag 1988:110-5.
49. Drumm B, Sherman P, Cutz E, Karmali M. Association of *Campylobacter pylori* on the gastric mucosa with antral gastritis in children. N Engl J Med 1987;316:1557-61.
50. Mahony MJ, Littlewood JM. *Campylobacter pylori* in pediatric. In: *Campylobacter pylori and Gastroduodenal Disease Populations*. Oxford: Blackwel Scientific publications, 1989:167-75.
51. Sullivan PB, Thomas JE, Wight DG, Neale G, Eastham EJ, Corrah T, Lloyd-Evans N, Greenwood BM. *Helicobacter pylori* in Gambian children with chronic diarrhoea and malnutrition. Arch Dis Child 1990;65:189-91.
52. Hill ID, Sinclair-Smith C, Lastovica AJ, Bowie MD, Emms M. Transient protein losing enteropathy associated with acute gastritis and *Campylobacter pylori*. Arch Dis Child 1987;62:1215-9.
53. Rokkas T, Pursey C, Uzoechina E, Dorrington L, Simmons NA, Filipe MI, Sladen GE. *Campylobacter pylori* and non-ulcer dyspepsia. Am J Gastroenterol 1987;82:1149-52.
54. Andersen LP, Elsborg L, Justesen T. *Campylobacter pylori* in peptic ulcer disease. III. Symptoms and paraclinical and epidemiologic findings. Scand J Gastroenterol 1988;23: 347-50.
55. Borsch G, Wegener M, Schmidt G, Sandmann M, Adamek R, Reitemeyer E. Prospective analysis of clinical and histologic factors associated with *Campylobacter pylori* colonization. Gastroenterology 1988; 94:A44(abstr).
56. McNulty CA, Gearty JC, Crump B, Davis M, Donovan IA, Melikian V. *Campylobacter pyloridis* and associated gastritis: investigator blind, placebo-controlled trial of bismuth salicylate and erythromycin ethylsuccinate. Br Med J 1986;293:645-9.
57. Rokkas T, Pursey C, Simmons NA, Filipe MI, Sladen GE. Non-ulcer dyspepsia and colloidal bismuth subcitrate therapy: the role of *Campylobacter pyloridis*. Gastroenterology 1987; 92:1599(abstr).
58. Rokkas T, Sladen GE. Bismuth: effects on gastritis and peptic ulcer. Scand J Gastroenterol 1988;23(suppl 142):82-6.
59. Glupczynski Y, Burette A, Labbé M, Deprez C, Dereuck M, Deltenre M. *Campylobacter pylori*-associated gastritis: a double-blind placebo-controlled trial with amoxycillin. Am J Gastroenterol 1988;83:365-72.

# 16

# Food allergy and the immune intestinal barrier: facts, doubts and fancy

J.-F. COLOMBEL(*), B. MESNARD(*), P. DESREUMAUX(**)

(*) Clinique des Maladies de l'Appareil Digestif, Hôpital Claude Huriez, 59037 Lille Cedex, France
(**) Unité Mixte INSERM U.167 — CNRS 624, Institut Pasteur de Lille, France

## Introduction

Food is the largest antigenic/allergenic challenge confronting the human body. An important adaptation of the gastrointestinal tract to this environment is the development of specific mechanisms to exclude luminal antigens from crossing the epithelial barrier and to control the systemic immune response to these foreign antigens [1, 2]. Disruption of this complex tolerance/reactiveness process could result in what is called food allergy, which is synonymous with food hypersensitivity (FHS) [3, 4]. The clinical definition of FHS must fulfil two criteria: the demonstration of a reproducible intolerance to food and evidence of an immunological reaction to food [5]. The subject of food allergy has suffered from contradictory information derived from clinical studies with methodological flaws. However, it has been clearly demonstrated that some adverse reactions to food are the result of immunological mechanisms. This chapter concentrates on recent experimental data in animals which have allowed a better understanding of the pathophysiology of FHS, but which have also highlighted the gap that remains between theory and fact in food allergy. The clinical relevance of food allergy in adults is further discussed.

*J.-F. Colombel, B. Mesnard, P. Desreumaux*

## Pathophysiology of food hypersensitivity reactions

### The theoretical model

The large surface area of the gastrointestinal tract, which represents a major interface between the external environment and internal milieu, is protected by a number of mechanisms. Non-immunological processes work in concert with the local mucosal immune system to constitute an effective barrier (the mucosal barrier) to the attachment and penetration of antigens. The secretory immunoglobulin (Ig) system is the best defined effector mechanism of mucosal immunity [1, 2]. Immunoglobulin A is well-known to be the predominant Ig of external secretions where it occurs predominantly (90%) in polymeric form linked to an epithelial cell glycoprotein, the secretory component. In adults more than 3g of IgA per day are selectively transported into the intestinal juice where they act as a first line defence [6]. In addition, the abundance of locally produced IgA antibodies is probably crucial for immunological homeostasis within the lamina propria. Immunoglobulin A may block the triggering of non-specific biological amplification mechanisms because it should lack potent effector functions such as classical complement activation [1].

When secretory antibodies are unable to perform adequate antigen exclusion, the internal body environment should preferably be protected against potentially harmful systemic types of immune reactions elicited by IgG, IgE or T-cell-mediated delayed-type hypersensitivity [1]. This phenomenon of decreased systemic immune responsiveness to orally administered antigens is called "oral tolerance" [7]. The mechanisms for oral tolerance are probably multiple, but antigen handling by an intact epithelium seems to be a critical induction event [8] and a predominant role of suppressor type intra-epithelial T8 cells is suspected [1]. In summary, immune mechanisms act, under normal conditions, in a coordinated fashion to ensure the proper handling and subsequent immune response to antigens (Fig. 1.A).

Food hypersensitivity might develop as a result of disruption of this complex tolerance/reactiveness process (Fig. 1.B) [4]. Initiation of hypersensitivity may occur as a result of increased intestinal permeability, IgA deficiency or interruption of oral tolerance. All these situations favour general stimulation of TH cells [1, 7]. T-cell activation can lead to increased production of IgA but also to excessive IgG and IgE response. Antibody-antigen binding is an important initiating event in FHS and is expressed as (1) binding of antigen to cell-surface-bound antibody (such as mast cell-bound IgE) with release of mediators; (2) formation of immune complexes that can initiate activation of inflammatory cells including mastocytes, eosinophils and neutrophils and also activate the complement system. In addition, antigen binding to specific receptors on T-cells can initiate activation, resulting in direct T-cell cytotoxicity as well as T-cell-mediated recruitment and activation of other cells via lymphokines. Finally, lymphocyte sensitization to food antigen could lead to T-cell-mediated delayed hypersensitivity reactions with chronic inflammation. Thus, in theory, pathological reactions to food antigens resulting from immune mechanisms can be divided into the four categories indicated in Table I [4, 9, 10].

### Experimental data in animals and humans

There is well-established evidence supporting a role for type I (IgE-mediated) reactions in some patients with food allergy. However, changes in intestinal function and

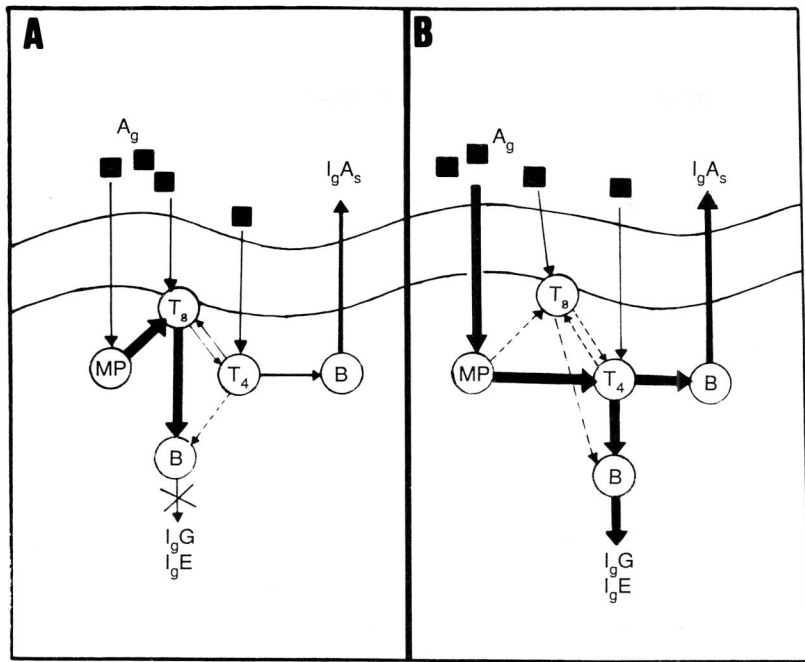

**Figure 1.** Hypothetical scheme for food hypersensitivity initiation. (Adapted from ref. [1]).
**A:** In normal conditions, presentation to T8 suppressor cells of antigen that has been processed by specialized mucosal macrophage or dendritic cell and/or by epithelial cell results in dominating signals of suppression. IgA synthesizing B cells receive help from T4 cells leading to secretory IgA secretion whereas no help is provided by T4 cells to IgG and IgE synthesizing B cells.
**B:** Food hypersensitivity initiation could result from an undue stimulation of antigen-presenting cells leading to overstimulation of T4 cells. The result is not only an increased production of IgA but also of IgG and IgE with onset of inflammatory reaction.

**Table I.** Different types of hypersensitivity [10].

| Reaction | Type | Mechanism |
| --- | --- | --- |
| Immediate hypersensitivity | I | Release of mediators from IgE sensitized mast cells |
| Antibody-mediated cytotoxicity | II | Cell injury caused by antibodies directed against cell surface Ag |
| Immune complex disorders | III | Cell damage from deposition of Ag-Ab complexes |
| Cell-mediated disorders | IV | T lymphocytes interact with Ag and release lymphokines |

Ag: antigen; Ab: antibody.

structure induced by anaphylaxis have mainly been studied in an animal model of rat sensitized to egg albumin [11]. Using an intestinal *in vivo* perfusion method, Perdue *et al.* have shown that intraluminal antigen challenge resulted in abnormalities of water and electrolyte absorption [12]. Epithelial cell damage was suggested by the findings of increased quantities of protein and DNA in the lumen despite the fact that light microscopy demonstrated little distortion of mucosal architecture [13]. Intestinal anaphylaxis also induced disturbances in motility with disruption of the migrating myoelectrical complex and clusters of aborally propagating contractions resulting in decreased transit time [14]. The intestinal response was shown to be specific for the sensitizing antigen and related to serum level of specific IgE-antibody [12]. The rapid onset of these changes and their persistence after the antigen was withdrawn were suggestive of an immediate IgE-mediated hypersensitivity reaction involving mediators released from mast cells [12]. Indeed, after antigen perfusion, histamine in mucosal homogenates and numbers of mast cells in the lamina propria of sensitized rats were increased [12]. Mast cell degranulation could also lead to the release of other preformed and newly formed mediators that have multiple significant biological effects such as 5-hydroxytryptamine, prostaglandins and leukotrienes [4, 9, 15]. Conversely, eosinophil counts and intraepithelial lymphocyte population were unaffected by antigen challenge in sensitized animals.

More recently, the stomach was added to the list of organs whose physiological function can be modulated by IgE-mediated reactions to food [16]. In sensitized animals, perfusion of the stomach with ovalbumin led to a significant increase in gastric acid output compared with perfusion with saline alone. Ovalbumin also produced a significant reduction in gastric emptying in sensitized animals. Gastric perfusion with specific antigen led to mast cell activation: challenge with ovalbumin increased the concentration of histamine in the stomach and histological examination showed significantly fewer granulated mast cells following antigen perfusion in sensitized rats.

Mast cells represent a heterogeneous population and in rodents two types of mast cells, termed connective tissue and mucosal, have been defined on differing morphological, compositional, functional and pharmacological properties [17, 18]. Recent work supports a selective role for mucosal mast cells during IgE-mediated mucosal reactions: gastric or jejunal perfusion with antigen caused a dramatic increase in serum (and intestinal perfusate) levels of rat mast cell protease which is specific for mucosal mast cells [19]; doxantrazole, an inhibitor of mast cell degranulation, but not sodium cromoglycate, an inhibitor of connective tissue mast cells, prevented mast cell degranulation and the subsequent intestinal dysfunction associated with intraluminal challenge [20].

The effect of chronic dietary antigen challenge on the intestine has also been examined in sensitized rats [21]. Chronic antigen challenge resulted in reduced food intake and weight gain. Nine days after antigen exposure, the proximal intestine showed decreased disaccharidase activity, brush border microvillus surface area and villus height. Here again, mast cells appeared to play a central role in the pathogenesis of the intestinal injury.

In man, the majority of immunologically-mediated adverse reactions to foods are thought to be mediated by classic type I hypersensitivity involving mucosal mast cells and food-specific IgE. Such reactions occur within minutes after the ingestion of a specific food to which a person is hypersensitive [3, 22, 23]. The target organs and characteristic reactions include the gastrointestinal tract (nausea, vomiting and diarrhoea), the skin (hives and angio-oedema), the respiratory tract (sneezing, rhinitis and asthma), and the circulatory system (hypotension and ultimately systemic anaphylaxis). The foods most commonly involved in FHS in France are given in Table II [24].

The pathological changes in the gastrointestinal tract associated with immediate type FHS have been poorly characterized in adults. Consequences of antigenic challenge have mainly been evaluated by measurement of intestinal permeability. The results have however been conflicting, depending on various probes and various clinical assessments of food allergy. André et al. [25, 26], using a solution of mannitol and lactulose, found normal absorption in basal conditions and an increase in lactulose absorption after food challenge. Intestinal permeation of polyethyleneglycol (MW 400, 600, 1000) and $^{51}$Cr-EDTA has been shown to be increased or normal in food-intolerant patients [27, 28]. Gastric mucosal reactions in FHS were more accurately studied in 30 patients with food allergy when allergens were applied to the gastric mucosa via an endoscope [29]. Immediate macroscopic changes ranged from erythema and swelling to frank bleeding. During the 24 h after provocation, all patients complained of symptoms and presented physical signs.

The participation of the mast cells in mucosal reactions to food is supported by a number of studies. During gastric challenge with antigen a significant decrease in tissue histamine concentrations and mast cell counts took place in association with the appearance of mucosal lesions [29]. Degranulation of *in vitro* passively sensitized mast cells in human jejunal mucosal biopsies upon exposure to the corresponding antigen has also been described [30]. Mast cells mostly degranulate in an IgE-dependent reaction. Increased numbers of mucosal IgE-containing cells have been reported in patients with food allergy and could be of diagnostic interest [31]. The interaction of food proteins with IgG or IgM leading to complement deposition in gastrointestinal tissues has also been postulated as a mean of triggering mast cell degranulation in the gut [9]. Finally, our understanding of mast cell heterogeneity in humans is also less clear than in rodents, though recent evidence indicates that distinct subtypes exist in humans as well [32, 33].

**Table II.** Most frequent food allergens encountered in France [24].

— *cow's milk*
— *fish*
— *shellfish:* shrimp, crab, crayfish, lobster
— *eggs:* egg white
— vegetables and umbellifers: *peanuts,* soya bean, garden peas, *celery,* tomatoes, beans, carrots...
— grains: corn, barley, rye
— meat: *pork,* chicken, horse
— fruits: *apple,* kiwi, banana, mango, orange, *peach,* strawberry, nuts, hazel nuts
— miscellaneous: mussel, radish, cabbage, mustard, onions, garlic

## What remains doubtful?

While a definite role for IgE-mediated hypersensitivity in food allergy is well documented, many aspects of the theoretical scheme proposed in part 1 remain unassessed.

First of all the mechanisms of initiation of food hypersensitivity are mostly unknown. It has been suggested that the pathological immune response in food-allergic subjects is caused by increased intestinal permeability [4]. The current hypothesis is that subjects develop food sensitivity when gastrointestinal permeation to intact food antigens leads to systemic absorption (macromolecular absorption) and immunization. In food-allergic patients an increased intestinal permeability has indeed been reported when lactulose/mannitol were administered as inert probes [25, 26]. But a recent study demonstrates that changes in intestinal permeability to sugars and large proteins are not correlated in any simple fashion in the rat [34]. Two recent studies have also cast doubt on this hypothesis. First, it was shown that transport of horseradish peroxidase (HRP, used as a protein marker) was only altered in biopsies of children with cow's milk allergy when infants were ingesting milk [35]. Once appropriate milk exclusion was implemented, HRP uptake was not different from that in normal controls, suggesting that increased permeability is a transient phenomenon and probably the result of gut inflammation. In a second study, ovalbumin was used as a marker of gut permeability and no evidence of increased ovalbumin uptake could be demonstrated in allergic patients compared with non-allergic patients [36].

Induction of hypersensitivity could also occur by a failure of another part of the normal immune response. A transient relative IgA deficiency may be important in initial sensitization in infants but this mechanism is unlikely in adults [4]. On the other hand, a defect in suppressor T-cell function, which might prevent induction of tolerance, has also been hypothesized in FHS [37]. However, the relevance of such a phenomenon in FHS remains to be proven.

Apart from anaphylactic reactions, involvement of other types of hypersensitivity in the pathogenesis of food allergy is doubtful. To date, there is no convincing evidence that type II reactions participate in food allergy. Type III reactions have been implicated in FHS, although most of the evidence is indirect. Immune complexes have been found in the circulation of normal and food-allergic patients, although the nature of the complex may differ in the two groups [38]. Immune complex deposition with evidence of complement activation has only been demonstrated in the small bowel of children with cow's milk allergy [10]. Along the same line, evidence for type IV cell-mediated hypersensitivity with activation of lymphocytes and lymphokine production has mostly been confined to this kind of infantile disease [10]. Finally there is accumulating evidence that food hypersensitivity is much more complex than was thought in the classic formulation of Gell and Coombs. In this regard, it has recently been demonstrated that mononuclear cells from patients with food allergy spontaneously produced a histamine-releasing factor capable of interacting with the IgE bound to the surface of basophils of other food-sensitive persons to provoke the release of histamine [39].

Most of the studies in food allergy have emphasized the role of mastcells. Conversely, little is known about the structure and function of intestinal eosinophils [40]. Eosinophils were once thought to be involved only in modulating hypersensitivity, but recent evidence suggests that they play a more active role in these responses [4]. Eosinophils are capable of causing tissue damage by the secretion of toxic mediators. If some features of gastrointestinal hypersensitivity are analogous to asthma, the most important factor released by eosinophils is perhaps major basic protein (MBP). A valuable model for evaluating the toxic potential of eosinophils could be allergic eosinophilic gastroenteritis (EG). Ultrastructural evidence for a selective release of MBP associated with ulcerated duodenal areas has been recently demonstrated in a patient with EG [41]. However it must be kept in mind that EG is a very uncommon disease and that in a recent study of 40 patients with EG, a past history of allergy was only reported in 50% [42].

## Food hypersensitivity reactions: clinical importance in adults

Some doctors and many members of the public have become convinced that adverse reactions to food are extremely frequent. It has been suggested that FHS is a common cause in adults of headache, insomnia, tinnitus, palpitations, breathlessness, ankle swelling, fatigue and various abdominal symptoms [43]. However, estimates of the prevalence of adverse food reactions are highly variable. No satisfactory epidemiological studies have been conducted in individuals of more than 6 years of age [44, 45]. Given an 8% prevalence of adverse reactions to food in children [44, 45] and the hypothesis that food hypersensitivity is often temporary [46], it is likely that food allergy is not so common in adults.

Nevertheless it is not surprising that several studies have tried to assign a role for food allergy in irritable bowel syndrome (IBS) [47-51]. Interest in this has recently been renewed by a study showing that dietary manipulations were effective in about half of patients with IBS, with prolonged symptomatic benefit [52]. In most of the studies, results of initial open exclusion diets with open food rechallenge were encouraging, being positive in 30-60% [47-49]. Objective evidence for food hypersensitivity, i.e. positive response to the double-blind placebo-controlled oral food challenge (DBPCFC), was however lacking [51, 52] or present in only few patients (20-30%) [48, 50]. Furthermore, the interpretation of the DBPCFC test was somewhat arbitrary in the absence of a clear correlation between IBS symptoms and test-induced manifestations [47, 49]. Finally the possibility of a bias because of patient selection was evident in some studies [49]. In general, the major concern when evaluating the role of FHS in digestive symptoms is the absence of a simple and reliable test for establishing the diagnosis. The DBPCFC has proved to be the "gold standard" [53], but it is time-consuming and the report of a high rate of symptomatic responses to placebo in adults is worrying [43]. Nonetheless, the importance of using appropriate diagnostic measures to evaluate FHS cannot be overemphasized. The paper from Pearson et al. [54] showing evidence of psychiatric disease in 18/23 patients referred to an allergy clinic for the assessment of probable food intolerance, claims that an objective evaluation is mandatory in FHS. Along the same line, recent reports have underlined the fact that incorrect diagnosis and treatment may delay diagnosis and treatment of serious organic disease [55, 56].

## Conclusion

Food hypersensitivity is perhaps a significant underdiagnosed condition. The issue has however been greatly blurred by extravagant claims based on tests lacking scientific validity, which have only served to arouse scepticism [57, 58]. Our understanding of the basic immunological mechanisms responsible for hypersensitivity reactions remains limited. The rigorous approach now being taken by several investigators in this field [59] provides hope that new information on immunopathogenic mechanisms, clinical relevance and better forms of therapy will become available. A desirable initial thrust could be a better analysis of *in situ* reactions provoked by food hypersensitivity in the digestive tract. Careful studies in well-characterized patients using endoscopy, histological examination and immunohistochemistry are clearly needed. In this regard, the intestinal perfusion technique, which allows direct antigenic challenge of the jejunal mucosa [60], might be a promising new tool.

**Acknowledgements.** The authors thank M. Capron (Unité Mixte INSERM U. 167-CNRS 624, Institut Pasteur de Lille) for manuscript revision.

## References

1. Brandtzaeg P, Halstensen TS, Kett K, Krajci P, Kvale D, Rognum TO, Scott H, Sollid LM. Immunobiology and immunopathology of human gut mucosa: humoral immunity and intraepithelial lymphocytes. Gastroenterology 1989;97:1562-84.
2. Fiocchi C. Mucosal immunity. Gastroenterology 1989;2:172-9.
3. Metcalfe DD. Diseases of food hypersensitivity. N Engl J Med 1989;321:255-7.
4. Lee TDG, Swieter M, Befus D. Mast cells, eosinophils, and gastrointestinal hypersensitivity. Immunol Allergy Clin North Am 1988;8:468-83.
5. Anderson JA. The establishment of common language concerning adverse reactions to foods and food additives. J Allergy Clin Immunol 1986;78:140-4.
6. Jonard PP, Rambaud JC, Dive C, Vaerman JP, Galian A, Delacroix DL. Secretion of immunoglobulins and plasma proteins from the jejunal mucosa. Transport rate and origin of polymeric immunoglobulin A. J Clin Invest 1984;74:525-35.
7. Mowat AM. The regulation of immune responses to dietary protein antigens. Immunol Today 1987;8:93-8.
8. Nicklin S, Miller K. Local and systemic immune responses to intestinally presented antigen. Int Arch Allergy Appl Immunol 1983;72:87-90.
9. Barrett KE, Metcalfe DD. Immunologic mechanisms in food allergy. In: Chiaramonte LT, Schneider AT, Lifshitz F, eds. *Food Allergy: a Practical Approach to Diagnosis and Management*. New York: M.Dekker, 1988: 23-44.
10. Wershil BK, Walker WA. Milk allergies and other food allergies in children. Immunol Allergy Clin North Am 1988;8:485-504.
11. Byars NE, Ferraresi RW. Intestinal anaphylaxis in the rat as a model of food allergy. Clin Exp Immunol 1976;24:352-6.
12. Perdue MH, Chung M, Gall DG. Effect of intestinal anaphylaxis on gut function in the rat. Gastroenterology 1984;86:391-7.
13. Perdue MH, Forstner JF, Roomi NW, Gall DG. Epithelial response to intestinal anaphylaxis in rats: goblet cell secretion and enterocyte damage. Am J Physiol 1984;247:G632-7.
14. Scott RB, Diamant SC, Gall DG. Motility effects of intestinal anaphylaxis in the rat. Am J Physiol 1988;255:G505-11.
15. Crowe SE, Sestini P, Perdue MH. Allergic reactions of rat jejunal mucosa. Ion transport responses to luminal antigen and inflammatory mediators. Gastroenterology 1990;99:74-82.

16. Catto-Smith AG, Patrick MK, Scott RB, Davison JS, Gall DG. Gastric response to mucosal IgE-mediated reactions. Am J Physiol 1989;257:G704-8.
17. Lee TD, Swieter M, Bienenstock J, Befus AD. Heterogeneity in mast cell populations. Clin Immunol Rev 1985;4:143-99.
18. Elson CO, Kagnoff MF, Fiocchi C, Befus AD, Targan S. Intestinal immunity and inflammation: recent progress. Gastroenterology 1986;91:746-68.
19. Patrick MK, Dunn IJ, Buret A, Miller HR, Huntley JF, Gibson S, Gall DG. Mast cell protease release and mucosal ultrastructure during intestinal anaphylaxis in the rat. Gastroenterology 1988;94:1-9.
20. Perdue MH, Gall DG. Transport abnormalities during intestinal anaphylaxis in the rat: effect of antiallergic agents. J Allergy Clin Immunol 1985;76:498-503.
21. Curtis GH, Patrick MK, Catto-Smith AG, Gall DG. Intestinal anaphylaxis in the rat. Effect of chronic antigen exposure. Gastroenterology 1990;98:1558-66.
22. Schreiber RA, Walker WA. Food allergy: facts and fiction. Mayo Clin Proc 1989;64:1381-91.
23. Sampson HA, Buckley RH, Metcalfe DD. Food allergy. JAMA 1987;258:2886-90.
24. Moneret-Vautrin DA, Grilliat JP. Vraies et fausses allergies alimentaires. Rev Prat 1982;32:1537-8.
25. André C. Allergie alimentaire. Diagnostic objectif et test de l'efficacité thérapeutique par mesure de la perméabilité intestinale. Presse Med 1986;15:105-8.
26. André C, André F, Colin L. Effect of allergen ingestion challenge with and without cromoglycate cover on intestinal permeability in atopic dermatitis, urticaria and other symptoms of food allergy. Allergy 1989;44(suppl 9):47-51.
27. Falth-Magnusson K, Kjellman NI, Odelram H, Sundqvist T, Magnusson KE. Gastrointestinal permeability in children with cow's milk allergy: effect of milk challenge and sodium cromoglycate as assessed with polyethyleneglycols (PEG 400 and PEG1000). Clin Allergy 1986;16:543-51.
28. Scadding G, Bjarnason I, Brostoff J, Levi AJ, Peters TJ. Intestinal permeability to $^{51}$Cr-labelled ethylene diaminetetraacetate in food-intolerant subjects. Digestion 1989;42:104-9.
29. Reimann HJ, Lewin J. Gastric mucosal reactions in patients with food allergy. Am J Gastroenterol 1988;83:1212-9.
30. Selbekk BH, Aas K, Myren J. *In vitro* sensitization and mast cell degranulation in human jejunal mucosa. Scand J Gastroenterol 1978;13:87-92.
31. André C, André F, Descos L, Cavagna S. Diagnosis of food allergy by enumerating IgE containing duodenal cells. Gut 1989;30:A751-2(abstr).
32. Befus D, Goodacre R, Dyck N, Bienenstock J. Mast cell heterogeneity in man.I. Histologic studies of the intestine. Int Arch Allergy Appl Immunol 1985;76:232-6.
33. Strobel S, Busuttil A, Ferguson A. Human intestinal mucosal mast cells: expanded population in untreated coeliac disease. Gut 1983;24:222-7.
34. Turner MW, Boulton P, Shields JG, Strobel S, Gibson S, Miller HR, Levinsky RJ. Intestinal hypersensitivity reactions in the rat.I. Uptake of intact protein, permeability to sugars and their correlation with mucosal mast-cell activation. Immunology 1988;63:119-24.
35. Heyman M, Grasset E, Ducroc R, Desjeux JF. Antigen absorption by the jejunal epithelium of children with cow's milk allergy. Pediatr Res 1988;24:197-202.
36. Powell GK, Mc Donald PJ, Van Sickle GJ, Goldblum RM. Absorption of food protein antigen in infants with food protein-induced enterocolitis. Dig Dis Sci 1989;34:781-8.
37. Bjorksten B. Atopic allergy in relation to cell-mediated immunity. Clin Rev Allergy 1984;2:95-106.
38. Kniker WT. Immunologically mediated reactions to food: state of the art. Ann Allergy 1987;59:60-70.
39. Sampson HA, Broadbent KR, Bemhisel-Broadbent J. Spontaneous release of histamine from basophils and histamine-releasing factor in patients with atopic dermatitis and food hypersensitivity. N Engl J Med 1989;321:228-32.

40. Mathieu-Chandelier C, Torpier G, Colombel JF, Capron M. Eosinophiles et pathologie du tube digestif. Gastroentérol Clin Biol 1991;(in press).
41. Torpier G, Colombel JF, Mathieu-Chandelier C, Capron M, Dessaint JP, Cortot A, Paris JC, Capron A. Eosinophilic gastroenteritis: ultrastructural evidence for a selective release of eosinophil major basic protein. Clin Exp Immunol 1988;74:404-8.
42. Talley NJ, Shorter RG, Phillips SF, Zinsmeister AR. Eosinophilic gastroenteritis: a clinicopathological study of patients with disease of the mucosa, muscle layer, and subserosal tissues. Gut 1990;31:54-8.
43. Sampson HA. Differential diagnosis in adverse reactions to foods. J Allergy Clin Immunol 1986;78:212-9.
44. Kajosaari M. Food allergy in Finnish children aged 1 to 6 years. Acta Paediatr Scand 1982;71:815-9.
45. Bock SA, Lee WY, Remigio LK, May CD. Studies of hypersensitivity reactions to foods in infants and children. J Allergy Clin Immunol 1978;62:327-34.
46. Pastorello EA, Stocchi L, Pravetonni V, Bigi A, Schilke ML, Incorvaia C, Zanussi C. Role of the elimination diet in adults with food allergy. J Allergy Clin Immunol 1989;84:475-83.
47. Jones VA, McLaughlan P, Shorthouse M, Workman E, Hunter JO. Food intolerance: a major factor in the pathogenesis of irritable bowel syndrome. Lancet 1982;2:1115-7.
48. Bentley SJ, Pearson DJ, Rix KJ. Food hypersensitivity in irritable bowel syndrome. Lancet 1983;2:295-7.
49. Petitpierre M, Gumowski P, Girard JP. Irritable bowel syndrome and hypersensitivity to food. Ann Allergy 1985;54:538-40.
50. Farah DA, Calder I, Benson L, MacKenzie JF. Specific food intolerance: its place as a cause of gastrointestinal symptoms. Gut 1985;26:164-8.
51. Zwetchkenbaum JF, Burakoff R. Food allergy and the irritable bowel syndrome. Am J Gastroenterol 1988;83:901-4.
52. Nanda R, James R, Smith H, Dudley CR, Jewell DP. Food intolerance and the irritable bowel syndrome. Gut 1989;30:1099-104.
53. Bock SA, Sampson HA, Atkins FM, Zeiger RS, Lehrer S, Sachs M, Bush RK, Metcalfe DD. Double-blind, placebo-controlled food challenge (DBPCFC) as an office procedure: a manual. J Allergy Clin Immunol 1988;82:986-97.
54. Pearson DJ, Rix KJ, Bentley SJ. Food allergy: how much in the mind? A clinical and psychiatric study of suspected food hypersensitivity. Lancet 1983;1:1259-61.
55. Robertson DA, Ayres RC, Smith CL, Wright R. Adverse consequences arising from misdiagnosis of food allergy. Br Med J 1988;297:719-20.
56. Labib M, Gama R, Wright J, Marks V, Robins D. Dietary maladvice as a cause of hypothyroidism and short stature. Br Med J 1989;298:232-3.
57. Jewett DL, Fein G, Greenberg MH. A double-blind study of symptom provocation to determine food sensitivity. N Engl J Med 1990;323:429-33.
58. Ferguson A. Food sensitivity or self-deception? New Engl J Med 1990;323:476-8.
59. Metcalfe DD, Sampson HA. Workshop on experimental methodology for clinical studies of adverse reactions to foods and food additives. J Allergy Clin Immunol 1990;86(suppl):421-42.
60. Lavo B, Knutson L, Loof L, Odlind B, Venge P, Hallgren R. Challenge with gliadin induces eosinophil and mast cell activation in the jejunum of patients with coeliac disease. Am J Med 1989;87:655-60.

# 17

# Abnormal perception of visceral pain

M. LÉMANN, J.-P. DEDERDING, B. FLOURIÉ, J.-C. RAMBAUD, R. JIAN

*Service de Gastroentérologie et INSERM U.290, Hôpital Saint-Lazare et Hôpital Saint-Louis, 75010 Paris, France.*

The cluster of symptoms referable to the upper gastrointestinal tract and not explained by a specific lesion or disease, known as non-ulcer or chronic idiopathic dyspepsia (CID), is very common in the general population and constitutes a frequent cause for consultation in outpatient care [1]. The only well-established anomalies in CID concern the motility of the upper digestive tract. These anomalies have been found either in gastric emptying studies [2], or by gastrointestinal manometry and electromyography [3, 4]. When these anomalies are present, their relief by prokinetic drugs may result in the improvement of symptoms [5]. However, the extent of gastric motility disorders is not clearly related to the intensity of symptoms [2]. Furthermore, in 30 to 50% of patients with CID, no motor anomalies can be found [2, 3]. These facts suggest that other kinds of disorders might be involved in CID. Several dyspeptic complaints, such as early satiety, or the sensation of epigastric discomfort or bloating after a normal meal, suggest an abnormal perception of gastric filling that might be due to increased visceral sensitivity. A similar abnormal perception of distension has been previously shown in other segments of the digestive tract in patients with dysphagia [6], non-cardiac chest pain [7], or irritable bowel syndrome [8-10]. If the sensory anomaly is present in patients with CID, it may be due: (1) to a defective accommodation of the proximal stomach, (2) to gastric motility anomalies, (3) to psychological disturbances, or (4) to a primitive disorder of the afferent sensory pathway.

## Sensory response to distension of the proximal stomach in patients with CID

Twenty-four CID patients were studied in our laboratory to investigate whether their symptoms might be related to a gastric sensory anomaly. CID was defined [2] by the presence for three months or more of at least two of the following symptoms: (a) early satiety, (b) postprandial epigastric tension or bloating, (c) sensation of prolonged digestion (i.e. of a non-emptied stomach lasting more than two hours after ingestion of a meal), and (d) nausea and/or vomiting. Patients were excluded if they had a history of peptic ulcer, previous gastric surgery or a specific disorder which might have caused dyspeptic symptoms. All patients underwent upper digestive tract endoscopy and routine laboratory tests which revealed no anomalies. A control group of 20 healthy volunteers was also studied. Volunteers were carefully selected on interview and persons with a history of dyspepsia or digestive disease were excluded.

A latex balloon, 7 cm long and 14 cm in diameter at maximum distension (800 ml), was mounted on the tip of a nasogastric tube and introduced into the proximal stomach under fluoroscopic control. Subjects were studied in the supine position after an overnight fast. Prior to the procedure, they were given a range of sensations to report (first sensation of discomfort, constant sensation of discomfort, or pain). They were informed that sensations might intensify, subside or disappear during the test. Patients were asked to compare the induced sensations to their spontaneous symptoms. The gastric balloon was then inflated by 100 ml increments of air to reach a maximum volume of 800 ml (or less if an intolerable pain occurred at a lower volume). Each distension volume was maintained for 5 minutes and between each volume increment, the balloon was completely deflated for 2 minutes to prevent gradual gastric accommodation to distension. Repeated distensions at the same volume and sham distensions were also performed to assess the reproducibility and specificity of the test.

Inflation of the balloon up to the maximum volume of 800 ml was possible in all the volunteers, but had to be stopped in 13 of the 24 patients at volumes ranging from 400 to 700 ml because of intolerable pain. Pain occurred at a lower volume of balloon distension in patients with CID than in controls (400 ml $vs$ 700 ml; $p<0.001$). The cumulative percentages of patients and controls experiencing pain during the stepwise balloon inflation are shown in Figure 1. The curve obtained in patients displayed a significant shift towards lower distension volumes compared to the control curve. Thirteen of the 24 patients experienced pain at a volume $\leq 400$ ml but only 1 of the 20 control subjects ($p<0.001$). This 400 ml threshold (corresponding to the 95th percentile of normal values) was therefore used to define a positive gastric distension test. When pain was induced, it was usually localized in the epigastric region, and was frequently associated with nausea and a sensation of bloating. In patients, the induced symptoms usually reproduced spontaneous complaints. No pain was induced by sham distension. Repeated distensions performed in the same subject gave identical pain thresholds. The occurrence of CID symptoms after distension of the stomach by a normal sized meal and the resemblance between symptoms induced by balloon distension and spontaneous complaints in our patients strongly suggest that this sensory anomaly has clinical significance. In contrast, intragastric balloon volumes corresponding to the first sensation of discomfort and to the constant painless sensation of discomfort were not different in patients and controls.

No difference in pain threshold was found between males and females either in patients or in controls. No correlation was shown between pain threshold and age in patients, whereas pain threshold increased with age in controls ($r=0.60$, $p=0.01$; Fig. 2). The increase of pain threshold with age found in controls may have led to an underestimation of the frequency of the sensory anomaly, since the patients were older than controls.

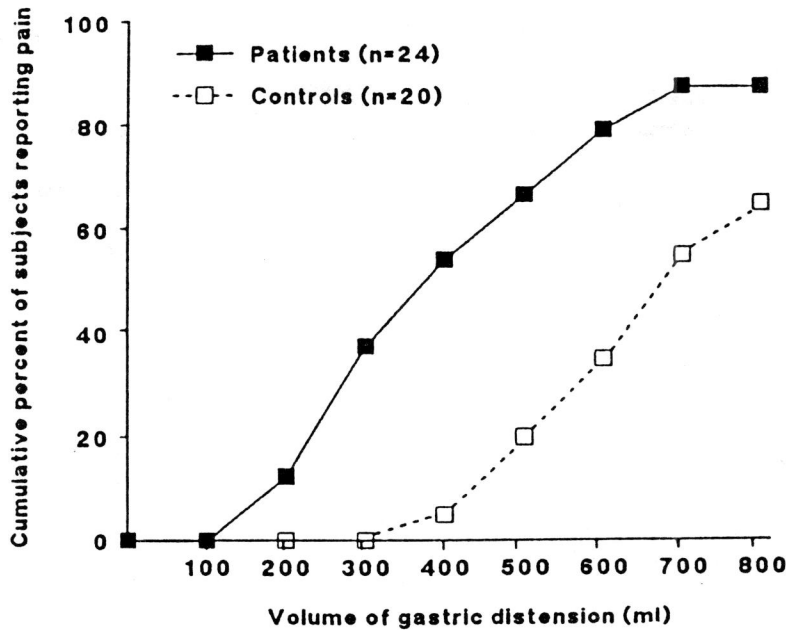

**Figure 1.** Cumulative percentages of patients and controls who experienced pain during the gastric distension test. The curve for the patients shows a significant shift towards lower volumes compared to the curve for the controls (Chi–2=15.18, df=7, $p<0.05$).

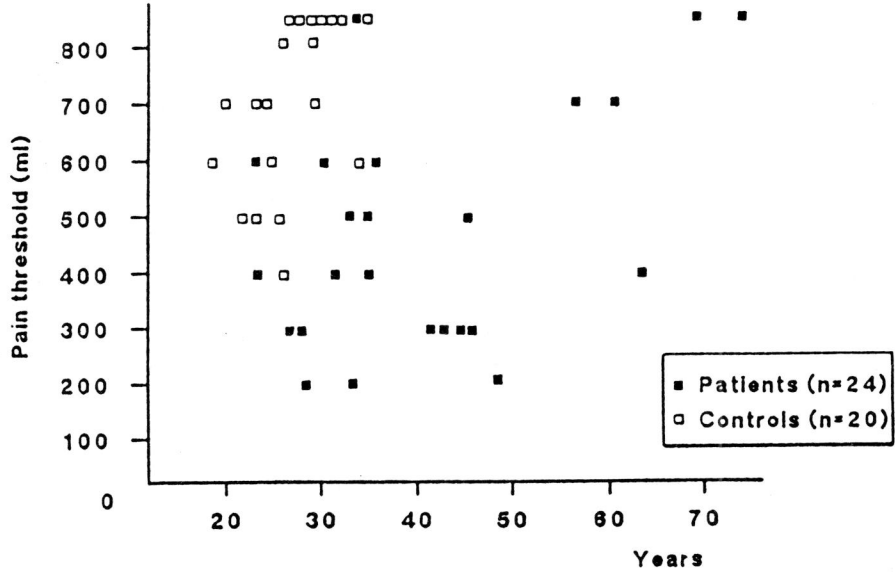

**Figure 2.** Relationship between age and pain threshold. In patients, no significant correlation was found; in controls, a positive correlation was found ($r=0.6$, $p<0.01$).

Our findings are in agreement with the recent results of Mearin et al. [11] obtained with the barostat technique. These workers found that during isobaric gastric distension, CID patients experienced more abdominal discomfort than controls.

## Accommodation of the proximal stomach to distension in patients with CID

Abnormal perception of gastric distension might be due to a defective accommodation of the proximal stomach to distension.

Such a defect has been shown after vagotomy or gastric surgery in patients who displayed symptoms similar to those of CID [12, 13].

During the gastric distension test in the same groups of dyspeptic patients and controls, intragastric balloon pressure was continuously recorded. After stabilization of the tracing, which took less than 1 min, the mean baseline pressure was determined for each level of distension tested. Pressure-volume curves were then modified by subtracting the pressure-volume curves generated by inflating the balloon in air to rule out the possibility that pressure changes were linked to the physical properties of the latex balloon.

Inflation of the balloon from 100 to 800 ml in the proximal stomach of our control subjects did not significantly increase intraballoon pressure, illustrating the previously described property of gastric accommodation to distension [14]. The intragastric pressure-volume curves obtained in patients and controls were not significantly different (Fig. 3). Furthermore, the pressure-volume curves were similar in patients with a normal or an abnormal pain threshold to gastric distension (Fig. 4).

These observations suggest that sensory anomaly was not due to a defective compliance of the proximal stomach. Mearin et al. [11] found similar results with the barostat. Basal gastric tone, gastric compliance and elasticity were not different in the dyspeptic patients and control groups. Similar abnormal perception of pain without compliance defect has been shown previously in other segments of the digestive tract in patients with dysphagia [6], non-cardiac chest pain [7], or irritable bowel syndrome [8-10].

## Relationship between sensory anomaly and gastric motility disturbances

The sensory anomaly might also be secondary to motility disturbances. Most of these anomalies can be revealed by delayed gastric emptying of liquids, solids or both [2, 5]. Gastric emptying was evaluated in 20 of the 24 patients, using a dual isotopic technique. Fasted subjects ingested a meal containing both a solid phase marker ($^{99m}$Tc sulphur colloid; 800 µCi) and a liquid phase marker ($^{111}$In DTPA; 150 µCi). Images were recorded for one minute every 30 minutes over a period of 3 h. Normal values were defined by the range of values obtained in 17 healthy controls (nine men and eight women, aged 20 to 35 years) previously studied under similar conditions [5]: $t\frac{1}{2}$ = 30 to 83 minutes for liquids; $t\frac{1}{2}$ = 51 to 172 minutes and β coefficient = 1.4 to 3.3 for solids.

The existence of gastric emptying anomalies was confirmed in the present work. Fourteen of the 20 patients (70%) had gastric stasis for solids in seven patients, liquids in 12, and both in five. However, the frequency of the sensory anomaly was not

# Abnormal perception of visceral pain

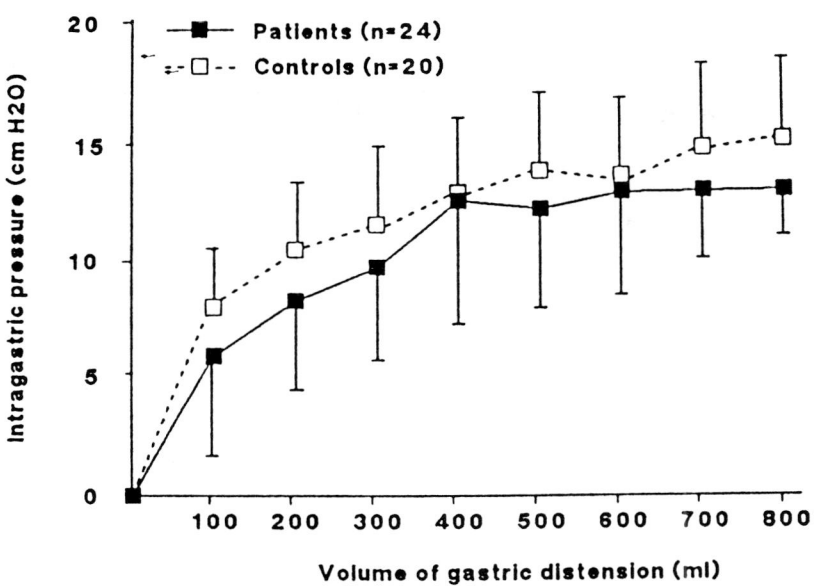

**Figure 3.** Intragastric pressure-volume curves obtained during stepwise balloon inflation in patients and controls. Curves do not differ significantly (analysis of variance).

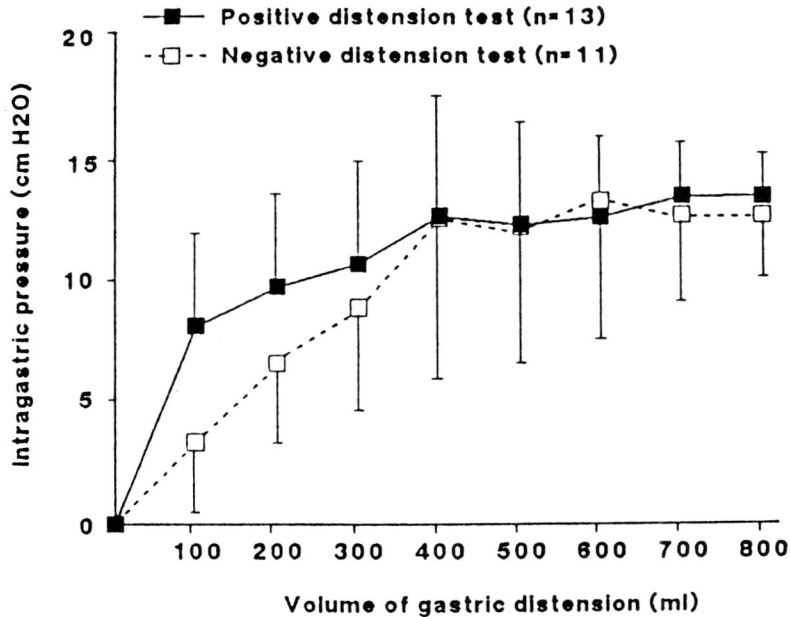

**Figure 4.** Intragastric pressure-volume curves in patients with a normal or an abnormal pain threshold to gastric distension. Curves do not differ significantly (analysis of variance).

different in patients with (7/14) and without (4/6) gastric emptying delay; no significant correlation was found between the pain threshold and the solid or liquid gastric emptying rates. Some of the patients with a very low pain threshold had normal gastric emptying.

As previously shown by others [3] and by our group [2], one third to one half of CID patients, studied either by radionuclide gastric emptying technique or antroduodenal manometry, have no motor disturbance. On the other hand, only half of the patients studied had an abnormal pain threshold, which was isolated (4/11) or more often associated with a delayed gastric emptying (7/11). It is therefore probable that disturbances in both motility and visceral pain perception are involved, either separately or together, in dyspeptic symptoms. A similar multifactorial pathophysiology has previously been reported in non-cardiac chest pain and irritable bowel syndrome [8, 15].

## Role of psychological disturbances in abnormal perception of pain

Since neither a defect of gastric accommodation nor motor abnormalities were related to the sensory anomaly, a psychological origin might be suspected. The perception of the verbally reported pain is a complex process dependent on factors such as anxiety, depression, individual cultural values and secondary gain [16]. Psychological status was evaluated in 18 of the 24 patients using the Mini-Mult test, a simplified version of the MMPI [17] which consists of 71 items and eight scales. Thirteen of the 18 patients (72%) had anomalies in one or more of the scales. Confirming the results obtained in previous studies [18, 19], patients with CID produced significantly higher scores than controls for hypochondriasis ($p<0.001$), depression ($p<0.001$), hysteria ($p<0.001$) and anxiety ($p<0.001$). However, sensory anomaly was significantly less frequent in patients with an abnormal psychological test (5/10) than in those with a normal test (8/8; $p<0.05$). This result argues against a psychological origin for the sensory anomaly. Moreover, the perfect reproducibility of the pain threshold when the patients were unaware of the magnitude or even the reality of distension is not compatible with a secondary gain attitude.

## Primitive disorder of the afferent sensorial pathway

All these facts combined with the unaltered sensation of discomfort (first and constant painless sensation), and the normal or even high cutaneous pain threshold found by others in similar functional disorders [20], strongly suggest that the pain threshold anomaly we evidenced in CID is due to a specific visceral disturbance affecting the perception of pain.

A primitive disorder of the afferent sensorial pathway seems the most probable explanation. Whether this is due to a reduced spinal "gate threshold" [21], to an increased sensitivity of nerve endings and muscular stretch or tension receptors, or to a hypersensitive (inflamed?) mucosa cannot be deduced from our study.

In conclusion, a low pain threshold in response to gastric distension is present in more than 50% of patients with CID and is not due to defective gastric compliance. This anomaly, either alone or combined with postprandial motility disorders, could play an important role in CID, and its presence suggests that, like the oesophagus and intestine, the stomach might also be irritable. The practical implications of this new concept should now be investigated by testing treatments that may affect visceral pain perception, such as drugs, relaxation or even biofeedback.

# References

1. Adami HO, Agenas I, Gustavsson S, Loof L, Nyberg A, Nyrén O, Tyllstrom J. The clinical diagnosis of "gastritis". Aspects of demographic epidemiology and health care consumption based on a nationwide sample survey. Scand J Gastroenterol 984;19:216-9.
2. Jian R, Ducrot F, Piedeloup C, Mary JY, Najean Y, Bernier JJ. Measurement of gastric emptying in dyspeptic patients: effect of a new gastrokinetic agent (cisapride). Gut 1985;26:352-8.
3. Malagelada JR, Stanghellini V. Manometric evaluation of functional upper gut symptoms. Gastroenterology 1985; 88:1223-31.
4. You CH, Chey WY. Study of electromechanical activity of the stomach in humans and in dogs with particular attention to tachygastria. Gastroenterology 1984;86:1460-8.
5. Jian R, Ducrot F, Ruskoné A, Chaussade S, Rambaud JC, Modigliani R, Rain JD, Bernier JJ. Symptomatic, radionuclide and therapeutic assessment of chronic idiopathic dyspepsia. A double-blind placebo-controlled evaluation of cisapride. Dig Dis Sci 1989;34:657-64.
6. Edwards DAW. "Tender esophagus": a new syndrome. Gut 1982;23:A919(abstr).
7. Richter JE, Barish CF, Castell DO. Abnormal sensory perception in patients with esophageal chest pain. Gastroenterology 1986;91:845-52.
8. Ritchie J. Pain from distension of the pelvic colon by inflating a balloon in the irritable colon syndrome. Gut 1973;14:125-32.
9. Swarbrick ET, Hegarty JE, Bat L, Williams CB, Dawson AM. Site of pain from the irritable bowel. Lancet 1980;2:443-6.
10. Stokes MA, Moriarty KJ, Catchpole BN. A study of the genesis of colic. Lancet 1988;1:211-5.
11. Mearin F, Cucala M, Azpiroz F, Malagelada JR. Origin of gastric symptoms in functional dyspepsia. Gastroenterology 1989; 96:A337(abstr).
12. Stadaas JO. Intragastric pressure/volume relationship before and after proximal gastric vagotomy. Scand J Gastroenterol 1975;10:129-34.
13. Azpiroz F, Malagelada JR. Gastric tone measured by an electronic barostat in health and postsurgical gastroparesis. Gastroenterology 1987;92:934-43.
14. Meyer JH. Motility of the stomach and gastroduodenal junction. In: Johnson LR, ed. *Physiology of the Gastrointestinal Tract*. Volume 1. 2nd ed. New York: Raven Press, 1987: 613-30.
15. Vantrappen G, Janssens J, Ghillebert G. The irritable oesophagus — A frequent cause of angina-like pain. Lancet 1987;1:1232-4.
16. Melzack R, Wall PD. *The Challenge of Pain*. New York: Basic Books, 1983.
17. Kincannon JC. Prediction of the standard M.M.P.I. scale scores from 71 items: the Mini-Mult. J Consult Clin Psychol 1968;32:319-25.
18. Talley NJ, Fung LH, Gilligan IJ, McNeil D, Piper DW. Association of anxiety, neuroticism and depression with dyspepsia of unknown cause. A case control study. Gastroenterology 1986;90:886-92.
19. Magni G, Di Mario F, Bernasconi G, Mastropaolo G, Naccarato R. Psychological distress in dyspepsia of unknown cause. Dig Dis Sci 1988;33:1052-3.
20. Cook IJ, Van Eeden A, Collins SM. Patients with irritable bowel syndrome have greater pain tolerance than normal subjects. Gastroenterology 1987;93:727-33.
21. Cervero F. Neurophysiology of gastrointestinal pain. Baillière's Clin Gastroenterol 1988;2:183-99.

# 18

# Psychosomatic heterogeneity in essential dyspepsia supports syndromatic clinical presentation

## S. BONFILS

*INSERM U.10, 170 Boulevard Ney, 75877 Paris Cedex 18, France*

Dyspepsia is a heterogeneous syndrome. This generic term designates various degrees of abdominal discomfort attributable to dysfunction of the upper digestive tract. Referred to variously as non-ulcerative dyspepsia, functional or essential dyspepsia, nervous dyspepsia, etc., the definition is essentially negative. The clinical profile can combine a sensation of immediate postprandial epigastric heaviness, potentially aggravated by certain types of food-stuffs, a burning median abdominal pain, nausea, vomiting (frequently of bile), eructation, abdominal distension and the inability to finish a normal meal.

The symptoms are non-specific, and can be seen in cases of organic pathology or can occur in conjunction with other functional pathologies [1]. A positive definition of dyspepsia would thus be very desirable; however this could not be based upon the apparently multifactorial pathogenesis of this disorder, which is highly variable between patients [2].

The poorly defined nature of the dyspeptic syndrome in conjunction with the multiplicity of possible pathogenic factors can account for the wide disparity of results of the various therapeutic studies which simply allow *a posteriori* classification of patients into various subgroups responsive or non-responsive to a given treatment [3], e.g. $H_2$-blockers, agents enhancing gastric motility such a cisapride; in relation to the present topic, the efficacy or the lack of efficacy of psychotropic agents or miscellaneous forms of psychotherapy might also allow an approach to the psychosomatic component of dyspepsia.

However, the psychosocial aspects of patients with functional disturbances of the digestive tract involve various psychosomatic links [4].

— Psychological stress exacerbates (if it does not create) gastrointestinal symptoms, just as it may to a smaller degree affect gastrointestinal function in healthy subjects.
— Psychological disturbance exists to a greater degree in patients with functional disorders than in those without such disorders, or in other medical populations, and in normal individuals.
— Having a functional digestive disorder may produce psychosocial effects.

Finally, independent of their possible aetiological role, psychological factors are considered to be of determining importance for the patients's well-being.

In this chapter these various aspects will be presented independently from their aetiological implications.

## Review of the literature

Whether a psychological stimulus is to become noxious (i.e., the individual cannot adapt to it and may even express stress-related disorders) or not depends upon many factors: genetic inheritance, earlier experiences, conditioning and social and cultural background. Wolf and associates [5] point out that it is not the external event or stimuli that are the determining factors but the individual's interpretation of them. In other words, the personality of the patients is of prime importance in functional digestive disorders, since it makes the subjects sensitive to psychological factors: personality is "permissive" for physical expression of a stimulus [6].

While keeping these considerations in mind, we shall study separately the environmental conditions and the personality patterns observed in dyspeptic patients.

### Environmental factors in dyspepsia

In a study from Talley and Piper [7], stress has been considered as assessable by major life events. The frequency of life events during the year before diagnosis of essential dyspepsia in 68 consecutive patients was compared with the frequency of these events over the same period of time in 68 randomly selected age- and sex-matched community controls. The mean number of events and the associated life changes and distress scores were similar for both groups.

The questionnaire technique used was unfortunately of very poor specificity as suggested by the fact that results similar to dyspepsia have been found in both duodenal and gastric ulcer patients [8, 9]. To improve the discriminative value of the self-report inventory, categorization of events was attempted: among the various selected categories, only bereavement gave significant differences, but unexpectedly with higher frequency in controls than in dyspeptic patients [7].

Evidence for stress-related dyspepsia is largely anecdotal. At variance with the findings of Talley and Piper, recent or unresolved bereavement has been reported among patients with unexplained abdominal pain [10]. A longitudinal investigation of air traffic controllers showed that these subjects are highly likely to develop dyspepsia and the trouble is rarely associated to peptic ulceration [11]. Finally, selection of patients is needed not only for a better categorization of the events but also for investigating the mental disturbance created by these events. In this respect it has been suggested that childhood factors are more revealing [12]. Talley therefore extended his work to father's occupation, education level, and childhood happiness, but none of these factors was found to be significantly different in dyspeptic patients from controls [12].

Words describe potentially disturbing events poorly. In Figure 1, we listed some environmental factors according to their duration; this clearly shows the lack of comparatibility between events commonly considered as stressful. Some people are unable to tolerate a chronic stress, even of mild grade: for others iterative acute stress (but not chronic stress) is psychologically highly damaging; hence comparisons between stresses considered to be identical in nature but different in duration is not likely to be relevant.

These remarks are in keeping with Talley's self-criticism underlying the fact that the methods he used cannot assess a particular individual's reaction to events and do not assess chronic stress [7]. Methodological shortcomings of check-list measures are

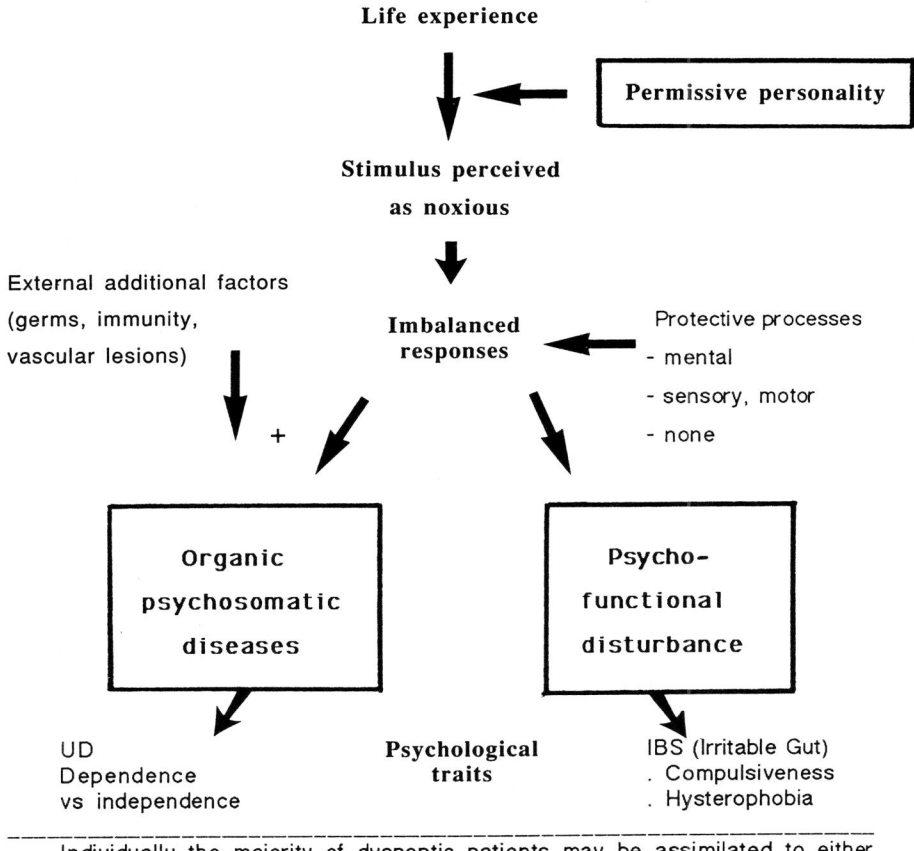

**Figure 1.** Working hypothesis for psychosomatic links in the two major aspects of psychosomatic digestive pathology. (Adapted from [6]).

so numerous that the use of these instruments in psychosomatic research should be abandoned. The belief that it is possible to assess the meaning of a particular event for an individual by using interviews is fallacious [13].

In conclusion, while emotional tension and stress in everyday life may produce a large range of gastrointestinal symptoms in the general population, it appears that there is a wide variety of response according to individual sensitivity.

**Personality patterns and mental symptoms in dyspepsia**

The presence of mental symptoms is far from constant in dyspeptic patients. This is not against the intervention of psychosomatic factors in essential dyspepsia, since somatization could be only one expression of a psychosomatic link when environmental factors are unconsciously perceived as noxious.

Evidence of permissive personality patterns, as defined above, might be obtained indirectly from the association between dyspepsia and other functional disturbances of the digestive tract, known to be frequently associated with mental symptoms. This is the case with aerophagia, a voluntary tic-like manoeuvre; it represents an exaggeration of the normal swallowing of air which occurs while eating and drinking. Belching is the process of expelling air accumulated in the stomach; it may be a repetitive compulsive process and should be regarded as an expression of psychoneurosis [14]. The prevalence of an association between dyspepsia and aerophagia is believed to be very high but exact figures have not been so far presented.

Irritable bowel syndrome (IBS) is another significant condition, believed to be a motor disorder that is not limited to the colon, but is also part of an entity called "irritable gut" [15]. In these patients, small bowel response to stress lends support to the concept of psychofunctional disturbance: in about half of a group of IBS patients, Kumar and Wingate [16] noticed that stress abolished the migrating motor complex (MMC) with a characteristic irregular motor activity associated to the usual clinical symptoms. Concerning psychological traits there is evidence that IBS patients differ from controls, and in particular with respect to anxiety levels, interpersonal sensitivity, depression, hostility and somatization of affect [17]. Prevalence of the combination of IBS and essential dyspepsia in the same patients was studied by Talley and Piper [1] in a large population of 327 consecutive patients who had at least one month of dyspepsia: 55% of these patients had IBS, associated with gastro-oesophageal reflux in about one half. Whether IBS and gastro-oesophageal reflux are responsible for dyspepsia is uncertain. But, as motility disturbances, these troubles should be considered in such patients as expressing at least in part the same mechanism of somatization as is present in essential dyspepsia.

Direct assessment of personality has been attempted by using psychometric tests. In a study by Talley *et al.* [18], a panel of such tests was used, yielding various scores concerning extraversion, neuroticism, anxiety, and depression. Tests were carried out in 76 essential dyspepsia patients and, as controls, in 76 randomly selected dyspepsia-free community subjects and 66 duodenal ulcer patients. In an initial study, the scores of dyspepsia and duodenal ulcer subjects showed that they were more neurotic, anxious and depressed than community controls. In a second study, dyspepsia patients were retested a mean of 3-6 months later: the abnormalities persisted on retesting and were not affected by the symptoms status. Author's conclusions underlined the fact that the numerical differences between the populations were small and that there is no evidence for a causal association between personality patterns and dyspepsia.

**Social behaviour in dyspepsia**

Under the heading of social behaviour we are concerned with the various aspects of human relationships; these may be considered to result from interaction between personality patterns and the various stresses from the daily life (excluding the massive physical and psychological stress triggered by accidents, war, life-threatening conditions, etc.).

Sickness absenteeism [19] was studied comparatively in an ulcer cohort of 74 patients and in a non-ulcer-dyspepsia cohort of 88 subjects. Although absenteeism was substantial in both cohorts, the proneness to report sick in dyspepsia patients was statistically greater than in ulcer patients. The patients with more sick-leave days were significantly younger than those with fewer such days. By contrast, no influence of sex was noted. The authors concluded that psychosocial factors seem to be of great importance in dyspepsia.

The ability (or the inability) to express emotions is another variable included in social behaviour. Control over anger, anxiety, unhappiness, and total emotional control over negative reactions were comparatively studied [20] in two populations with either essential dyspepsia (82 cases), or duodenal ulcer (53 cases), and randomly selected community controls (82 cases). No difference was found between the three populations using a self-report scale mailed to the patients after telephone contact. I personally am reluctant to use a method which is expected to assess patient's behaviour without any direct contact with the physician.

**Biological correlates with psychosomatic implications in dyspepsia**

Subgroups of dyspepsia have been suggested according to the predominant pathophysiological factor involved. So, independently from symptomatology, we should envisage three aspects of this condition with potential links between biological disturbance and psychological factors: acid secretion, motor disturbance (i.e. slow gastric emptying), and visceral perception.

*Acid secretion*

Gastric acidity as pathogenic factor in dyspeptic pain may act in two ways: (1) acidity could be directly algogenic for a damaged mucosa; (2) acidity could cause mucosal lesions.

Correlation between acid secretion changes and psychological factors have been shown in duodenal ulcer patients [21, 22]. According to personality types, acid secretion can be high or low, however, without demonstrating causality. Assuming that dyspeptic patients might have "ulcer-type" personality patterns, and even that non-ulcer dyspepsia, with or without duodenitis and duodenal ulcer, might be a continuum of the same disease [23, 24], gastric tests were carried out in a comparative manner in non-ulcer dyspepsia patients with or without duodenitis, and in duodenal ulcer patients. In duodenal ulcer patients, basal acid secretion was significantly higher than in the two other populations. Although not fully conclusive, these results do not suggest that a distinction exists between non-ulcer dyspepsia and duodenal ulcer in relation to psychic stimulation of acid secretion. However, we have demonstrated [22] that in a subpopulation of duodenal ulcer patients, presenting with major dependence traits, gastric secretion is lower than in the remaining cases. Thus high basal acidity is far from being specific for duodenal ulcer.

*Motor disturbances*

Slow gastric emptying has been observed in approximately 40% of dyspeptic patients [25], while psychological interference with gastric emptying has also been shown [26]. The most revealing data result from purely experimental research. Acoustic stress delays gastric emptying in a variety of animals [27, 28]. Injection of corticotrophin releasing factor (CRF) mimics these inhibitory effects on gastric motility and anti-CRF prevents the CRF effects [26]. This suggests that hypothalamic pathways may mediate the motor gastric dysfunction induced by acoustic stress.

Few experiments on stress-induced motor gastric disturbance have been carried out in man. In normal volunteers psychological stress induced by a dichotomous listening test succeeded in inducing acceleration of the mouth-to-caecum transit in normal volunteers, but no consistent or significant effect on gastric emptying was observed [29]. This is at variance with results obtained in a non-controlled study using double-labelling ($^{99}$M-Technicium and $^{113}$Indium) of a solid-liquid meal, in which it was shown that acoustic stress in healthy men resulted in an increased speed of stomach emptying. Conversely, physical stress induced by cold was associated with slowed gastric emptying both from the total stomach and from the proximal stomach [30].

In essential dyspepsia, the influence of stress on antral motility was studied in patients undergoing transcutaneous electrical nerve stimulation. When given 70 minutes after the end of the meal, this stress allowed subjects to be classified into two types: first, those with postcibal antral hypomotility that was not changed during stress; second, patients with normal postcibal motility which was suppressed by stress. Worthy of mention is the fact that clinical presentation, personality traits, autonomic (pulse, blood pressure, etc.) and humoral (plasma β-endorphin and catecholamine levels) functions were not different in the two groups [31]. The authors' conclusions emphasized that the first group appeared to be afflicted by a form of gastroparesis and was thus unable to respond to stress. The second group was strictly normal so far as the various measured indices were concerned: it is unlikely that a stress-induced motility disturbance was the cause of symptoms in this group.

Anorexia nervosa is usually considered to be an important psychosomatic disease. Digestive symptoms are very common, including nausea and gastric fullness. Specific psychological traits are present in this disorder, particularly a disturbance of body image. A multidisciplinary study of eight patients with anorexia nervosa and eight age- and sex-matched controls was undertaken by Abell *et al.* [32], which aimed at quantifying gastrointestinal motor functions in these patients. In anorexia nervosa most patients have abnormal gastric electromechanical activity secondary to abnormalities in hormonal responses to a meal (disturbed norepinephrine and neurotensin response, but not gastrin, CCK and HPP), and in autonomic functions (blood pressure, skin conductance). Delayed gastric emptying with a normal early emptying phase is the most relevant observation in relation to dyspepsia; but the gastric electrical dysrhythmia and depressed postprandial phasic pressure activity observed in these patients may be responsible for this slowing [32].

Applying a renutrition programme to patients with anorexia nervosa (and without using any drug known to modify gastric emptying) Rigaud *et al.* [33] succeeded in obtaining improvement in gastrointestinal symptoms and, at the same time, better emptying of both liquid and solid phases of a test meal. This study suggests that a purely nutritional and psychological approach of anorexia nervosa can improve gastric motility.

In conclusion there seems to exist in anorexia nervosa a close relationship between dyspeptic symptoms and delayed gastric emptying and for both there is a possible link with the psychological traits associated to the disease. But there is no evidence that, in essential dyspepsia, such a psychosomatic interrelationship exists as a rule.

*Visceral perception*

In dyspepsia the appearance and/or intensity threshold of tolerance to functional disturbances or simply to pain may be of importance. This has been largely proved for IBS [34, 35] and was recently studied in patients with essential dyspepsia [36]. Progressive gastric distension was induced in dyspeptic patients and in controls with measurement of symptomatic responses and pressures at the gastric fundus and the lower oesophageal sphincter. Patients had a significantly lower threshold both to the initial symptomatic recognition and to perception of pain during gastric distension. Domperidone might have an effect on the threshold of these conscious visceral sensations. These increased visceral perceptions might explain dyspepsia symptoms alone or on a background of functional motor abnormalities.This would make dyspepsia a potential member of the "irritable gut" syndrome [15] with its well-known psychosomatic implications. However, it is likely that this hypersensitivity is not the cause of symptoms in every case of dyspepsia.

**Psychotherapeutic approach**

The feasibility and the benefit of psychotherapy in essential dyspepsia has never been fully assessed. Svedlund's positive judgement concerning the benefit of psychotherapy in some digestive diseases was wrongly extended to dyspepsia. The distinction of dyspeptic symptoms in IBS, as suggested by Dotevall [37], is purely artificial.

Sjödin and Svedlund [38] honestly underlined the difficulty of approaching dyspepsia: "It is an impossible question to answer in a meaningful way, chiefly because of the undefined nature of this clinical concept". This negative statement is puzzling since the title of these authors' paper was "Psychological aspects of non-ulcer dyspepsia".

The most recent publication on psychological treatment for IBS strongly exemplifies the methodological and interpretation problems raised by functional digestive disorders [39].

**Personal approach**

Obviously from the literature, there is great difficulty in adequately defining essential dyspepsia in the realm of psychosomatic disturbances. This is not exclusively due to the lack of relevance and accuracy of the methods used, although application of questionnaires devoted to psychiatric studies or to sociology might yield bias and fallacies — psychosomatic research needs methods which simultaneously take into consideration psychological and physical (i.e. related to the organ trouble) dimensions.

Since essential dyspepsia is unanimously recognized as a heterogeneous syndrome with various pathophysiological mechanisms, there is no hope of obtaining homogeneous psychosomatic information. A significant example of heterogeneity is given by Magni's work [40] comparing essential dyspepsia patients with matched controls suffering from dyspepsia of organic cause (gallstones, hiatus hernia). While both populations scored identically for compulsiveness and phobic traits, significant differences were obtained for sleep disturbance, paranoid ideation, somatization and anxiety.

With respect to psychosomatic causation, the symptoms observed in essential dyspepsia need to be compared to pathological conditions inducing complaints of the same type. We proposed in 1962 [41] a classification of psychosomatic troubles in two main patterns: psychosomatic diseases (such as peptic ulcer, ulcerative colitis) and psychofunctional disturbances, one type of which is the irritable bowel syndrome or more largely irritable gut. These concepts cover clinical aspects easily recognizable with respect to psychological traits, behaviour, operatory thinking (alexithymia), target organ fixity, precipitating factors, etc [42]. The two patterns are summarized in Table I.

Comparison of patients suffering from either pattern with dyspeptic patients was attempted. In a period of 6 months, consecutive patients presenting with either dyspepsia, duodenal ulcer or IBS were selected: they underwent a psychological interview and were asked to answer a questionnaire derived from that used in preceding study on ulcer patients [43]. Since we expected to receive only rough indications from this pilot study, we did not match these subpopulations. Findings in control subjects (duodenal ulcer and IBS) were largely in accordance with previously described schemes (Table II): duodenal ulcer patients with dependence *vs* independence tensions (17/20); IBS patients with compulsive features (16/22). Dyspeptic patients clearly did not show a predominance of either mental structure.

Table I. Some comparative psychosomatic parameters in the two major aspects of psychosomatic digestive pathology (DU: duodenal ulcer; IBS: irritable bowel syndrome; both conditions are presented as examples with their general and specific features).

|  | Psychosomatic disease (DU) | Psychofunctional disturbances (IBS) |
|---|---|---|
| Target organ fixity | + | − |
| Precipitating factors | Symbolic | Casual |
| Personality pattern | Well-defined Dependence *vs* independence | Variable From compulsiveness to phobia |
| Alexithymia (Operatory thinking) | + | − |
| Psychotherapy | Difficult and not harmless | Useful |

**Table II.** Comparison of various psychological traits (see Table I) in consecutive patients consulting the same physician (DU: duodenal ulcer; IBS: irritable bowel syndrome).

|  | Dyspepsia n=12 | DU n=20 | IBS n=22 |
|---|---|---|---|
| Psychofunctional traits | | | |
| — Compulsive feature | 2 | 2 | 16 |
| — Aggressivity | 3 | 4 | 4 |
| — Precipitating factors | | | |
| • Casual | 4* | — | 13 |
| Psychosomatic traits (organic) | | | |
| — Precipitating factors | | | |
| • Symbolic | 5* | 8 | 2 |
| — Operatory thinking (Alexithymia) | 4 | 12 | 2 |
| — Target organ fixity | 8 | 15 | 0 |
| — Dependence vs independence | 4 | 17 | 2 |

* "Stress": 9=75%

On this small number of patients, clinical and psychological features allow three groups to be identified:
— Irritable gut-like:     4 cases
— Peptic ulcer-like:      5 cases
— Autonomous-dyspeptic:   3 cases

Although these data should be considered only as indicative of psychological heterogeneity in dyspepsia, they are not fully in keeping with the conclusions drawn from published reports, as presented above. They suggest that:

(1) There is no dominant psychological pattern in dyspepsia.

(2) Dyspepsia is not included, as a whole, in the concept of "irritable gut" even if in many patients symptomatic presentation is that of purely functional digestive trouble.

(3) In the therapeutic approach to dyspepsia, psychological support may be of importance but should be modulated according to case; indeed ulcer-like, irritable gut-like and autonomous presentations might need different kinds of support.

# Conclusions and suggestions

The general difficulty in drawing significant conclusions from studies on essential dyspepsia (whatever the variable studied, aetiological, clinical or biological), is obviously related to the heterogeneity of the underlying functional trouble(s). Pathophysiological classification [44] is of little help in resolving this problem: when considering true essential dyspepsia, symptoms are not easily attributable to one specific disturbance.

**Table III.** A tentative classification of essential dyspepsia including psychosomatic parameters.

| | |
|---|---|
| Type I | Irritable gut-like |
| | Epigastric fullness, bloating; tic-like manoeuvres (aerophagia) |
| | Psychofunctional mental structure |
| Type II | Ulcer-like |
| | Abdominal pain; epigastric burning; well-defined food-intolerance |
| | Predominance of dependence *vs* independence conflictual traits |
| | (psychosomatic mental structure) |
| Type III | Anorexia nervosa-like |
| | Vomiting; alimentary restriction |
| | Lack of appetite, "cannot face food" |
| | Alteration of body image |
| Type IV | Nervous dyspepsia |
| | Chronic stress, anecdotal influences on dyspepsia intensity |
| | Benefit from rest and vacation |
| | No dominant psychological structure |
| Type V | Casual types (autonomous dyspepsia) |

Large-scale statistical evaluation enabled by the high frequency of cases of essential dyspepsia gives no more information than a few cases adequately studied... and rather less. This is particularly the case for psychosomatic studies.

If psychosomatics means the simultaneous involvement of mind and body, classification of psychosomatic troubles should take into consideration parameters from both sides. On this basis we propose (Table III) various subgroups of dyspeptic patients, which must be distinguished by individual examination and psychological assessment by the same physician, at least for initial screening.

We hope that this classification, if validated, could help in designing studies on essential dyspepsia using a comprehensive and relevant approach; methods adequately selected according to subgroups of patients might suppress the feelings of frustration which generally arise from meetings and symposia on dyspepsia.

## References

1. Talley NJ, Piper DW. The association between non-ulcer dyspepsia and other gastrointestinal disorders. Scand J Gastroenterol 1985;20:896-900.
2. Read NW. Functional gastrointestinal disorders: building castles in the air. Gastroenterol Int 1990;3:182-3.
3. Bonfils S, Phuoc KN, René E. La dyspepsie "non ulcéreuse". Pour un abord rationnel des études thérapeutiques. Gastroentérol Clin Biol 1988;12:187-92.
4. Drossman DA, Thompson WG, Talley NJ, Funch-Jensen P, Janssens J, Whitehead WE. Identification of sub-groups of functional gastrointestinal disorders. Gastroenterol Int 1990;3:159-72.
5. Wolf S, Goodell H. *Stress and Disease*. Springfield: Charles Thomas Publisher, 1968.
6. Bonfils S. Personality in functional digestive disorders: a permissive factor. In: Taché Y, Wingate D, eds. *Brain Gut Interactions*. Boca Raton: CRC Press, 1991:351-61.

7. Talley NJ, Piper DW. Major life event stress and dyspepsia of unknown cause: a case control study. Gut 1986;27:127-34.
8. Piper DW, McIntosh JH, Ariotti DE, Calogiuri JV, Brown RW, Shy CM. Life events and chronic duodenal ulcer: a case control study. Gut 1981;22:1011-7.
9. Thomas J, Greig M, Piper DW. Chronic gastric ulcer and life events. Gastroenterology 1980;78:905-11.
10. Gomez J, Dally P. Psychologically mediated abdominal pain in surgical and medical outpatients clinics. Br Med 1977;1:1451-3.
11. Rose RM, Jenken CD, Hurst MW. Airtraffic controller health change study. Report to a Federal Aviation Administration under Contract N° FA7 3WA-3211, August 1978.
12. Talley NJ, Jones M, Piper DW. Psychosocial and childhood factors in essential dyspepsia. A case-control study. Scand J Gastroenterol 1988;23:341-6.
13. Bass C. Life events and gastrointestinal symptoms. Gut 1986;27:123-6.
14. Malagelada JR. Rumination, aerophagia, and other functional upper gut disturbances. GI report 1986;1(volume 12):1-7.
15. Richter JE, Obrecht WF, Bradley LA, Young LD, Anderson KO. Psychological comparison of patients with nutcracker esophagus and irritable bowel syndrome. Dig Dis Sci 1986; 31:131-8
16. Kumar D, Wingate DL. The irritable bowel syndrome: a paroxysmal motor disorder. Lancet 1985;2:973-7.
17. Whitehead WE, Engel BT, Schuster MM. Irritable bowel syndrome: physiological and psychological differences between diarrhoea-predominant and constipation-predominant patients. Dig Dis Sci 1980;25:404-13.
18. Talley NJ, Fung LH, Gilligan IJ, Mcneil D, Piper DW. Association of anxiety, neuroticism, and depression with dyspepsia of unknown cause. A case-control study. Gastroenterology 1986;90:886-92.
19. Nyrén O, Adami HO, Gustavsson S, Lööf L. Excess sick-listing in non-ulcer dyspepsia. J Clin Gastroenterol 1986;8:339-45.
20. Talley NJ, Ellard K, Jones M, Tennant C, Piper DW. Suppression of emotions in essential dyspepsia and chronic duodenal ulcer. A case-control study. Scand J Gastroenterol 1988;23:337-40.
21. Bonfils S. Psychosomatic parameters in duodenal ulcer. Theoretical basis and practical interest of an original classification. In: Domschke W, Wormsley UG, eds. *Magen und Magenkraukheitem*. Stuttgart: George Thieme, 1981:103-11.
22. Mazet P, Bonfils S. Actions des facteurs psychologiques et psychosomatiques sur la sécrétion gastrique chez l'homme. Biol Gastroentérol (Paris) 1970;1:77-86.
23. Joffe SN. Relevance of duodenitis to non-ulcer dyspepsia and peptic ulceration. Scand J Gastroenterol 1982;17(suppl 79):88-97.
24. Myren J. Gastric secretion in duodenitis. Scand J Gastroenterol 1982;17 (suppl 79):98-101.
25. Jian R, Ducrot F, Piedeloup C, Mary JY, Najean Y, Bernier JJ. Measurement of gastric emptying in dyspeptic patients: effect of a new gastrokinetic agent (cisapride). Gut 1985;26:352-8.
26. Bueno L, Gue M. Evidence for the involvement of corticotropin-releasing factor in the gastrointestinal disturbances induced by acoustic and cold stress in mice. Brain Res 1988;441:1-4.
27. Gue M, Fioramonti J, Bueno L. Comparative influences of acoustic and cold stress on gastrointestinal transit in mice. Am J Physiol 1987;253:G124-8.
28. Gue M, Peeters T, Deppoortere I, Vantrappen G, Bueno L. Stress-induced changes in gastric emptying, postprandial motility, and plasma gut hormone levels in dogs. Gastroenterology 1989;97:1101-7.
29. Cann PA, Read NW, Cammack J, Childs H, Holden S, Kashman R, Longmore J, Nix S, Simms N, Swallow K, Weller J. Psychological stress and the passage of a standard meal through the stomach and small intestine in man. Gut 1983;24:236-40.

30. Fone DR, Horowitz M, Maddox A, Akkermans LM, Read NW, Dent J. Gastroduodenal motility during the delayed gastric emptying induced by cold stress. Gastroenterology 1990;98:1155-61.
31. Camilleri M, Malagelada JR, Kao PC, Zinsmeister AR. Gastric and autonomic responses to stress in functional dyspepsia. Dig Dis Sci 1986;31:1169-77.
32. Abell TL, Malagelada JR, Lucas AR, Brown ML, Camilleri M, Go VL, Azpiroz F, Callaway CW, Kao PC, Zinsmeister AR et al. Gastric electromechanical and neurohormonal function in anorexia nervosa. Gastroenterology 1987;93:958-65.
33. Rigaud D, Bedig G, Merrouche M, Vulpillat M, Bonfils S, Apfelbaum M. Delayed gastric emptying in anorexia nervosa is improved by completion of a renutrition program. Dig Dis Sci 1988;33:919-25.
34. Ritchie J. Pain from distension of the pelvic colon by inflating a balloon in the irritable colon syndrome. Gut 1973;14:125-32.
35. Cann PA, Read NW, Brown C, Hobson N, Holdsworth CD. Irritable bowel syndrome: relationship of disorders in the transit of a single solid meal to symptom patterns. Gut 1983;24:405-11.
36. Bradette M, Pare P, Douville P, Morin A. Visceral perception in health and functional dyspepsia. Cross-over study of gastric distension with placebo and domperidone. Dig Dis Sci 1991; 36:52-8.
37. Dotevall G. Stress and common gastrointestinal disorders; a comprehensive approach. New York: Praeger, 1985.
38. Sjödin I, Svedlund J. Psychological aspects of non-ulcer dyspepsia: a psychosomatic view focusing on a comparison between the irritable bowel syndrome and peptic ulcer disease. Scand J Gastroenterol 1985;20(suppl 109):51-8.
39. Guthri E, Creed F, Dawson D, Tomenson B. A controlled trial of psychological treatment for the irritable bowel syndrome. Gastroenterology 1991;100:450-7.
40. Magni G, Di-Mario F, Bernasconi G, Mastropaolo G, Naccarato R. Psychological distress in dyspepsia of unknown cause. Dig Dis Sci 1988;33:1052-3.
41. Bonfils S. Maladies psychosomatiques et troubles psychofonctionnels. Nécessité d'un démembrement de la pathologie psychogène en gastroentérologie. Arch Fr Mal App Dig 1962;51:825-34.
42. Bonfils S, Hachette JC, Danne O. L'Abord psychosomatique en gastroentérologie. Paris: Masson, 1982.
43. Bonfils S, Hachette JC, Cukier S, Mignon M. Proximal gastric vagotomy compared with long-term cimetidine treatment: influence of psychosomatic factors in patients with duodenal ulcer. In: Baron JH, Alexander-Williams J, Allgower M, Muller C, Spencer J, eds. *Vagotomy in Modern Surgical Practice* (Proceedings of the Symposium, Basel, February 1981). London: Butterworths, 1982:299-304.
44. Colin-Jones DG, Bloom B, Bodemar G, Crean G, Freston J, Gugler R, Malagelada JR, Nyrén O, Petersen H, Piper D. Management of dyspepsia: report of a working party. Lancet 1988;1:576-9.

# SESSION IV

# Management of non-ulcer dyspepsia

Chairman: P. BERNADES

# 19

## An introduction to the management of non-ulcer dyspepsia. Is a rational approach currently available?

M. MIGNON, Ph. RUSZNIEWSKI

*Service d'Hépato-Gastroentérologie, CHU Bichat - Claude Bernard, 75877 Paris Cedex 18, France*

It is somewhat hazardous to dare introduce, in a symposium devoted to non-ulcer dyspepsia (NUD), a session aiming at defining the treatment of this syndrome. Indeed, there remain so many unresolved problems that the task is obviously of paramount difficulty.

These problems can be summarized as follows:

1 — Absence of an unequivocal definition of NUD and a clear delineation of clinicians' objective: definite exclusion of organic disease, or alleviation of patients' symptoms considered as purely functional?

2 — Lack of concordance between symptoms and pathophysiological abnormalities when present.

3 — Uncertainty concerning the primitive or secondary nature of lesions or dysfunctions evidenced by investigations of the upper GI tract, e.g. erosions in ulcer-like dyspepsia or delayed gastric emptying in dysmotility-like dyspepsia.

4 — Scarcity of valid clinical trials, due to numerous shortcomings, especially in patients' selection and methodological problems.

5 — Difficulty in assessing the benefit of a psychosomatic approach in these patients, although the implication of stress(es) as precipitating factor(s) is often suspected.

Lack of consensual definition of NUD is obvious as emphasized by R. Jian's introductory remarks [1]. Indeed, summarizing the three most recent attempts at delimitating the clinical relevance of NUD [1-3] clearly illustrates that, with the exception of patients with dysmotility-like dyspepsia, major discrepancies exist. Fortunately, almost half of the patients belong to this latter category. They usually complain of an abdominal distress which is described in various ways: epigastric fulness or heaviness, early satiety, sensation of slow digestion, bloating, nausea, vomiting... Clearly such a definition fits adequately to the actual etymological significance of dyspepsia which originates from the association of the Greek prefixe δυσ (difficult, bad) and the Greek verb πεπτειν (to digest).

In a large proportion of these patients (usually more than 50%), delayed gastric emptying has been documented [4]. Even if no straight correspondence exists between symptoms and objective anomalies in gastric emptying, the latter findings provide at least some rationale for initiating a therapeutic strategy. It is indeed in this category of patients that prokinetic agents are providing uniquevocal benefit [5-7]. According to Galmiche and Vallot, cisapride could represent, among the prokinetic agents, a first choice drug in the treatment of NUD, should long term clinical experience and further trials confirm its efficacy and safety [8]. Obviously, however, further research is needed to clarify and unravel better the underlying pathophysiological and aetiological mechanisms of NUD.

Individuals with epigastric pain, whether it is suggestive of gastro-œsophageal reflux (GOR) or of peptic ulcer (PU), represent a second category of patients, although their aggregation to the previously described category could be questioned from a strictly semantic point of view. They constitute, however, an interesting subset of NUD patients both for pragmatical and therapeutical considerations. Pragmatically indeed these individuals, in case of recurring or persisting pain, will receive some form of investigation of the upper digestive tract aiming at excluding organic diseases and at ascertaining the diagnosis of reflux-like dyspepsia [9] or of ulcer-like dyspepsia [10].

In case of reflux-like dyspepsia, a rationale for therapy is also present. It may consist, if postural recommendations are not effective, in the prescription, at demand, of an alginate-antacid mixture, or $H_2$-antagonists to protect the mucosa and reduce gastric juice agressivity, or of a prokinetic agent in order to strengthen the lower oesophageal sphincter tone and accelerate gastric emptying.

In most cases, and for many investigators, ulcer-like dyspepsia does not appear to raise difficult therapeutic choices. Although, indeed, gastric acid secretion is often normal in these patients [11], the majority of medical trials has demonstrated the efficacy of $H_2$-blockers in this condition (Fig. 1). This could be particularly true when upper GI endoscopy discloses erosions in the stomach and/or the duodenum; ranitidine leads to healing these lesions in about 80% of the cases [12]. Mucosal protecting agents such as sucralfate can also be of therapeutic interest in these patients. Dietetic recommendations, dietary and hygienic advice could be advocated to these patients as well as avoidance of NSAIDs and restrictions of tobacco-smoking and coffee-drinking as well as alcohol consumption.

Finally, a last and ill-defined group of patients remains and raises the most difficult therapeutic options. This group would encompass:

a — Patients who experience symptoms of ulcer-or dysmotility-like dyspepsia, without demonstration of any endoscopic mucosal abnormality or gastric motor disturbance. These patients could be defined as having purely essential dyspepsia. Whether they have a lowered threshold of gastric sensory mechanisms or not remains an open question [13]. Non-responders to gastrokinetic or antisecretory drugs and protective agents might be included in this subset.

b — Patients whose symptoms mimic other types of diseases of the upper part of the abdomen, arising from biliary, pancreatic and colonic organs. In these particular individuals, the notions of alarm symptoms and age threshold are of prime importance in deciding the extent of investigations and the type of therapy [8-9]. A psychosomatic approach may be of benefit for some patients [14].

One cannot dissimulate that the treatment of non-ulcer dyspepsia has raised more questions than it actually did offer clear answers. A restrictive definition of NUD covering only dysmotility-, reflux- and ulcer-like dyspepsia is but an oversimplification of the dramatic diagnostic and therapeutic challenges that the clinician has to face at every moment.

No doubt that new concepts and avenues for basic and clinical research as thoroughly discussed by R.C. Heading later in this book [15], will contribute to alleviate patients' complaints as well as physicians' intellectual trouble.

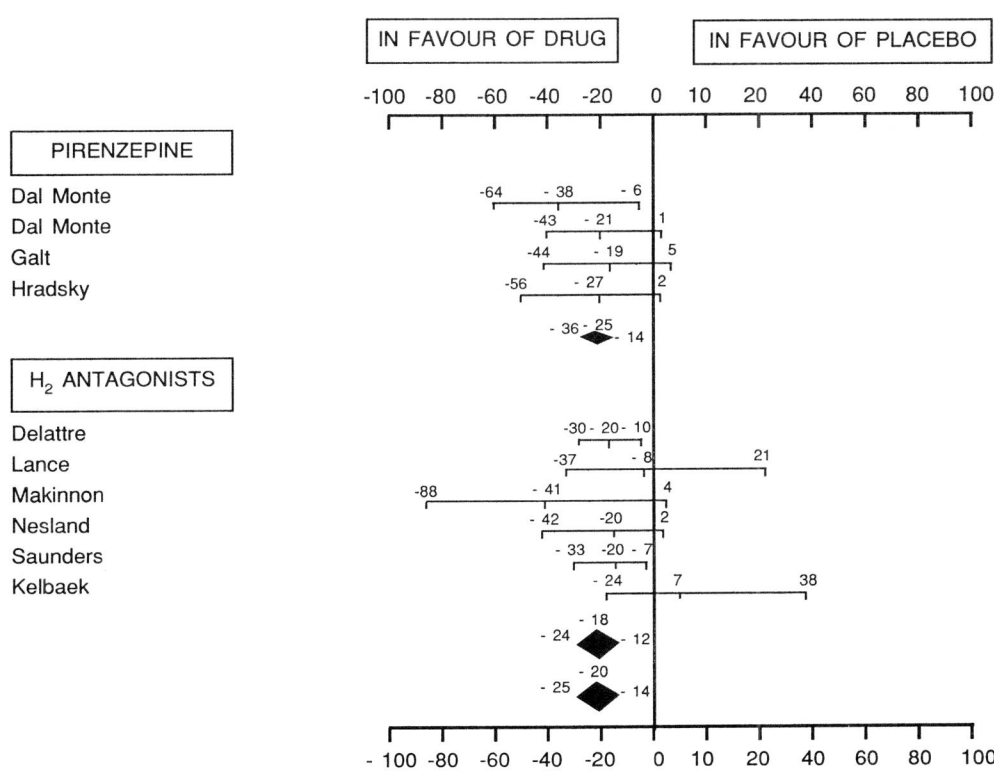

**Figure 1.** Differences in success rates between patients treated with placebo and those treated with anti-secretory drugs. Numbers at midpoints of lines are percent differences. Numbers at endpoints indicate 95% confidence limits. (From ref. [7]).

## References

1. Jian R. Non-ulcer dyspepsia: from the iceberg to the tower of Babel. In: Galmiche JP, Jian R, Mignon M, Ruszniewski Ph, eds. *Non-ulcer Dyspepsia: Therapeutic and Pathophysiological Approaches*. Paris: John Libbey Eurotext, 1991:3-5.
2. Colin Jones DG, Bloom B, Bodemar G et al. Management of dyspepsia: report of a working party. Lancet 1988; 1: 576-9.
3. Barbara L, Camilleri M, Corinaldesi GP. Definition and investigation of dyspepsia. Consensus of an international *ad hoc* working party. Dig Dis Sci 1989; 34: 1272-6.
4. Bruley des Varannes S. Disturbances of gastric emptying. In: Galmiche JP, Jian R, Mignon M, Ruszniewski Ph, eds. *Non-ulcer Dyspepsia: Therapeutic and Pathophysiological Approaches*. Paris: John Libbey Eurotext, 1991:105-20.
5. Rosch W. Cisapride in non-ulcer dyspepsia. Results of a placebo-controlled trial. Scand J Gastroenterol 1987; 22: 161-4.
6. Jian R, Ducrot F, Ruskoné A, Chaussade S, Rambaud JC, Modigliani R, Rain JD, Bernier JJ. Symptomatic radionuclide and therapeutic assessment of chronic idiopathic dyspepsia. A double-blind placebo-controlled evaluation of cisapride. Dig Dis Sci 1989; 34: 657-64.
7. Dobrilla G, Comberlato M, Steele A, Vallaperta P. Drug treatment of functionnal dyspepsia. A meta-analysis of randomized controlled clinical trials. J Clin Gastroenterol 1989; 11: 169-77.
8. Galmiche JP, Vallot T. Therapeutic strategy. In: Galmiche JP, Jian R, Mignon M, Ruszniewski Ph, eds. *Non-ulcer Dyspepsia: Therapeutic and Pathophysiological Approaches*. Paris: John Libbey Eurotext, 1991:247-64.
9. Vantrappen G. Diagnostic strategy. In: Galmiche JP, Jian R, Mignon M, Ruszniewski Ph, eds. *Non-ulcer Dyspepsia: Therapeutic and Pathophysiological Approaches*. Paris: John Libbey Eurotext, 1991:239-45.
10. Petersen H. Role of acid and pepsin. In: Galmiche JP, Jian R, Mignon M, Ruszniewski Ph, eds. *Non-ulcer Dyspepsia: Therapeutic and Pathophysiological Approaches*. Paris: John Libbey Eurotext, 1991:121-7.
11. Collen MJ, Loebenberg MJ. Basal gastric acid secretion in non-ulcer dyspepsia with or without duodenitis. Dig Dis Sci 1989; 34: 246-50.
12. Ruszniewski P, Mignon M et Groupe Multicentrique. Etude prospective randomisée en double aveugle de l'efficacité de la ranitidine (R) dans les érosions gastroduodénales (EGD). Gastroentérol Clin Biol 1991; 15: A110 (abstr.).
13. Lémann M, Dederding JP, Flourié B, Rambaud JC, Jian R. Abnormal perception of visceral pain. In: Galmiche JP, Jian R, Mignon M, Ruszniewski Ph, eds. *Non-ulcer Dyspepsia: Therapeutic and Pathophysiological Approaches*. Paris: John Libbey Eurotext, 1991:175-81.
14. Bonfils S. Psychosomatic heterogeneity in essential dyspepsia supports syndromatic clinical presentation. In: Galmiche JP, Jian R, Mignon M, Ruszniewski Ph, eds. *Non-ulcer Dyspepsia: Therapeutic and Pathophysiological Approaches*. Paris: John Libbey Eurotext, 1991:183-94.
15. Heading RC. Prospects and priorities for research in non-ulcer dyspepsia. In: Galmiche JP, Jian R, Mignon M, Ruszniewski Ph, eds. *Non-ulcer Dyspepsia: Therapeutic and Pathophysiological Approaches*. Paris: John Libbey Eurotext, 1991:265-73.

# 20

# Pharmacological bases of therapeutics

C. SCARPIGNATO

*Institute of Pharmacology, School of Medicine and Dentistry, University of Parma, Parma, Italy*

> The desire to take medicines is perhaps the greatest feature which distinguishes man from animals.
>
> Sir William Osler
> 1904
> *Science and Immortality*

## Introduction

Dyspepsia, an ill-defined collection of upper abdominal symptoms [1], affects 25 to 30% of the community and accounts for 3 to 4% of the general practitioner consultations [2, 3]. However, for most people the symptoms are mild and transient, requiring no treatment, or are adequately controlled by over-the-counter remedies. Non-ulcer dyspepsia (NUD), for which no focal lesion or systemic disease can be found responsible, is a common syndrome. It is heterogeneous [4, 5] and has arbitrarily been subdivided into several categories such as reflux-like dyspepsia, ulcer-like dyspepsia and dysmotility-like dyspepsia [6].

Despite a substantial decline in the prevalence of peptic ulceration over the past 20 years, the incidence of dyspepsia has remained constant [3]. This syndrome continues to be a dilemma for doctors posing a diagnostic and therapeutic challenge [7]. Many patients presenting with dyspeptic symptoms have one or more clearly apparent aggravating or precipitating factors. Removal of causative agents is therefore worthwhile. Giving up smoking and reducing alcohol consumption, attempting to modify or discontinue treatment with drugs likely to cause symptoms, particularly NSAIDs, and simple dietary changes [8] may all help to ameliorate symptoms. Reassurance is also likely to prove helpful, since most patients will not have any serious underlying cause for their symptoms, and fear is likely only to perpetuate the problem.

If these lifestyle modifications fail, drug treatment is clearly indicated. Due to the heterogeneity of this syndrome and the multifactorial nature of its pathogenesis, no single drug is suitable for all patients. As a consequence, many different compounds have been used in different groups of patients. In this review the drugs currently employed in the medical treatment of NUD will be discussed, giving special emphasis to human pharmacology.

## Acid lowering drugs

Acid lowering compounds include antacids, alginates, selective muscarinic antagonists, $H_2$-receptor antagonists, substituted benzimidazoles and synthetic prostaglandins.

### Antacids

Antacids are among the most widely used medicines. Often, to be sure, they are taken as a result of self-diagnosis and self-treatment, and the trigger for buying and taking an antacid is not based on structural abnormalities but on symptoms. Patients take antacids to feel better rather than to heal an ulcer or oesophagitis.

Antacids are preparations (commonly based on aluminium compounds) that are primarily designed to neutralize gastric acid. As a consequence of the increase in gastric pH, an irreversible inactivation of pepsin occurs. Many formulations incorporate magnesium salts that counteract the constipating effect of aluminium and contribute to the acid-binding capacity [9]. It is now clear that the pharmacological actions of antacids are far beyond their acid neutralizing activity. These compounds indeed display a mucosal protective activity, mainly connected with increased synthesis and release of endogenous prostaglandins [10].

Antacids have been the backbone of the medical therapy of gastro-oesophageal reflux disease and peptic ulcer for many years and they could theoretically be useful in patients with ulcer-like dyspepsia and reflux-like dyspepsia. Surprisingly, however, the analysis of controlled clinical trials reveals that they are no more effective than placebo in all forms of NUD [11].

### Alginate containing preparations

These pharmaceutical preparations, of which the most widely known is Gaviscon®, contain alginic acid combined with small doses of antacids. In the stomach, alginic acid creates a viscous foamy raft that floats on the surface of the gastric pool, providing a mechanical barrier to reflux at the cardia. Compared with antacids, alginate containing preparations float and show a selective retention in the fundus (Fig. 1). The antacid component does not alter the pH of the gastric contents below the foam barrier and has no real neutralizing capacity [12]. By using a dual-isotope scintigraphic technique, Malmud *et al.* [13] first showed that most of the ingested alginic acid is located in the upper half of the stomach in both normal subjects and patients with gastro-oesophageal reflux. In those subjects in whom reflux did occur after treatment

*Pharmacological bases of therapeutics*

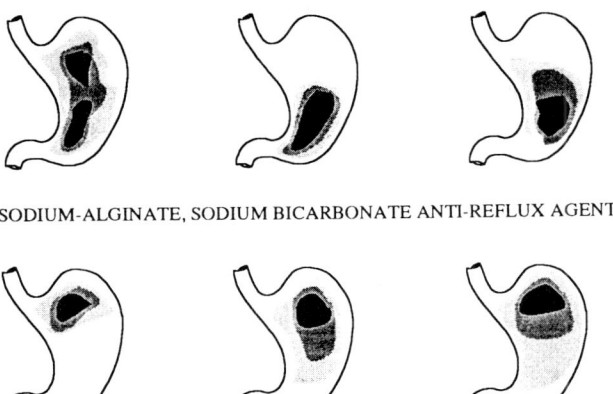

**Figure 1.** Flotation and selective retention in the fundus of the stomach of an alginate-containing anti-reflux agent compared to a conventional antacid formulation. (Redrawn from ref. [16]).

with alginic acid, the labelled compound refluxed into the oesophagus preferentially compared with the liquid content of the stomach. Therefore, when reflux occurs, this viscous foam comes into contact with the oesophageal mucosa first.

Commercial anti-reflux preparations use a wide range of alginate materials. It is difficult to correlate their properties with those of the alginate, since the alginate used is rarely specified by the manufacturer, and a wide range of particulates are added to many formulations (e.g. particulate antacids). The alginates used in the anti-reflux formulations fall into two groups; the soluble salts (sodium and potassium alginates), which form a gel by reaction with gastric acid, and the insoluble alginates (alginic acid, calcium and magnesium alginate) which primarily form a gel by rehydration. Often these two types of material may be mixed in a particular formulation. Even in the same formulation the composition varies greatly from country to country (Table I). This is the case of liquid Gaviscon®, which is manufactured under licence by different pharmaceutical companies. An interesting study [14] compared four international preparations of liquid Gaviscon® and found that each formulation possesses markedly different raft strength (Fig. 2) and neutralization profiles. The inclusion of antacids into the formulation increased the neutralization capacity within the raft, but decreased the breaking strength and hence the ability of the raft to form a viscous "plug" in the opening of the oesophagus as a barrier to reflux. This suggests that the modes of action may be different even though the trade names of the formulations are the same. And this, of course, complicates comparison of the results obtained in different clinical trials from different countries.

Another component of these anti-reflux formulations critical for raft formation is the gas-producing agent. Without it, the formulation would mix and empty with the

**Table I.** Liquid Gaviscon® formulations in various countries.

| Formulation | U.K. | Canada | U.S.A. | Sweden |
|---|---|---|---|---|
| Sodium alginate | 500 mg | 500 mg | 267 mg | 500 mg |
| Sodium bicarbonate | 267 mg | * | — | 170 mg |
| Aluminium hydroxide | — | 200 mg | 63.3 mg | 1 g |
| Magnesium carbonate | — | — | 275 mg | — |
| Calcium carbonate | — | — | — | 150 mg |

* Quoted as 60 mg of sodium/10 ml which is equivalent to 219 mg of sodium bicarbonate/10 ml.

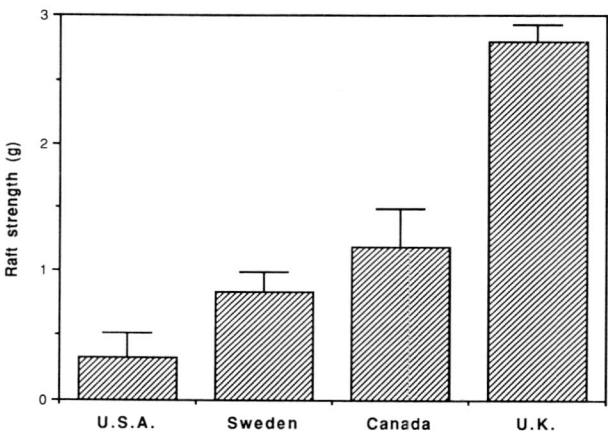

**Figure 2.** Raft strengths of the minimum recommended doses of liquid Gaviscon® available in four different countries. (From ref. [14]).

meal [15]. Its concentration is crucial, too. Indeed, too much gas formation can disrupt and weaken the raft, while gas, which is generated too rapidly or too slowly, will not be trapped in the gel. The rate at which the gas-producing agent can react with the gastric content will depend on many factors such as the quantity of particulate antacid present in the formulation, and the acid available in the stomach, which in turn depends on the type, volume and buffering capacity of the meal present. There will be a competition for free $H^+$ ions available within the stomach between the gas-producing agent, particulate antacid and food. Generally, the gas-producing agent is sodium bicarbonate. In an attempt to reduce the sodium content of some formulations, potassium salt has been substituted to it, but these formulations have less buoyancy than those containing sodium bicarbonate [16]. A novel method of incorporating the gas-producing agent is the use of an aerosol device to inject gas in order to produce a foam prior to administration (Topaal Whip®). The foam is ejected onto a spoon and is then swallowed. This formulation does not rely on the erratic quantity of acid present in the stomach to ensure flotation.

Anti-reflux preparations do not have an inherent capacity to be retained in an empty stomach for prolonged periods of time and it is essential that they are given *after a meal* to ensure gastric flotation [17]. When the anti-reflux agent is taken on an empty stomach, the formulation sinks to the base of the greater curvature and 50% is emptied within 20 min of administration. When the formulation is taken 30 min before, the anti-reflux agent does not float on a meal ingested subsequently, but the food actually displaces the anti-reflux agent from the fundus to the antrum as it is ingested. Once in the antrum, which has virtually no capacity for acid secretion, the anti-reflux agent is caught up by the mixing and grinding action of this region. It will then become diluted with the fluid from the meal and thus it empties ahead of the meal *without forming a raft*. This elegant scintigraphic study demonstrates the importance of the correct dosing regimen of anti-reflux agents with respect to meals.

Several studies, by using pH-monitoring of the distal oesophagus, have demonstrated a significant decrease in episodes or quantity of reflux after administration of alginate containing preparations [18]. Quite recently, Washington [19] used an oesophageal pH probe coupled with a small gamma-detector strapped to the chest wall and, by using a radiolabelled meal, was able to show that 20 ml of liquid Gaviscon®, administered 30 min after the meal, significantly reduced the amount of both acid and food reflux into the oesophagus (Fig. 3).

Several placebo-controlled trials have demonstrated that these alginate containing preparations are effective in relieving heartburn and reflux symptoms [20] and therefore suggest their use for symptomatic relief in patients with reflux-like dyspepsia.

**Combined alginate/$H_2$-antagonist formulations**

A combined formulation of this kind is commercially available in the U.K. (i.e. Algitec®). Each tablet of Algitec® contains 500 mg alginic acid and 200 mg cimetidine. The recommended daily dosage for adults is 1-2 tablets four times daily after meals for 4 or 8 weeks. The combined alginate-cimetidine formulation has no additional benefit over cimetidine alone in the healing of oesophagitis, but it does produce better symptomatic relief [21], despite the fact that there is only half the dose of cimetidine in the alginate-cimetidine formulation compared to the standard cimetidine treatment. Cimetidine-alginate combinations are also reported to provide better symptomatic relief than alginic acid-antacid combinations [22]. According to the manufacturer's data sheet, the absorption of cimetidine is not significantly affected by the presence of alginic acid. However, there is some evidence that the absorption of the $H_2$-antagonist from the combined formulation is decreased and slowed [23], although co-administration of cimetidine with liquid Gaviscon® in two separate formulations does not affect the availability of cimetidine [24].

**Selective muscarinic antagonists**

Compounds which display a selective high affinity for $M_1$-receptors are termed selective muscarinic antagonists. $M_1$-receptors, like nicotinic receptors, are located

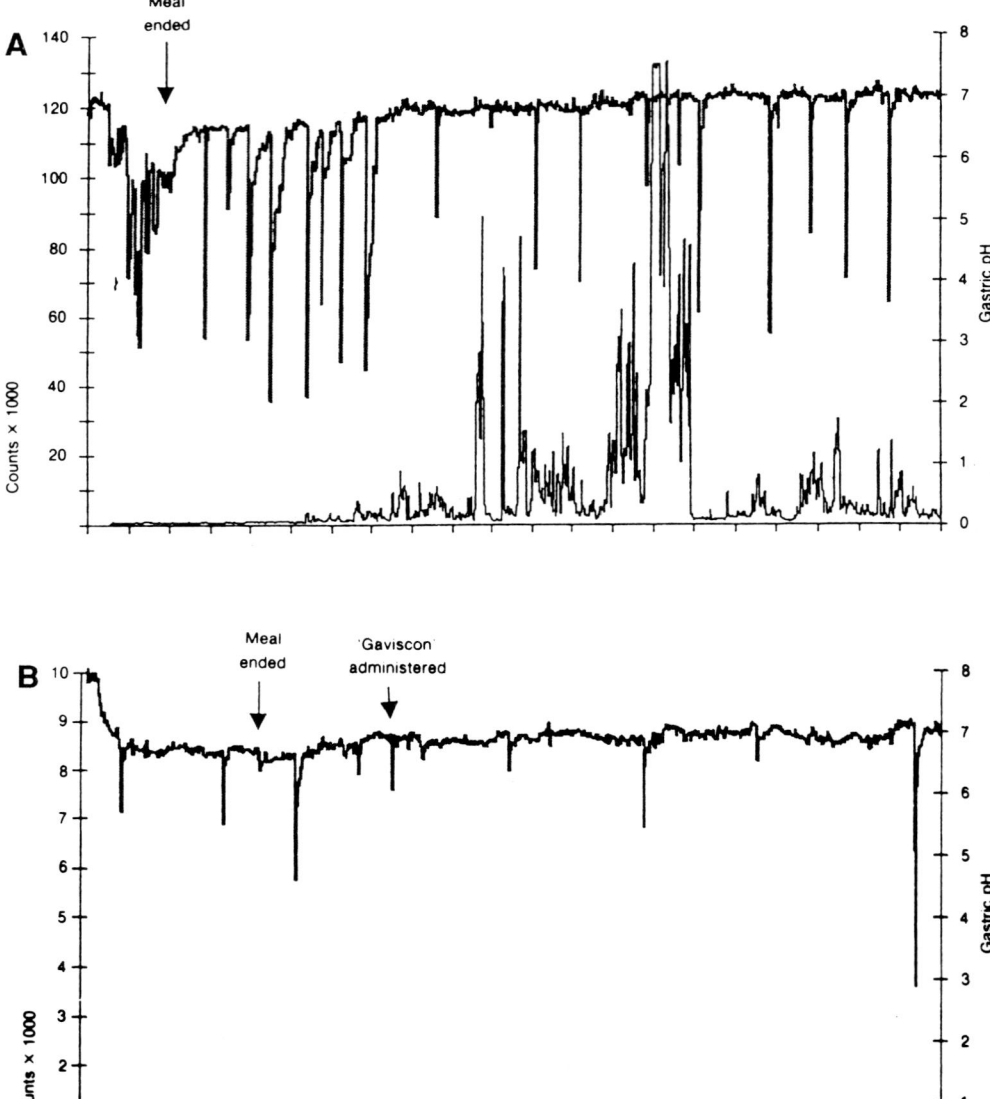

**Figure 3.** Postprandial reflux of acid (top tracing) and radiolabelled food (bottom tracing) into the oesophagus. **A.** untreated control; **B.** after 20 ml of liquid Gaviscon® (UK). (From ref. [19]).

mainly in sympathetic ganglia, whereas $M_2$-receptors exist in sympathetic nerve endings (where they inhibit noradrenaline release) and in gastrointestinal and possibly vascular smooth muscle [25]. The first and best known member of this class of drugs is pirenzepine to which telenzepine, an analogue having an altered tricyclic structure and an unchanged side-chain, was recently added.

Oral therapeutic doses of pirenzepine have no adverse effect on oesophageal and gastric motility [26]. Due to its antisecretory activity, the compound was found to be capable of significantly reducing oesophageal exposure to acid [27], an effect not shared by telenzepine [28] most probably because of the strong inhibition of salivary secretion with consequent reduction of oesophageal clearing.

The efficacy of pirenzepine in NUD has been evaluated in several trials. Although a recent meta-analysis showed an overall therapeutic gain of 25% [29], the high percentage (i.e. about 50%) of patients experiencing untoward effects (mainly dry mouth) renders this compound not a first choice drug in patients with NUD.

## $H_2$-receptor antagonists

Five compounds belonging to this class of drugs (namely cimetidine, ranitidine, nizatidine, famotidine and roxatidine) are currently available. These drugs are extremely safe and effective for the treatment of various acid-related disorders [30-31]. Although their chemical structures are different, the mechanism of their antisecretory action is identical, i.e. a competitive inhibition of $H_2$-receptors located on the parietal cells, with the consequent reduction of intracellular cyclic AMP concentrations and reduction of acid secretion (Fig. 4). However, they possess non-antisecretory effects that may be connected to $H_2$-receptor blockade (specific effects) or be independent of this main action (non-specific effects) [26]. The first are class-dependent, whereas the second are mainly connected with the structure of the single molecules of the family.

Although intravenous administration of some $H_2$-blockers was found capable of modifying lower oesophageal sphincter pressure and gastric emptying in humans [18], effective oral doses of these compounds do not significantly affect the motor activity of the gastrointestinal tract.

The usual dose regimen varies for the different compounds according to their antisecretory potency. The relative potencies of the five $H_2$-blockers in inhibiting the secretion of gastric acid vary from 20 to 50-fold, cimetidine and famotidine being the least and the most potent, respectively. Pharmacokinetic parameters (Table II) are not dissimilar among the different compounds [32, 33], with the exception of oral bioavailability which is higher for nizatidine and roxatidine. This last compound also displays the longest half-life. With ordinary doses, the duration of a serum concentration above the level of 50% inhibition ranges from approximately 6 h for cimetidine to approximately 10 h for the other $H_2$-antagonists.

When equiactive antisecretory doses are employed, the efficacy of the different compounds is virtually identical. Many different factors, however, can influence the extent and the duration of antisecretory action [34]. These include the dose, the frequency of administration, the time of dosing and the effect of food and smoking. In summary, to produce a substantial effect on intragastric acidity during the day, $H_2$-antagonists must be administered frequently and in high dosage. Increasing the dose is more effective than adding an anticholinergic drug. The duration of their nocturnal

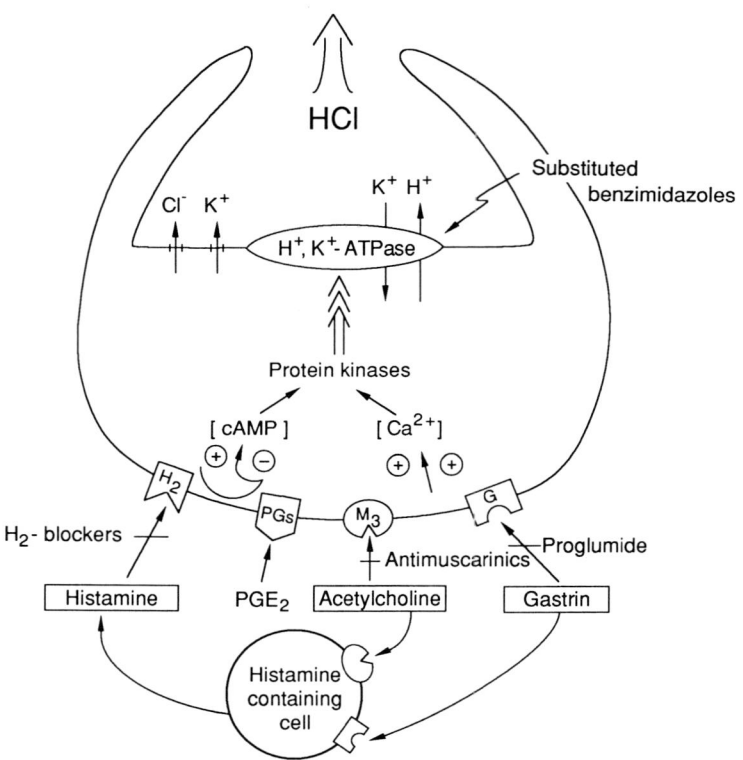

**Figure 4.** Receptors, mediators and drugs involved in the physiopharmacological control of acid secretion by the parietal cell.

antisecretory effect can be prolonged by giving them in the early evening rather than at bedtime. However, it is probably of more importance that food is avoided after the last dose of the day.

$H_2$-receptor antagonists (especially cimetidine) have been tested in many randomized clinical trials. These compounds usually reduce the severity of dyspeptic symptoms and have been employed successfully in patients with reflux-like or ulcer-like dyspepsia [11], although some trials have shown them to be no more effective than placebo [5]. In any event, the meta-analysis performed by Dobrilla and coworkers [29] found for this class of drugs an overall therapeutic gain of 18%.

**Substituted benzimidazoles**

These drugs represent a new class of antisecretory agents. Omeprazole, the first member of the class, was recently introduced in clinical practice, and other derivatives

**Table II.** Pharmacokinetic parameters of the currently available $H_2$-receptor antagonists*.

| Variable | Cimetidine | Ranitidine | Nizatidine | Famotidine | Roxatidine |
|---|---|---|---|---|---|
| **Absorption** | | | | | |
| Bioavailability (%) | 30-80 (60) | 30-88 (50) | 75-100 (98) | 37-45 (43) | 90-99 (95) |
| Time to peak serum concentration (h) | 1-2 | 1-3 | 1-3 | 1-3.5 | 1-3 |
| **Distribution** | | | | | |
| Volume (l/kg of body weight) | 0.8-1.2 | 1.2-1.9 | 1.2-1.6 | 1.1-1.4 | 1.7 |
| Protein binding in serum (%) | 13-26 | 15 | 26-35 | 16 | 6-7 |
| CFS: serum ratio [1] | 0.18 | 0.06-0.17 | Unknown | 0.05-0.09 | 0-0.09 |
| Breast milk: serum ratio | 4.6-11.8:1 | 1.9-23.8:1 | Unknown | 0.41-1.78:1 | 0.0022:1 |
| Fetal: maternal ratio | 0.4-0.8:1 | Unknown | Unknown | 0.06:1 | Unknown |
| **Elimination** | | | | | |
| Total systemic clearance (ml/min) | 450-650 | 568-709 | 667-850 | 417-483 | 327-379 |
| Half-life in serum (h) | 1.5-2.3 | 1.6-2.4 | 1.1-1.6 | 2.5-4 | 5.7-6.3 |
| Hepatic clearance (%) | | | | | |
| Oral | 60 | 73 | 22 | 50-80 | 47 |
| Intravenous | 25-40 | 30 | 25 | 25-30 | 33 |
| Renal clearance (%) | | | | | |
| Oral | 40 | 27 | 57-65 | 25-30 | 53 |
| Intravenous | 50-80 | 50 | 75 | 65-80 | 67 |

\* Average values are shown in parentheses.   [1] CSF denotes cerebrospinal fluid.

(i.e. lansoprazole, pantoprazole, etc.) are under extensive clinical investigation. Their mechanism of action represents a new principle, as they interact with gastric $H^+$, $K^+$-ATPase, the enzyme constituting the final step in the formation of gastric acid (Fig. 4) [35]. This specific inhibitory action on the "proton pump" offers a unique and highly selective means of controlling acid secretion. When given in single morning doses of 20 mg or greater, omeprazole significantly reduces acid secretion for as long as 24 h, despite its short half-life (about 1 h) [36]. This behaviour can be easily explained taking into account that omeprazole concentrates in the parietal cell, where it is converted into the active metabolite, sulfenamide, which irreversibly inactivates the $H^+$, $K^+$, ATPase, located in the region of the secretory canaliculus. Omeprazole is therefore the most potent and long-acting antisecretory compound today available. As a result, its efficacy on dyspectic symptoms is of a magnitude never seen before. But, as with all potent drugs, the danger for indiscriminate and inappropriate use calls for careful diagnostic evaluation before starting treatment. This drug should therefore be reserved for severe peptic diseases with resistant dyspectic symptoms and should not be used for the trivial symptomatology of NUD.

Due to the virtual suppression of acid secretion achieved with this compound, omeprazole could be employed as a "pharmacological tool" to investigate further the role of acid in the pathogenesis of NUD.

## Synthetic prostaglandins

Prostaglandins (PGs) are a family of polyunsaturated oxygenated fatty acids endowed with gastroprotective, antisecretory and anti-ulcer actions [37]. The natural PGs require parenteral administration and their duration of action does not exceed 1 h. In order to obtain PGs with oral and long-acting properties, analogues have been synthesized. In contrast to the natural ones, synthetic PGs do not have adverse effects on gastrointestinal motility [38]. Due to their pharmacological properties, these compounds should be useful in patients with NUD. However, a recent double-blind, placebo-controlled, multicentre study [39] showed that misoprostol treatment had a significant worsening effect on epigastric pain, nausea, meteorism, lower abdominal pain and diarrhoea as compared with placebo in patients with NUD and erosive prepyloric changes. Since many trials [5, 40, 41] suggest that aspirin and other NSAIDs induce acute dyspepsia more often than placebo, PGs should be reserved to patients taking NSAIDs in whom misoprostol (and probably other synthetic derivatives) improves dyspeptic symptoms and prevents mucosal lesions [42].

## Mucosal protective compounds

These agents include sucralfate, colloidal bismuth subcitrate (CBS) and sulglicotide. Sucralfate and CBS are non-antisecretory compounds which also display *site-protective actions,* i.e. they adhere to the mucosa and form a mechanical layer that insulates the underlying mucosa from luminal acid and pepsin. Both compounds possess gastroprotective properties which are partially prostaglandin-dependent.

Sucralfate is a basic aluminium salt of sulphated sucrose that forms stable complexes with protein molecules, which in turn are resistant to the proteolytic action of pepsin. It also inhibits peptic activity by adsorbing pepsin itself. When exposed to gastric acid, it turns into a highly condensed, viscous, adhesive substance which retains most of its acid-buffering capacities. The affinity of sucralfate for inflamed mucosa is explained by the drug's viscous adhesiveness and the formation of polyvalent bridges between the negatively charged sucralfate polyanions and the positively charged proteins present in high concentrations in mucosal lesions [43]. In summary, almost all the mechanisms involved in mucosal protection are affected by sucralfate. The basis for the *acute protective action* of sucralfate is its effect on the normal gastric mucosa enhancing the natural defensive mechanisms, stimulating mucus, bicarbonate and prostaglandin release as well as mucus cell renewal. The *therapeutic action* of sucralfate is most likely the result of: (a) a local action on ulcerated areas of the mucosa by formation of a protective barrier reducing pepsin and acid injury to the mucosa; (b) binding of pepsin and bile acids; and (c) a trophic effect on the entire mucosa which facilitates healing and re-epithelization. The *long-term prophylactic efficacy* of sucralfate is probably due to its chronic trophic action on the gastric mucosa.

The above-cited pharmacological properties provide the rationale for the use of sucralfate in dyspeptic patients with erosive and non-erosive gastritis, especially those taking NSAIDs in whom the compound seems to be particularly effective [11].

Colloidal bismuth subcitrate (De-Nol®), a complex bismuth salt of citric acid, exhibits strong mucosal protective activity in both animals and man. It prevents gastric mucosal damage induced by a variety of noxious agents in laboratory animals and displays high efficacy in healing gastroduodenal ulceration in humans [43]. In the stomach, CBS is rapidly converted to bismuth oxyde and oxychloride and combines with proteinaceous material at the ulcer base to form a mechanically stable coating. The action of CBS is however rather complex and has been clarified only recently. Many of the mechanisms involved in mucosal protection are affected by the drug. The mechanisms involved in its a*cute protective action* (i.e. experimentally-induced lesions in animals and NSAID-induced gastric damage in humans) are likely to be the stimulation of mucus, bicarbonate, and prostaglandin release, whereas those implicated in the *therapeutic action* (healing of gastric and duodenal ulcers) are mainly the formation of a mechanical layer that insulates the underlying mucosa from luminal acid and pepsin and stimulates reparative processes, as well as the bactericidal action against *Helicobacter pylori*. This last action, which gives rise to eradication of bacteria and clearing of associated histological gastritis, is also believed to be important in the prevention of ulcer relapse. CBS inhibits the growth of *H. pylori in vitro* with MICs ranging between 2 and 64 mg/litre. Other anti-ulcer preparations are ineffective. In contrast with other antimicrobials (i.e. ofloxacine or metronidazole), no *H. pylori* resistance to CBS has been reported, as yet. In patients with *H. pylori* colonization, the compound produced marked changes in the organisms and their relationship with the epithelium. Between 60 and 95 min after ingestion, the organisms were mostly in the gastric mucus layer rather than beneath it. Most of the bacterial profiles were irregular or fragmented, with structural degradation ranging from focal vacuolation beneath the cell wall to gross vacuolation with retraction and condensation of the bacterial contents. Deposits of electron-dense material, presumably bismuth, were present in the external surfaces and within the bacteria [44] (Fig. 5).

There is now growing evidence suggesting that *H. pylori* and associated histological gastritis may play a role in NUD [45-47]. Clearance of the bacteria and histological improvement is often associated with a significant decrease in symptoms [45]. Although the correlation between symptomatic improvement and bacterial clearance is not always high, a recent meta-analysis [48] concluded that a treatment leading to clearance of *H. pylori* in at least 75% of patients is followed by a significant symptom relief. CBS on its own is very effective at clearing the organism, but eradication is more difficult. Antibacterial combinations (like for instance CBS with amoxicillin or/and a nitro-imidazole drug) will be more successful, with triple therapy achieving 90% eradication [49].

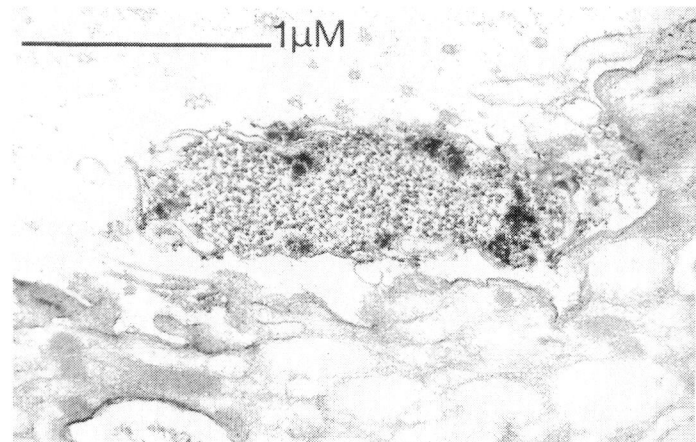

**Figure 5.** Marked structural degradation with selective deposition of particulate bismuth complex in and on the surface of *H. pylori* organisms in a biopsy specimen taken 2 hours after oral administration of CBS. (Courtesy of Professor G.N.J. Tytgat, Academic Medical Centre, Amsterdam).

The best strategy for bismuth therapy would be to give it with meals so as to keep the drug in the stomach as long as possible, as well as to distribute it widely within the stomach. Administration of CBS in the fasting patient may result in most of the agent passing into the small intestine before the formulation can dissolve or disperse. Administration with meals may provide for prolonged residence in the stomach. The grinding and mixing functions of the stomach may also ensure wide dispersal. Eating is associated with desquamation of surface cells and discharge of mucus, possibly exposing the organisms to higher concentrations of the agent [50].

The best formulation is unknown, but one would predict that the formulation (tablet, capsule, liquid, etc.) may have a profound influence on agents that are expected to act topically. Subtle differences in formulation may result in marked differences in effectiveness, and studies are needed comparing dosage formulations, salts, and administration in relation to meals. Frequency of administration is also important whereas the duration of treatment seems not to be so crucial. Indeed, whereas a q.i.d. dose appears more effective than a b.i.d. dose, an 8-week treatment has no advantage over one of 4 weeks [49].

Among patients with NUD, those positive for *H. pylori* and with active antral gastritis will have the better chance of symptomatic improvement under De-Nol® therapy. The decision to initiate anti-*H. pylori* treatment should not be undertaken lightly. One popular image is that anti-*H.pylori* therapy will cure *H. pylori* related diseases. This is not always true because the clinical and bacteriological outcomes of the therapy are not necessarily parallel and the results of treatment are therefore unpredictable.

Sulglycotide (Gliptide®) is an extractive polysulphated glycopeptide, isolated from pig duodenum, endowed with anti-ulcer and prostaglandin-dependent gastroprotective activity [51]. It also displays a lysosomal membrane stabilizing activity [52] and stimulates gastric bicarbonate secretion in man [53].

Due to its peculiar pharmacological activity, this compound could be useful in patients with NUD and those taking NSAIDs. Preliminary data seem to suggest that — in the above-cited clinical conditions — sulglycotide has an effectiveness similar to that of sucralfate [11].

## Motor stimulating compounds

The consistency with which positive effects have been reported in studies on patients with NUD indicated that there is place for motor stimulating compounds in the treatment of this syndrome. These compounds have been extensively used in the past for the treatment of various actual or alleged gastrointestinal motility disorders, and their popularity precedes the recognition of any consistent abnormalities.

Schematically, and oversimplicistically of course, one could envisage the motor functions as the expression of a balance at the level of the smooth muscle cells between inhibitory mechanisms mainly regulated by dopamine levels and stimulatory events mainly regulated through release of acetylcholine [18]. It follows from this balance that gastrointestinal motility can be stimulated both by dopamine antagonists, such as metoclopramide, domperidone and L-sulpiride, or by substances which release acetylcholine such as metoclopramide or cisapride, or directly by cholinergic drugs which bind and act on muscarinic receptors of the smooth muscle cell, for example bethanechol [18]. A true prokinetic agent is one that not only enhances motility, but also coordinates the activity between the different segments of the gastrointestinal tract. In this respect, only a narrow choice is available. Among the existing prokinetic compounds, dopamine antagonists, on the one hand, and cholinomimetic drugs, on the other hand, should be distinguished (Table III). Since compounds endowed with dopamine antagonism have the disadvantage of causing neuro-endocrine side-effects and/or extrapyramidal dyskinetic reactions (seen especially after metoclopramide), the recently developed non-cholinergic non-antidopaminergic compound, cisapride, seems to be the most promising one. Its *main* mechanism of action is considered to be the stimulation of myenteric cholinergic nerves with consequent increase of acetylcholine release [54, 55]. An interaction of the drug with serotonin receptors (i.e. inhibition of $5-HT_3$ receptors and stimulation of $5-HT_4$) was recently reported [56, 57].

Prokinetic compounds have been found to be capable of counterbalancing the motor derangements often present in functional dyspepsia and may therefore be useful in the medical treatment of this syndrome. In this connection a recent meta-analysis of the trials conducted with these drugs showed a distinct overall superiority for this class of drugs as compared with placebo with a therapeutic gain of 46%. It must be pointed out however that, although positive results have been reported with all the available drugs [11, 58, 59], the use of small and rather ill-defined patients populations (sometimes including patients with various organic disorders) and of multiple end-point variables in many trials, suggests that some caution is needed in interpreting the results and in transferring them to clinical practice.

## A look to the future

### CCK-antagonists

Although the pancreas and gallbladder are the principal target organs of cholecystokinin (CCK) in the gastrointestinal tract, CCK receptors are found to be

**Table III.** Currently available motor stimulating compounds.

| Mechanism of action | Compound |
| --- | --- |
| Direct action on muscarinic receptors | Bethanechol |
|  | Metoclopramide |
| Dopamine-receptor ($D_2$) antagonism | Metoclopramide |
|  | Clebopride |
|  | L-Sulpiride |
|  | Domperidone |
| Enhanced acetylcholine release | Metoclopramide |
|  | Cisapride |
| Interaction with serotonin receptors ($5-HT_3$ antagonism*/$5-HT_4$ agonism) | Cisapride |

\* Metoclopramide and clebopride also display $5-HT_3$ antagonist activity at very high doses (as those used to prevent chemotherapy-induced emesis).

present throughout the gut, and on the smooth muscle of the stomach, gallbladder, small intestine and colon. It is therefore conceivable that CCK has a physiological role not only in the stimulation of pancreatic and biliary secretions, but also in the regulation of gastrointestinal motility. Inhibition of lower oesophageal sphincter pressure and gastric emptying are among the physiological actions of CCK [60]. The recent discovery of potent and specific CCK-receptor antagonists has stimulated a broad array of investigations into the physiological actions of this hormone and to examine its putative pathophysiological role in certain diseases [61]. Among the available compounds, a glutaramic acid derivative (i.e. the compound CR1505 called loxiglumide) has been studied in humans.

Although no effect on basal lower oesophageal sphincter pressure was evident, the compound was able to counteract the meal-induced decrease in sphincter's pressure [62]. It could therefore be able to prevent or reduce postprandial reflux. Loxiglumide was also found to accelerate gastric emptying of radiopaque markers after a *liquid* test meal [63] and to improve the delayed gastric emptying of a *solid-liquid* meal in patients with non-ulcer dyspepsia [64]. Corazziari and his coworkers [65], however, by using a solid meal were unable to confirm the gastrokinetic effect of loxiglumide. This peculiar pharmacological effect, which may also be useful in the treatment of gastro-oesophageal reflux disease, needs to be further investigated.

*Motilin-receptor agonists*

Motilin seems to affect mainly, but not exclusively, the proximal part of the gastrointestinal tract [66]. The peptide has no significant influence upon the contractile activity of the gut during the digestive state. Conversely, in the interdigestive state, it induces the cyclic recurrent episodes of caudal moving bands of strong contractions that move from the lower oesophageal sphincter to the terminal ileum. Exogenous motilin infusion was shown to increase LOS pressure and gastric emptying in humans [66], but this peptide is obviously not suitable for use as a gastrokinetic because of its short half-life and the need of intravenous administration.

Recent studies have shown that erythromycin mimics the effect of motilin on gastrointestinal motility [67]. Erythromycin and related 14-member macrolide compounds inhibit the binding of motilin to its receptors on gastrointestinal smooth muscle membranes and may therefore act as motilin agonists [68, 69]. The contractile activity of these drugs is similar to that induced by motilin and cannot be blocked by atropine or TTX, thus suggesting a direct effect upon smooth muscle cells [69]. As with motilin, their action on gastrointestinal smooth muscle is $Ca^{++}$-dependent [70]. In fact, recent papers have shown erythromycin to be capable of accelerating emptying rate in diabetic gastroparesis (Fig. 6) [71, 72] and increasing lower oesophageal sphincter pressure in healthy volunteers (73), thus confirming that this antibiotic behaves as a gastrokinetic compound. Since the drug is active when given orally, long-term, placebo-controlled studies of the oral administration of erythromycin should be undertaken to determine its therapeutic efficacy in patients with disordered motility. Further development of this class of drugs, now called *motilides,* will depend on the development of compounds devoid of antibiotic activity (like for instance ME-34 and EM-523) and the absence of fading of the gastrokinetic effect during prolonged administration.

# Pharmacological bases of therapeutics

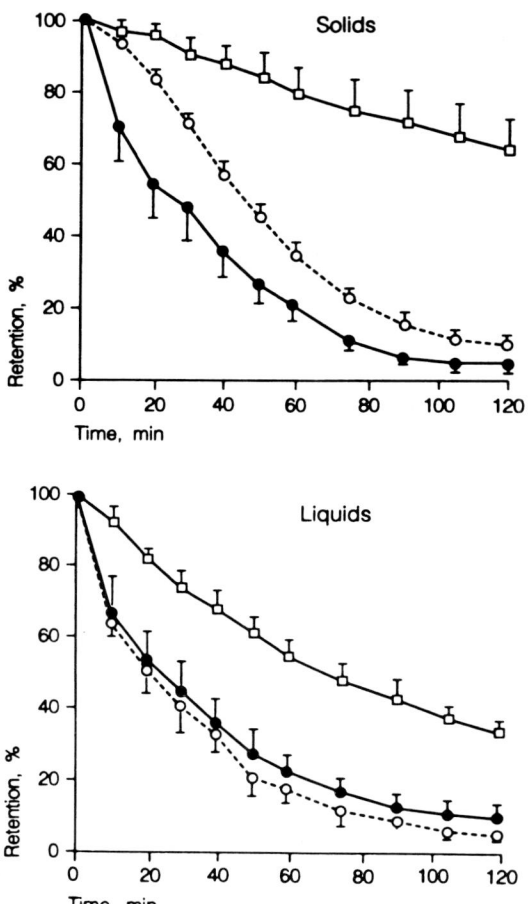

**Figure 6.** Dual isotope gastric emptying study of the effect of erythromycin in diabetic gastroparesis. Curves show the retention of the different phases of the meal for the diabetics given placebo (□), the diabetics given erythromycin (●) and healthy controls (○). (From ref. [71]).

## 5-HT$_3$-receptor antagonists

It is well-known that metoclopramide is an effective, albeit weak, antagonist of 5-HT$_3$-receptors which have been found only to be associated with peripheral autonomic, afferent and enteric neurones [74]. The effectiveness — as antiemetic and motor stimulating compounds — of some selective 5-HT$_3$ antagonists (ICS 205-930, Ondansetron, Granisetron, MDL 72222 and BRL 24924), *devoid of any effect on dopamine receptors,* suggested that the blockade of these sites plays an important role in the mechanism of action of metoclopramide [75]. As a consequence, the potential of 5-HT$_3$-antagonists as gastrokinetic drugs has been explored in both animals and humans. In accordance with results obtained in laboratory animals [76], one of these compounds (i.e. ICS 205-930) was found to increase lower oesophageal sphincter pressure [77] and gastric emptying [78] in normal subjects. Provided this gastrokinetic profile can be confirmed in patients with upper digestive motility disorders, these compounds will deserve to be tested in clinical trials to evaluate their clinical potential.

**Summary and perspectives**

Drugs enhancing gastrointestinal motility and coordination are now available. These compounds are not only able to correct the underlying pathophysiological disorder (i.e. deranged upper gut motility in NUD) but also to improve the associated symptoms. Further work is needed to determine the predictive value of objective anomalies for the efficacy of a drug in the individual patient. This is the crucial point to define a rational strategy in clinical practice, especially to establish if functional investigation is needed before a gastrokinetic drug be given.

## Pancreatic enzymes

The clinically accepted indication for pancreatic enzyme therapy is restricted to a small group of patients with steatorrhoea due to pancreatic exocrine insufficiency [79, 80]. Pancreatic enzymes, however, are often prescribed to patients with various dyspeptic complaints. The rationale for such a liberal prescription of pancreatic enzymes is incomplete.

Experimental studies have shown that, in some species including man, intestinal trypsin controls pancreatic secretion via a negative cholecystokinin (CCK)-mediated feedback mechanism [81, 82]. Since pancreatic enzymes have also been reported to relieve pain and other dyspeptic symptoms in patients with chronic pancreatitis in the absence of steatorrhoea [79], their efficacy was also tested in patients with NUD. Although old investigations [83] and anecdotal reports have suggested some benefit, a recent well-conducted placebo-controlled study [84] failed to show any advantage. The study was, however, restricted to short-term (4 days) periods of treatment and therefore the possibility that a longer treatment with pancreatic enzymes could have a beneficial effect cannot be ruled out.

## Biliary acids

It was only a few years after the advent of chenodeoxycholic acid (CDCA) for medical cholesterol gallstone therapy that ursodeoxycholic acid (UDCA) was introduced in oral cholelitholysis and proved to be as effective as CDCA. Some 60-80% of all gallstone patients treated with UDCA or CDCA are free of symptoms within a couple of weeks following the onset of therapy. Non stone-related dyspeptic complaints can be improved under UDCA therapy as well. Masuda et al. [85] were first to publish a controlled study of 104 patients where UDCA (150 or 600 mg/day) proved to be better than placebo, with the lower dose being more efficacious. Similar results were reported recently by Pazzi and his coworkers [86].

Modification of bile acid composition by UDCA may explain its favourable effect on dyspeptic symptoms [87]. It is well-known indeed that — in contrast to the other endogenous biliary acids — UDCA is virtually devoided of damaging effects on the gastro-oesophageal mucosa [88]. This rationale of use should however rely on a clear demonstration of an abnormal duodenogastric reflux (DGR) in patients with NUD. Fournet and his coworkers [89, 90] recently showed that this is not the case. Indeed they found no evidence of increased DGR, either in the postprandial [90] or in the interdigestive [89] period, in NUD patients compared with control (healthy) subjects. As a result, drug therapy *specifically* directed to control DGR (i.e. bile acids sequestrants, UDCA) should not routinely be used in NUD and should be reserved for the individual patient in whom a *quantitatively pathological* DGR can be demonstrated.

UDCA also affects gallbladder motility. Gallbladder contraction in response to exogenous CCK is reduced after treatment with UDCA [91]. This could explain the remarkable symptomatic improvement in patients with *painful* NUD.

## Adsorbing and defoaming agents

Dyspeptic symptoms are frequently attributed to abnormal development of gas in the gastrointestinal tract, but the nature and importance of this phenomenon are difficult to evaluate. The origin of gastrointestinal gas is schematically represented in Figure 4. Intraluminal gas, including methane, which is produced in appreciable amounts only in 30% of the population, can spread freely through the mucosa [92, 93]. The only factor determining the direction of the gas flow (blood-lumen or lumen-blood) is the partial-pressure gradient.

Although it may be possible that defective swallowing and abnormal output of gas are among the causes of disorders contributing to the overall symptomatology of dyspepsia, it is very difficult to provide confirmation of this hypothesis on the basis of objective data. Some studies [94, 95] have indeed failed to show any difference in gastric gas content between patients with flatulent dyspepsia and control subjects, either in the fasting condition or after a meal. In dyspeptic patients, however, gut sensitivity to distension by intraluminal gas could be more pronounced than in healthy subjects [96-98].

Besides avoiding gas-producing foods [93], administration of simethicone and/or activated charcoal may also contribute to relief of abdominal discomfort in patients with flatulent dyspepsia. Activated charcoal, an odourless, tasteless fine black powder, is the residue from the destructive distillation of various organic materials, treated to increase its adsorptive power. The adsorptive capacity of various brands of activated charcoal differs enormously; a finely powdered activated charcoal with high adsorptive capacity is satisfactory. Some double-blind randomized trials have shown that activated charcoal is effective in controlling dyspeptic symptoms (mainly pain and flatulence) and in decreasing the amount of expired hydrogen, but these results have not been confirmed in other investigations [93]. Although the compound is relatively non-toxic when given by mouth, gastrointestinal disturbances such as vomiting and constipation have been reported. It may also colour the faeces black.

Simethicone, a mixture of dimethylpolysyloxanes, is a gastric defoaming agent. By reducing their surface tension, it causes gas bubbles to be broken or to coalesce into a form that can be eliminated more easily by belching or passing flatus. It has no activity as an antacid. Although its effectiveness has been questioned [99], this compound may also be useful in patients with reflux-like dyspepsia by decreasing intragastric pressure [100]. Lower oesophageal sphincter competence is indeed dependent on intragastric pressure [101, 102].

Simethicone is used alone or in combination with antacids. It must be pointed out, however, that simethicone defoaming activity is greatly reduced when combined with aluminium hydroxide [103]. The observed low activity suggests that the defoaming agent is adsorbed onto antacid, rendering both substances less available. Therefore, the combination of simethicone with antacids, at least those containing aluminium, is questionable.

## Sodium cromoglycate and other anti-allergic compounds

Food allergy is a complex syndrome. Different pathophysiological mechanisms are involved and a broad variety of organs and apparati can be affected [104]. The incidence of dyspeptic symptoms in patients with food allergy is relatively high, approaching 20% [105]. As a consequence, allergic mechanisms should be looked for in patients with NUD. Diagnosis of food allergy is difficult but, once made, calls for appropriate treatment. This includes avoidance of suspected food(s) and pharmacological therapy.

Preventive treatment is usually made with oral sodium cromoglycate whereas symptomatic treatment involves the use of classic antihistamines ($H_1$-receptor antagonists), antiserotonin compounds and even steroids. The primary action of sodium cromoglycate is considered to be stabilization of mast cells and consequent inhibition of the release of preformed and membrane-derived mediators. It also displays some anti-inflammatory and calcium antagonistic actions [106]. The compound (250-500 mg), which is well tolerated and has no side effects, is given half-an-hour before the meals.

## Psychotropic drugs

Emotional factors are often presumed to influence functional disorders of the gut because stress alters secretion, motility and vascularization [107]. Since NUD is suspected to be a disorder of function, emotional factors have been thought to be important and psychotropic drugs have been proposed in patients with NUD. The compounds most often employed are benzodiazepines and tricyclic antidepressants. Besides their central action, these drugs inhibit nocturnal and stimulate diurnal acid secretion [108-110], an effect which could be beneficial in patients with ulcer-like dyspepsia. The lower oesophageal sphincter pressure lowering effect of benzodiazepines [111] and the anticholinergic effect of tricyclic compounds make them unsuitable for those patients who fall in the group of reflux-like dyspepsia. Benzodiazepines also possess a remarkable muscle-relaxant activity and can reduce gastrointestinal motility. *In vitro* experiments [Scarpignato, unpublished observations] have actually shown high dose diazepam to be capable of inhibiting both basal and stimulated gut motility.

Although psychotropic drugs are frequently prescribed to patients with NUD, no double-blind trial has been performed as yet. Due to possibility of abuse and dependence, their use should be restricted to the individual patient with a clear-cut psychosomatic trait.

## Placebo and placebo effect

There is no doubt that placebos can exert positive pharmacological actions which in some instances appear to be significantly more potent than accepted active drugs for a given indication. This is confirmed by the fact that placebos display characteristics which are considered to be exclusive of active drugs. It is well-known, for instance, that a relatively constant proportion of patients (about 30%) obtain significant pain relief from a placebo [112]. Over a period, tolerance is produced to placebo analgesia and there is a tendency to increase the dosage. An abstinence syndrome can also appear if the placebo is suddenly withdrawn [112]. Not only do these facts imply a true pharmacological action of placebo in certain clinical conditions, but they may also indicate the existence of a possible chemical component of the mode of placebo action. In this connection, Levine et al. [113] found that placebo-induced analgesia could be blocked by naloxone and therefore suggested that the placebo effect may be mediated by endorphin release.

Placebos do not only have a therapeutic effect on symptoms or disease; they can also provoke adverse reactions, sometimes even of such severity that the treatment must be interrupted. The incidence of complaints after placebo is generally higher among healthy subjects than that observed in patients. Symptoms present before treatment often disappear during placebo, while new symptoms arise [114].

It is now well established that any treatment, involving use of a drug or not, carries the possibility of a placebo effect. It follows from this that any observed effects of a drug do not necessarily reflect its true intrinsic pharmacodynamic activity. In addition, it may be difficult to show a statistically significant difference between a new drug and an old therapy in a clinical condition, like NUD, where the placebo effect is pronounced. In order to assess any true activity, it is therefore mandatory to make a direct comparison between drug and placebo [115]. The only method by which the placebo-effect of a drug therapy can be precisely ascertained is direct and simultaneous comparison of drug and placebo in very similar groups of patients under very similar circumstances. Ideally, these groups should be "crossed over" and the drug and placebo compared again. Physical features of placebos may be significant and, consequently, in the controlled trials placebo and active drugs must be matched in physical form as closely as possible. Such matching, of course, applies not only to physical features but also to dosage regimens. This is usually done by using the so-called "double-dummy" technique.

The placebo effect is the only single action that all drugs have in common, and in some instances it is the only useful action that medications exert. Due to placebo effect, drugs are reported effective four to five times more frequently in uncontrolled studies than in controlled ones. Therefore only a placebo-controlled trial allows one to isolate the intrinsic effect of active therapy and only drugs successful in double-blind, placebo-controlled trials must be considered truly effective.

## Conclusions

There is a natural tendency for NUD to improve at least in the short-term [116], and the large placebo response in this group of patients makes evaluation of different treatments difficult. Although no specific medication, drug, or group of drugs appears effective in all patients with dyspepsia, classification of patients with dyspeptic symptoms into a number of groups, based largely on symptoms, may help the choice of the drug for the individual patient.

Various drugs to manage NUD are available today. The very fact that so many compounds have been tested is evidence that no single drug is effective in all patients and emphasizes once more the heterogeneity of the syndrome. New remedies are under development and will be available in the future. They are unlikely to offer any major advantage over the existing ones but they will be surely more expensive. If one looks for a cheap and effective remedy, one should rely on banana powder [117].

**Acknowledgements.** I am indebted to Professor J.-P. Galmiche (Nantes, France) for his criticism and useful suggestions. I am also grateful to Dr. Cinzia Corradi for checking the references and to Miss Sabina Cavagni for her help in the preparation of the manuscript.

## References

1. Barbara L, Camilleri M, Corinaldesi R, Crean GP, Heading RC, Johnson AG, Malagelada JR, Stanghellini V, Wienbeck M. Definition and investigation of dyspepsia. Consensus of an international *ad hoc* working party. Dig Dis Sci 1989;34:1272-6.
2. Tibblin G. Introduction to the epidemiology of dyspepsia. Scand J Gastroenterol 1985;20(suppl 109):29-33.
3. Jones R, Lydeard S. Prevalence of symptoms of dyspepsia in the community. Br Med J 1989;298:30-2.
4. Greydanus MP, Vassalo M, Camilleri M, Nelson DK, Hanson RB, Thomforde GM. Neurohormonal factors in functional dyspepsia: insights on pathophysiological mechanisms. Gastroenterology 1991;100:1311-8.
5. Talley NJ, Phillips SF. Non-ulcer dyspepsia: potential causes and pathophysiology. Ann Int Med 1988;108:865-79.
6. Colin-Jones DG, Bloom B, Bodemar G, Crean GP, Freston J, Gugler R, Malagelada JR, Nyrén O, Petersen H, Piper D. Management of dyspepsia: report of a working party. Lancet 1988;1:576-9.
7. Heatley RV, Rathbone BJ. Dyspepsia: a dilemma for doctors? Lancet 1987;2:779-82.
8. Dobrilla G, Amplatz S. Dietetic approach to patients with functional dyspepsia. In: Barbara L *et al.*, eds. *Nutrition in Gastrointestinal Disease*. New York: Raven Press, 1987:27-39.
9. Washington N, Wilson CG. Antacids: physiology versus pharmaceutics. Int J Pharm 1986;28:249-60.
10. Scarpignato C. Antacid protection of the gastric mucosa: an overview. In: Cheli R *et al.*, eds. *Gastric Protection*. New York: Raven Press, 1988:253-70.

11. Galmiche JP, Vallot T. Therapeutic strategy. In: Galmiche JP, Jian R, Mignon M, Ruszniewski Ph, eds. *Non-Ulcer Dyspepsia: Pathophysiological and Therapeutic Approaches*. Paris: John Libbey Eurotext, 1991:247-64.
12. Beckloff GL, Chapman JH, Shiverdecker P. Objective evaluation of an antacid with unusual properties. J Clin Pharmacol 1972;12:11-21.
13. Malmud LS, Charkes ND, Littlefield J, *et al*. The mode of action of alginic acid compound in the reduction of gastroesophageal reflux. J Nucl Med 1979;20:1023-8.
14. Washington N, Washington C, Wilson CG, Davis SS. What is "Liquid Gaviscon"? A comparison of four international formulations. Int J Pharmaceutics 1986;34:105-9.
15. Moss HA, Washington N, Greaves JL, Clive G, Wilson. Anti-reflux agents: stratification or flotation? Eur J Gastroenterol Hepatol 1990;2:45-51.
16. Washington N. *Handbook of Antacids and Anti-Reflux Agents*. Boca Raton: CRC Press, 1991 (in press).
17. Washington N, Greaves JL, Wilson CG. Effect of time of dosing relative to a meal on the raft formation of an anti-reflux agent. J Pharm Pharmacol 1990;42:50-3.
18. Scarpignato C. Pharmacological bases of the medical treatment of gastroesophageal reflux disease. Dig Dis 1988;6:117-48.
19. Washington N. Investigation into the barrier action of an alginate gastric reflux suppressant, liquid Gaviscon®. Drug Invest 1990;2:23-30.
20. Galmiche JP, Scarpignato C. Antacids in gastroesophageal reflux disease. In: Bianchi Porro G, Richardson CT, eds. *Antacids in Peptic Ulcer Disease. State of the Art*. Verona/New York: Cortina International/Raven Press, 1988:53-65.
21. Kennedy N, Keeling PWN. Comparison of cimetidine with a cimetidine/alginic acid combination in the treatment of oesophageal reflux disease. Gastroenterology Int 1988;1(suppl 1):682A.
22. Lennox B, Snell C, Lamb Y. Response of heartburn symptoms to a new cimetidine/alginate combination compared with an alginic acid/antacid. Br J Clin Pract 1988;42:503-5.
23. Boyko D., Lamb Y. Comparison of the availability of cimetidine from a cimetidine/alginate combination tablet and from standard cimetidine. Gastroenterology Int 1988;1(suppl 1):680A.
24. Britton AM, Nichols JD, Draper PR. The comparative bioavailability of cimetidine-alginate treatments. J Pharm Pharmacol 1991;43:122-3.
25. Hammer R, Giachetti A. Muscarinic receptor subtypes: $M_1$ and $M_2$. Biochemical and functional characterization. Info Sci 1982;31:2991-8.
26. Scarpignato C. Antisecretory drugs in the medical treatment of gastroesophageal reflux disease (GERD): why, which and how? In: Mignon M, Galmiche JP, eds. *Safe and Effective Control of Acid Secretion*. Paris: John Libbey Eurotext, 1988:203-24.
27. Garcia-Albarran A, Ruiz de Leon A, Diaz Rubio M. Gastroesophageal reflux. Study of the treatment with pirenzepine (Gastrozepin). Dig Dis Sci 1986;31(suppl):467S.
28. Stöckbrugger RW, Armebrecht U, Reul W. The effect of $M_1$-selective antimuscarinic drug telenzepine on gastroesophageal reflux in healthy volunteers. In: *Abstract Book of the XI International Symposium on Gastrointestinal Motility*, 7th-11th September, Oxford 1987:56.
29. Dobrilla G, Comberlato M, Steele A, Vallaperta A. Drug treatment of functional dyspepsia. A meta-analysis of randomized controlled clinical trials. J Clin Gastroenterol 1989;11:69-77.
30. Feldman M, Burton ME. Histamine$_2$-receptor antagonists. Standard therapy for acid peptic diseases (First of two parts). N Engl J Med 1990;323:1672-80.
31. Feldman M, Burton ME. Histamine$_2$-receptor antagonists. Standard therapy for acid peptic diseases (Second of two parts). N Engl J Med 1990;323:1749-55.
32. Lauritsen K, Laursen LS, Rask-Madsen J. Clinical pharmacokinetics of drugs used in the treatment of gastrointestinal diseases (Part I). Clin Pharmacokinet 1990;19:11-31.
33. Lauritsen K, Laursen LS, Rask-Madsen J. Clinical pharmacokinetics of drugs used in the treatment of gastrointestinal diseases (Part II). Clin Pharmacokinet 1990;19:94-125.

34. Howden CW. What is potent acid suppression and how can this be best achieved? In: Williams JG, ed. *Potent Acid Suppression: When it is Appropriate?* London: Royal Society of Medicine, 1990:1-11.
35. Sachs G, Munson K, Hall K, Hersey S. Gastric H+, K+-ATPase as a therapeutic target in peptic ulcer disease. Dig Dis Sci 1990;35:1537-44.
36. Howden CW. Clinical pharmacology of omeprazole. Clin Pharmacokinet 1991;20:38-49.
37. Scarpignato C, Villardel F. Prostaglandins: their role in gastric mucosal defence. In: Cheli R, ed. *Treatment and Prevention of NSAID-induced Gastropathy*. London: Royal Society of Medicine, 1989;25-33.
38. Dajani E. Prostaglandins and the integrity of the esophageal mucosa. In: Scarpignato C, ed. *Advances in Drug Therapy of Gastroesophageal Reflux Disease*. Basel: Karger, 1991 (in press).
39. Hauksen T, Stene-Larsen G, Lange O, Aronsen O, Nerdrum T, Hegbom P, Schulz T, Berstad A. Misoprostol treatment exacerbates abdominal discomfort in patients with non-ulcer dyspepsia and erosive prepyloric changes. A double-blind, placebo-controlled, multicentre study. Scand J Gastroenterol 1990;25:1028-33.
40. Avila MH, Walker AM, Romieu I, Spiegelman DL, Perera DR, Jick H. Choice of non-steroidal anti-inflammatory drugs in persons treated for dyspepsia. Lancet 1988;2:556-9.
41. Shallcross TM, Heatley RV. Effect of non-steroidal anti-inflammatory drugs on dyspeptic symptoms. Br Med J 1990;300:368-9.
42. Naves J, Morales I, Santoyo R. Prophylactic effects of misoprostol on gastric lesions and symptoms induced by the ingestion of aspirin: are symptoms predictive of lesions? In: Cheli R, ed. *Treatment and Prevention of NSAID-induced Gastropathy*. London: Royal Society of Medicine, 1989;55-61.
43. Scarpignato C, Galmiche JP. Mucosal coating agents: pharmacology and clinical use. In: Bianchi Porro G, ed. *Topics in Digestive Disease*. Vol. 1, Verona/New York: Cortina International/Raven Press, 1988:73-133.
44. Tytgat GNJ, Rauws EAJ, Langebberg W, Houthoff HJ. Significance of *Campylobacter pyloridis*. In: Bianchi Porro G, ed. *Topics in Digestive Disease*. Vol. 1, Verona/New York: Cortina International/Raven Press, 1988:59-71.
45. Lambert JR, Dunn K, Borromeo M, Korman MG, Hansky J. *Campylobacter pylori* — A role in non-ulcer dyspepsia ? Scand J Gastroenterol 1989;24(suppl 160):7-13.
46. Gad A, Hradsky M, Furugard K, Malmodin B, Nyberg O. *Campylobacter pylori* and non-ulcer dyspepsia. A prospective study in a Swedish population. Scand J Gastroenterol 1989;24(suppl 167):44-88.
47. Greenberg R, Bank S. The prevalence of *Helicobacter pylori* in non-ulcer dyspepsia. Importance of stratification according to age. Arch Intern Med 1990;150:2053-5.
48. Lamouliatte H, Cayla R, Bernard PH, Quinton A, Boulard A. Meta-analyse des essais randomisés dans les dyspepsies non ulcéreuses associées à *Helicobacter pylori*. Gastroentérol Clin Biol 1991;15:119A(abstr).
49. Axon ATR. *Campylobacter pylori* — therapy review. Scand J Gastroenterol 1989;24(suppl 160):35-8.
50. Graham DY, Borsch GMA. The who's and when's of therapy for *Helicobacter pylori*. Am J Gastroenterol 1990;85:1552-5.
51. Niada R, Mantovani M, Prino G, et al. Sulglycotide displays cytoprotective activity in rat gastric mucosa. Int J Tissue Reac 1983;5:285-8.
52. Porta R, Niada R, Pescador R, et al. Gastroprotection and lysosomal membrane stabilization by sulglycotide. Arzneim-Forsch/Drug Res 1986;36:1079-82.
53. Guslandi M, Nannini D, Tittobello A. Effect of sulglycotide on gastric bicarbonate secretion in humans. Drugs Exp Clin Res 1985;11:683-5.
54. McCallum RW, Prakash C, Campoli-Richards DM, Goa KL. Cisapride. A preliminary review of its pharmacodynamic and pharmacokinetic properties, and therapeutic use as a prokinetic agent in gastrointestinal motility disorders. Drugs 1988;36:652-81.

55. Fraitag B, Cloarec D, Galmiche JP. Le cisapride: pharmacologie, résultats thérapeutiques actuels et perspectives d'avenir. Gastroentérol Clin Biol 1989;3:265-76.
56. Tonini M. An appraisal of the action of cisapride and other substituted benzamide prokinetics on myenteric neurones. In: *Abstract Book of the Second International Cisapride Investigators' Meeting*. Nice, December 3-4. 1990:23.
57. Andrews PLR, Bingham S. Gastrointestinal motility effects of cisapride mediated by non-adrenergic non-cholinergic (N.A.N.C.) mechanisms. In: *Abstract Book of the Second International Cisapride Investigators' Meeting*. Nice, December 3-4. 1990:24.
58. Guslandi M. Drugs for upper digestive disorders. Drugs of Today 1989;25:101-13.
59. Galmiche JP, Bruley des Varannes S, Le Bodic L. Les médicaments prokinétiques en gastroentérologie. Gastroentérol Clin Biol 1991;15:T7-T10.
60. Bertaccini G. Cholecystokinin. In: Bertaccini G, ed. *Handbook of Experimental Pharmacology*. Vol. 59/II, Berlin: Springer-Verlag, 1982:40-70.
61. Scarpignato C. CCK-receptor antagonists: digestive pharmacology and therapeutic potential. In: Scarpignato C, ed. *Advances in Drug Therapy of Gastroesophageal Reflux Disease*. Basel: Karger, 1991 (in press).
62. Koppelberg T, Wank U, Adler G, Rovati L, Arnold R. CCK plays a role as a physiological regulator of human esophageal motility. Gastroenterology 1990;98:365A.
63. Meyer BM, Werth BA, Beglinger C, Hildebrand P, Jansen JBMJ, Zach D, Rovati LC, Stalder GA. Role of cholecystokinin in regulation of gastrointestinal motor functions. Lancet 1989;2:12-5.
64. Li Bassi S, Rovati LC, Giacovelli G, Bolondi L, Barbara L. Effects of loxiglumide, a cholecystokinin antagonist, in non-ulcer dyspepsia. Gastroenterology 1990;98:77A.
65. Corazziari E, Ricci R, Biliotti D, Bontempo I, De' Medici A, Pallotta N, Torsoli A. Oral administration of loxiglumide (CCK antagonist) inhibits postprandial gallbladder contraction without affecting gastric emptying. Dig Dis Sci 1990;35:50-4.
66. McIntosh CHS, Brown JC. Motilin: isolation, secretion, actions and pathophysiology. In: Scarpignato C, Bianchi Porro G, eds. *Clinical Investigation of Gastric Function*. Basel: Karger, 1990:307-52.
67. Tomomasa T, Kuruome T, Arai H, Wakabayashi K, Ito Z. Erythromycin induces migrating motor complex in human gastrointestinal tract. Dig Dis Sci 1986;31:157-61.
68. Kondo Y, Torii K, Itoh Z, Omura S. Erythromycin and its derivatives with motilin-like biological activities inhibits the specific binding of $^{125}$I-motilin to duodenal muscle. Biochem Biophys Res Comm 1988;150:877-82.
69. Peeters T, Matthijs G, Depoortere I, Cachet T, Hoogmartens J, Vantrappen G. Erythromycin is a motilin receptor agonist. Am J Physiol 1989;257:G470-G474.
70. Peeters TL, Matthijs G, Vantrappen G. $Ca^{2+}$ dependence of motilide-induced contractions in rabbit duodenal muscle strips *in vitro*. Naunyn Schmiedebergs Arch Pharmacol 1991;343:202-8.
71. Janssens J, Peeters TL, Vantrappen G, Tack J, Urbain JL, De Roo M, Muls E, Rouillon R. Improvement of gastric emptying in diabetic gastroparesis by erythromycin. N Engl J Med 1990;322:1028-31.
72. Pouliquen B, Bizais Y, Murat A, Galmiche JP. L'erythromycine accélère de façon spectaculaire la vidange gastrique (VG) des patients atteints de gastroparesie diabétique (GP). Gastroentérol Clin Biol 1990;14:47A(abstr).
73. Michopoulos S, Chaussade S, Guerre J, Couturier D. Effet de l'erythromycine (ERY) sur la motricité œsophagienne chez l'homme normal. Gastroentérol Clin Biol 1990;14:44A(abstr).
74. Fernandez AG, Massingham R. Peripheral receptor populations involved in the regulation of gastrointestinal motility and the pharmacological actions of metoclopramide-like drugs. Life Sci 1985;36:1-14.
75. Fozard JR. 5-HT$_3$ receptors and cytotoxic drug-induced vomiting. Trends Pharmacol Sci 1987;8:44-5.

76. Gamse R, Buchheit KH. 5HT$_3$-receptor antagonists: pharmacology and potential in the treatment of GORD. In: Scarpignato C, ed. *Advances in Drug Therapy of Gastro-oesophageal Reflux Disease*. Basel: Karger, 1991 (in press).
77. Stacher G, Steiner G, Gaupmann G, *et al.* Effects of the 5-HT$_3$-receptor antagonist, ICS 205-930, on oesophageal motor activity and on lower oesophageal sphincter pressure: a double-blind cross-over study. Hepatogastroenterology 1990;37(suppl 2):118-21.
78. Akkermans LMA, Vos A, Hoekstra A, Roelofs JMM, Horowitz M. Effect of ICS 205-930 (a specific 5-HT$_3$-receptor antagonist) on gastric emptying of a solid meal in normal subjects. Gut 1988;29:1249-52.
79. Dobrilla G. Management of chronic pancreatitis. Focus on enzyme replacement therapy. Int J Pancreatol 1989;5:17-29.
80. Di Luca Sidozzi A, Corradi C, Pititto A, Scarpignato C. Pancreatic enzymes. In: Braga PC, Guslandi M, Tittobello A, eds. *Drugs in Gastroenterology*. New York: Raven Press, 1991 (in press).
81. Ihse I, Lija P, Lundquist I. Feedback regulation of pancreatic enzyme secretion by intestinal trypsin in man. Digestion 1977;15:303-8.
82. Liener IE, Godale RL, Deshmukh A, *et al.* Effect of trypsin inhibitor from soybeans (Bowman-Birk) on the secretory activity of human pancreas. Gastroenterology 1988;94:419-27.
83. Rider JA. The use of bile acids and pancreatic enzyme substitutes in the treatment of "functional indigestion". Am J Gastroenterol 1960;33:734-9.
84. Kleveland PM, Johannessen T, Kristensen P, Loge I, Sandbakken P, Dybdahl J, Petersen H. Effect of pancreatic enzymes in non-ulcer dyspepsia. A pilot study. Scand J Gastroenterol 1990;25:298-301.
85. Masuda M, Hosoda S, Baba T, *et al.* Double-blind trial of ursodeoxycholic acid in maldigestive malabsorption syndrome (chronic biliary tract and pancreatic disease). Clin Rep 1976;10:85-102.
86. Pazzi P, Stabellini G, Trevisani L, Arlotti A, Massari M, Alvisi V. Effect of ursodeoxycholic acid (UDCA) on "biliary dyspepsia" in patients without gallstones. Curr Ther Res 1985;37:685-94.
87. Stefaniwsky AB, Tint GS, Speck J, *et al.* Ursodeoxycholic acid treatment of bile reflux gastritis. Gastroenterology 1985;89:1000-4.
88. Leuschner U, Kurtz W. Pharmacological aspects and therapeutic effects of ursodeoxycholic acid. Dig Dis 1990;8:12-22.
89. Bost R, Hostein J, Valenti M, Bonaz B, Payen N, Faure H, Fournet J. Is there an abnormal fasting duodenogastric reflux in non-ulcer dyspepsia? Dig Dis Sci 1990;35:193-9.
90. Bonaz B, Caravel JP, Bost R, Fournet J, Hostein J. Gallbladder emptying and duodenogastric reflux in non-ulcer dyspepsia. Hepatogastroenterology 1988;35:177.
91. Forgacs IC, Hilson AJW, Maisey MN, Murphy GM, Dowling RH. Ursodeoxycholic acid treatment reduces gallbladder contraction in response to exogenous CCK. A possible explanation for relief of biliary pain during therapy. Clin Sci 1982;62:21A.
92. Levitt MD, Bond JH. Intestinal gas. In: Sleisinger MH, Fordtran JS, eds. *Gastrointestinal Disease: Pathophysiology, Diagnosis, Management*. Philadelphia: Saunders, 1989:257-63.
93. Cloarec D, Flourié B, Marteau P, Galmiche JP. Les gaz digestifs: aspects physiopathologiques et thérapeutiques au cours des troubles fonctionnels. Gastroentérol Clin Biol 1990;14:641-50.
94. Lasser RB, Bond JH, Levitt MD. The role of intestinal gas in functional abdominal pain. N Engl J Med 1975;293:524-6.
95. Lasser RB, Levitt MD, Bond JH. Studies of intestinal gas after ingestion of a standard meal. Gastroenterology 1976;70:906A.
96. Richter JE, Barish CF, Castell DO. Abnormal sensory perception in patients with esophageal chest pain. Gastroenterology 1986;91:845-52.

97. Lémann M, Dederling JP, Jian P, Flourié B, Franchisseur C, Rambaud JC. Abnormal sensory perception to gastric distension in patients with chronic idiopathic dyspepsia. The irritable stomach. Gastroenterology 1989;96:294A(abstr).
98. Ritchie J. Pain from distension of the pelvic colon by inflating a balloon, in the irritable colon syndrome. Gut 1973;14:125-32.
99. Jain NK, Patel VP, Pitchumoni CS. Activated charcoal, simethicone, and intestinal gas: a double-blind study. Ann Intern Med 1986;105:61-2.
100. Bernstein JE, Schwartz SR. An evaluation of the effectiveness of simethicone in acute upper gastrointestinal distress. Curr Ther Res 1974;16:617-20.
101. Müller-Lissner SA, Blum A. Fundic pressure rise lowers lower esophageal sphincter pressure in man. Hepatogastroenterology 1982;29:151-2.
102. Holloway RH, Hongo M, Berger K, et al. Gastric distension: a mechanism for postprandial gastroesophageal reflux. Gastroenterology 1985;89:779-84.
103. Stead JA, Wilkins A, Ashford JJ. In vitro and in vivo defoaming action of three antacid preparations. J Pharm Pharmacol 1978;30:350-2.
104. Ciprandi G, Scordamaglia A, Cheli R, Canonica GW. Food allergy and digestive pathology: pathophysiological, diagnostic and therapeutic aspects. Dig Dis 1990;8:89-98.
105. Canonica GW, Ciprandi G. Food allergy and dyspepsia. Lancet 1988;1:1233.
106. Foreman JC, Pearce FL. Cromolyn. In: Middleton E et al., eds. Allergy. Principles and Practice. St Louis: The C.V. Mosby Co., 1988:766-81.
107. Talley NJ, Fung LH, Gilligan IJ, McNeil D, Piper DW. Association of anxiety, neuroticism, and depression with dyspepsia of unknown cause. A case control study. Gastroenterology 1986;90:886-92.
108. Birnbaum D, Karmeli F, Toefera M. The effect of diazepam on human gastric secretion. Gut 1971;12:616-8.
109. Murie JA, MacKay C. The effect of lorazepam on human gastric secretion. Clin Ther 1980;2:387-9.
110. Berardi RR, Caplan NB. Agents with tricyclic structures for treating peptic ulcer disease. Clin Pharm 1983;2:425-31.
111. Scarpignato C. Is there any effect of neuromuscular blocking agents on the lower esophageal sphincter pressure? In: Giuli R. et al., eds. Primary Motility Disorders of the Esophagus, Paris: John Libbey Eurotext, 1991:228-30.
112. Haegerstam G, Huitfeldt B, Nillson BS, Siövall J, Syvälahti E, Wahlén A. Placebo in clinical drug trials — a multidisciplinary review. Meth Find Exptl Clin Pharmacol 1982;4:261-8.
113. Levine JD, Gordon NC, Fields HL. The mechanism of placebo analgesia. Lancet 1978;1:654-7.
114. Green DM. Pre-existing conditions, placebo reactions, and "side effects". Ann Intern Med 1964;60:255-65.
115. Dobrilla G. Placebo and placebo effect: general aspects and the extent of the problem. In: Dobrilla G, ed. Controlled Therapeutic Trials in Gastroenterology. Verona/New York: Cortina International/Raven Press, 1986:11-6.
116. Talley NJ, McNeil D, Hayden A, Colreavu C, Piper DW. Prognosis of chronic unexplained dyspepsia. Gastroenterology 1987;92:1060-6.
117. Arora A, Sharma MP. Use of banana in non-ulcer dyspepsia. Lancet 1990;1:612-3.

# 21

# Randomized clinical trials in patients with dyspepsia

T. POYNARD, B. MORY, D. LEVOIR, J.-P. PIGNON, S. NAVEAU, J.-C. CHAPUT

*Service d'Hépato-Gastroentérologie, Hôpital Antoine Béclère, 157 rue de la Porte-de-Trivaux, 92141 Clamart Cedex, France*

## Introduction

Dyspepsia is a common medical disease and its costs to society are very high because of the price of treatment prescribed and because of absenteeism. As there is no consensus for the definition of dyspepsia(s), the criteria of inclusion in clinical trials are heterogeneous. Therefore populations of patients included and treatments tested are very different. The aim of this review was to identify the randomized clinical trials (RCTs) of medical treatment in patients with dyspepsia, to describe these RCTs and to evaluate their clinical and methodological qualities. Particular attention has been paid to describing the clinical heterogeneity of patients included in these RCTs.

## Methods

### Literature search for RCTs

For the literature search we used computer searches (Medlars), bibliographies of reviews, and references in the papers found. We also reviewed systematically the contents of Index Medicus from 1980 to 1990, the contents of Gastroenterology, Digestive Diseases and Sciences, Gastroentérologie Clinique et Biologique and Gut from 1988 to 1990. We did not confine ourselves to a Medlars search because we and others have previously demonstrated its inefficacy in retrieving all RCTs in subspecialties [1].

**Criteria of inclusion and exclusion of RCTs**

To be included RCTs must be randomized. RCTs not clearly randomized were excluded unless the trial was double-blind. Only RCTs dealing with dyspepsia were included. Dyspepsia was defined as upper abdominal or retrosternal pain or discomfort, heartburn, nausea, vomiting, or any other symptom considered to be referable to the proximal alimentary tract and lasting for more than 4 weeks, unrelated to exercise and for which no focal lesion or systemic disease can be found responsible. Only RCTs with initial endoscopy or where more than 50% of patients were endoscoped were included (only one RCT with 70 % of endoscopy has been identified). Only RCTs dealing with minor abnormalities at initial endoscopy were included. Minor abnormalities were defined as gastritis (erosive or otherwise, with or without histological assessment), duodenitis, and gastro-oesophageal reflux without erosive oesophagitis was also included. RCTs with *Helicobacter pylori*-associated gastritis without duodenal ulcer were included. Only RCTs published as scientific articles or chapters in books were included. When a RCT was published in several articles the overall information available was taken into account but only one reference was given. RCTs published in French, English, Spanish, Portuguese, German or Italian were accepted. RCTs published in other languages were included only if a translation was available. RCTs dealing with organic diseases at initial endoscopy were excluded. Organic diseases were defined as ulcer (duodenal or gastric) and erosive oesophagitis, carcinoma, cholelithiasis and pancreatitis. RCTs concerning post gastrectomy or other post digestive surgical patients were excluded. Poor methodological quality was not a criterion of exclusion. All RCTs included and excluded have been reviewed by two of the authors. RCTs were excluded only if the two observers agreed, without any consideration of the results or the quality of the trial.

**Clinical evaluation of RCTs**

For each RCT a questionnaire assessing the clinical description was completed. A first version of this questionnaire was tested in a random sample of 10 RCTs. Afterwards a revised version was elaborated. This questionnaire included 41 items.

**Methodological evaluation of RCTs**

We elaborated a questionnaire [2] which is derived from that of Chalmers *et al.* [3] but with fewer items (n=14) and only three possible responses for each item. One item concerns the end point, four items the description of the population of patients, three items the blindness of the trial and six items the statistical methods. For 13 items, the score is 2 points for a correct answer, 1 point for a partial answer and 0 for no or an unknown answer. For the last item concerning the power of the trial, negative points are given for negative trials with less than 100 patients per group; 1 point between 30 and 100 patients and 2 points if the number of patients per group is less than 30. No points are subtracted for positive trials. Thus, the total score of the methodological assessment can range from 0 to 26 points. Each questionnaire is filled in independently by two authors and the discordances are resolved in conference.

## Meta-analysis

We have pooled only treatments for which more than 10 RCTs were published, that is $H_2$-blockers, cisapride and domperidone. Methods described by Yusuf and Peto were used.

## Results

Between 1978 and 1990 a total of 54 RCTs have been identified in the treatment of dyspepsia [4-57]. Eighty percent of these RCTs have been published in the last 5 years. Seventy percent were published by European centres, and only 5% by US centres. France has published only one RCT. Table I gives the type of symptoms accepted for patients inclusion. Several symptoms were given for each RCT leading to a total of 35 different associations of symptoms. The median of the minimum duration of symptoms accepted for inclusion was 3 months (range 1 to 6). Characteristics of patients included are given in table II. Only 21 RCTs noted whether or not patients with previous history of gastroduodenal ulcer were excluded; six did not exclude these patients. Ultrasonography was systematically performed in 23 RCTs, colonoscopy in four and a search for *Helicobacter pylori* in 10. Treatments tested are given in table III. Only one RCT compared a combination of treatments (amoxycillin plus bismuth) with a single treatment. Prescription of antacids was described in 24 RCTs, of which 18 allowed antacids in both groups (75%). Only two RCTs described analgesic prescriptions which were allowed in one of them. Designs of the RCTs are given in table IV. One third were cross-over RCTs. Only 25% were analysed using the intention-to-treat method. At least one significant ($p<0.05$) result was observed in 64% of RCTs. Assessment of methodological quality is given in table V. The median methodological score was 15 (range 3-22) for an ideal total score of 26.

**Table I.** Description of RCTs in the treatment of dyspepsia: type of symptoms accepted for inclusion.

| Type of symptom accepted for inclusion | Number of RCTs which included patients with this symptom | % |
|---|---|---|
| Epigastric pain or burning | 41 | 93 |
| Nausea or vomiting | 32 | 74 |
| Heartburn | 29 | 65 |
| Meteorism | 25 | 58 |
| Belching | 20 | 47 |
| Early satiety | 16 | 37 |
| Meal provocation | 12 | 28 |
| Regurgitation | 11 | 26 |
| Nocturnal pain | 8 | 19 |
| Meal relief | 8 | 19 |
| Antacid relief | 5 | 12 |
| Irritable bowel syndrome | 3 | 7 |

**Table II.** Characteristics of patients included in RCTs in the treatment of dyspepsia.

| Characteristics | Number of RCTs with data | Median | Range |
|---|---|---|---|
| Epidemiological data | | | |
| male (%) | 36 | 50 | 30-84 |
| age (year) | 39 | 40 | 31-56 |
| smokers (%) | 19 | 46 | 9-57 |
| alcohol users (%) | 13 | 40 | 0-80 |
| Clinical symptoms (%) | | | |
| epigastric pain or burning | 23 | 85 | 3-100 |
| nausea or vomiting | 17 | 57 | 16-90 |
| heartburn | 15 | 58 | 0-100 |
| meteorism | 12 | 80 | 17-100 |
| belching | 12 | 58 | 0-100 |
| early satiety | 7 | 68 | 0-100 |
| meal provocation | 7 | 52 | 0-100 |
| regurgitation | 5 | 30 | 0-80 |
| nocturnal pain | 7 | 45 | 0-50 |
| meal relief | 5 | 27 | 0-54 |
| antacid relief | 2 | 50 | 0-50 |
| irritable bowel syndrome | 5 | 22 | 0-52 |
| Mean duration of symptoms before inclusion (months) | 21 | 36 | 3-120 |
| Endoscopic signs (%) | | | |
| erosive gastritis | 9 | 11 | 0-60 |
| erosive duodenitis | 5 | 10 | 0-13 |
| non-erosive gastritis | 9 | 49 | 4-100 |
| non-erosive duodenitis | 5 | 9 | 8-28 |
| gastritis* | 14 | 67 | 0-100 |
| duodenitis* | 6 | 20 | 0-100 |
| gastritis* or duodenitis* | 7 | 22 | 0-97 |

* no precise description of endoscopic abnormalities.

**Table III.** Treatment tested by RCTs in patients with dyspepsia.

| Treatment | Number of RCTs | References |
|---|---|---|
| Placebo | 39 | [4 - 42] |
| Cimetidine | 13 | [4], [5], [9-11], [20-23], [30], [39], [43] |
| Ranitidine | 3 | [44], [36], [50] |
| Cisapride | 15 | [7], [9], [10], [12], [24], [25], [28], [29], [32], [40-42], [46], [51], [52] |
| Bismuth | 7 | [26], [27], [33], [34], [37], [39], [43] |
| Sucralfate | 5 | [8], [35], [39], [44], [47] |
| Domperidone | 9 | [14], [19], [48], [49], [53-57] |
| Pirenzepine | 5 | [16-18], [38], [49] |
| Metoclopramide | 2 | [21], [45] |
| Antibiotics | 3 | [31], [33], [39] |
| Antacids | 4 | [18], [20], [30], [48] |
| Sulpiride | 1 | [6] |
| Sulglycotide | 1 | [47] |

**Table IV.** Design of RCTs in the treatment of dyspepsia.

| Item | Number of RCTs with data | Median | Range |
| --- | --- | --- | --- |
| Duration of treatment (week) | 47 | 4 | 1-16 |
| Total number of patients randomized | 47 | 70 | 16-500 |
| Number of arms | 47 | 2 | 2-6 |
| Number of patients analysed in the smaller group | 42 | 24 | 5-109 |
| Number of patients excluded after randomization | 40 | 7 | 0-49 |

**Table V.** Methodological quality of RCTs.

| Item | Yes n (%) | Partial n (%) | No or unknown n (%) |
| --- | --- | --- | --- |
| End point | | | |
| — Is (are) the major end point(s) clearly stated? | 14 (32) | 28 (68) | 0 (0) |
| Description of the population | | | |
| — Are the criteria of inclusion and exclusion clearly stated? | 33 (78) | 7 (17) | 2 (5) |
| — Is the number of patients seen and rejected given? | 9 (20) | 9 (22) | 24 (59) |
| — Is the number of patients randomized clearly stated for both groups? | 27 (63) | 14 (34) | 1 (2) |
| — Are the numbers of patients who were withdrawn and dropped out given and reasons clearly stated? | 24 (56) | 10 (24) | 8 (20) |
| Blindness of the trial | | | |
| — Are the patients blind to treatment? | 33 (78) | 3 (7) | 6 (15) |
| — Are the caring physicians blind to treatment? | 34 (81) | 2 (5) | 6 (15) |
| — Are the persons assessing major end points blind to treatment? | 35 (78) | 4 (10) | 5 (12) |
| Statistical method | | | |
| — Is the method of randomization given and is this randomization blind? | 3 (5) | 0 (0) | 39 (95) |
| — Is the necessary sample size pre-calculated? | 2 (5) | 4 (10) | 36 (85) |
| — Are pre-treatment variables adequately analysed and discussed? | 18 (44) | 21 (49) | 3 (7) |
| — Are statistical tests used appropriate? | 24 (59) | 9 (22) | 8 (20) |
| — Is handling of withdrawals correct? | 3 (7) | 30 (71) | 9 (22) |

| | n (%) |
| --- | --- |
| — Trial positive or negative with at least 100 subjects per group | 26 (61) |
| — Negative trial with 30 to 100 subjects per group | 4 (10) |
| — Negative trial with less than 30 subjects per group | 12 (29) |

Meta-analysis of $H_2$-blockers, cisapride and domperidone efficacy *versus* placebo are given in table VI, VII and VIII respectively. They were highly significant (p<0.0001) without statistical heterogeneity.

**Discussion**

This overview of RCTs in the treatment of dyspepsia has shown that these trials are very heterogeneous. This heterogeneity was observed for at least four factors:

**Table VI.** Meta-analysis of RCTs comparing $H_2$-blockers to placebo.

| First author | Placebo | | $H_2$-blockers | |
|---|---|---|---|---|
| | Improved / Total | (%) | Improved / Total | (%) |
| Delattre | 115 / 205 | (56.1) | 152 / 209 | (72.7) |
| Kolbaeck | 16 / 26 | (61.5) | 13 / 24 | (54.2) |
| Lance | 12 / 33 | (36.4) | 21 / 34 | (61.8) |
| MacKinnon | 5 / 10 | (50.0) | 10 / 11 | (90.9) |
| Nesland | 15 / 46 | (32.6) | 22 / 44 | (50.0) |
| Olubuyide | 1 / 22 | (4.5) | 1 / 23 | (4.3) |
| Saunders | 70 / 136 | (51.5) | 82 / 115 | (71.3) |
| Total | 234 / 478 | (49.0) | 301 / 460 | (65.4) |

Odds ratio = 0.48 (95% CI: 0.37 - 0.63) p<0.0001
Heterogeneity test = 5.79 (NS)

**Table VII.** Meta-analysis of RCTs comparing cisapride to placebo.

| First author | Placebo | | Cisapride | |
|---|---|---|---|---|
| | Improved / Total | (%) | Improved / Total | (%) |
| Creytens | 9 / 16 | (56.3) | 15 / 16 | (93.8) |
| Goethals | 7 / 24 | (29.2) | 15 / 24 | (62.5) |
| Milo | 1 / 16 | (6.3) | 12 / 16 | (75.0) |
| Deruyttere | 31 / 56 | (55.4) | 42 / 56 | (75.0) |
| François | 17 / 34 | (50.0) | 29 / 34 | (85.3) |
| Rosch | 17 / 55 | (30.9) | 44 / 54 | (81.5) |
| Van Ganse | 1 / 8 | (12.5) | 7 / 8 | (87.5) |
| Coutant | 2 / 8 | (25.0) | 14 / 20 | (70.0) |
| Total | 85 / 217 | (39.2) | 178 / 228 | (78.1) |

Odds ratio = 0.19 (95% CI: 0.13 - 0.28) p<0.0001
Heterogeneity test = 9.4 (NS)

**Table VIII.** Meta-analysis of RCTs comparing domperidone to placebo.

| | Placebo | | Domperidone | |
|---|---|---|---|---|
| First author | Improved / Total | (%) | Improved / Total | (%) |
| Milo | 1 / 10 | (10.0) | 9 / 10 | (90.0) |
| Bekhti | 4 / 20 | (20.0) | 13 / 20 | (65.0) |
| Van de Mierop | 2 / 15 | (13.3) | 12 / 17 | (70.6) |
| Van Ganse | 5 / 21 | (23.8) | 19 / 23 | (82.6) |
| De Loose | 22 / 71 | (31.0) | 62 / 68 | (91.2) |
| Total | 34 / 137 | (24.8) | 115 / 138 | (83.3) |

Odds ratio = 0.09 (95% CI: 0.06 - 0.15) $p<0.0001$
Heterogeneity test = 1.6 (NS)

symptoms accepted for inclusion, characteristics of patients, treatment and methodological quality. From the symptoms accepted for inclusion (table I) different categories of dyspepsia were treated: (1) heartburn and regurgitation which are symptoms close to gastro-oesophageal reflux, (2) meteorism which is closely linked to irritable bowel syndrome, (3) early satiety which is closely linked to "mechanical" dyspepsia, (4) pain relief by a meal or by antacids which is closely linked to non-ulcer dyspepsia. The characteristics of patients effectively included in RCTs were not sufficiently detailed (table II), especially for symptoms and endoscopic signs. Less than half of RCTs gave details. There was a wide range of symptoms observed as detailed in table II. For example, some RCTs included no patients with heartburn and in others all were affected. Some RCTs included 52% of patients with irritable bowel syndrome and others included 54% of patients with pain relieved by a meal. Lack of information and high heterogeneity were also observed for endoscopic signs. Some RCTs included erosive disease such as erosive gastritis or duodenitis and other excluded all types of gastritis. The heterogeneity was also observed for the treatment. Thirteen different drugs were evaluated but only seven in at least four RCTs. From this small number of RCTs per drug and from the *clinical* heterogeneity meta-analysis of RCTs is extremely difficult to perform without risk. Dobrilla *et al.* [58] have presented a meta-analysis of RCTs into patients with dyspepsia. They arbitrarily classified RCTs into two groups, flatulent dyspepsia and ulcer-like dyspepsia. From our data we have not been able to perform such a classification.

As in other fields of hepatology or gastroenterology the methodological quality of RCTs is far from perfect. The items most often incorrect or not given are a description of patients seen and not included, the number and reasons for drop-outs in each group, the absence of precalculation of the sample size, and the absence of analysis using the intention-to-treat method. The number of patients analysed is too small with a median of 24, which leads to too low a power. With this sample size only a difference of 50% between treatments can be assessed. Overall the median quality was greater than in other digestive diseases, mainly because most of these RCTs have been conducted in a double-blind fashion.

Because of the clinical heterogeneity of patients included in these RCTs we have limited our meta-analyses to $H_2$-blockers, cisapride and domperidone for which more than 10 RCTs were identified. From the results of these three meta-analyses it is clear that these three treatments are effective. There was no significant statistical heterogeneity. However from these RCTs it is impossible to know exactly which patients could benefit the more from these treatments. For this type of conclusions, individual data with all prognostic covariables by patient should be analysed. Cisapride and domperidone should be effective in patients with "mechanical" dyspepsia, and $H_2$-blockers in those with reflux-like dyspepsia and ulcer-like dyspepsia, and in patients with dyspepsia plus erosive gastritis/duodenitis.

The main conclusion from this overview is that new RCTs must include more homogeneous dyspeptic patients. These new RCTs must include more patients and editors should refuse small RCTs with negative results. The following new RCTs are probably the most interesting: $H_2$-blockers in erosive gastritis, erosive duodenitis and ulcer-like dyspepsia and prokinetics only in patients with mechanical dyspepsia. Because of lack of clinical information per patient included and because of observed clinical heterogeneity no definitive conclusions can be drawn from meta-analyses of these RCTs.

## References

1. Poynard T, Conn HO. The retrieval of randomized clinical trials in liver disease from the medical literature: a comparison of Medlars and manual methods. Controlled Clin Trials 1985;6:271-9.
2. Poynard T. Evaluation de la qualité méthodologique des essais thérapeutiques randomisés. Press Med 1988;17:315-8.
3. Chalmers TC, Smith H, Blackburn B, Silverman B, Schroeder B, Reitman D, Ambroz A. A method for assessing the quality of a randomized control trial. Controlled Clin Trials 1981;2:31-49.
4. Hui WM, Lam SK, Lok ASF, Mataing M, Wong KL, Fok KM. Sulpiride improves functional dyspepsia; a double-blind controlled study. J Gastroenterol Hepatol 1986;1: 391-9.
5. Lance P, Wastell C, Schiller KFR. A controlled trial of cimetidine for the treatment of non-ulcer dyspepsia. J Clin Gastroenterol 1986;8:414-8.
6. Kelbaek M, Linde J, Eriksen J, Munkgaard S, Moesgaard F, Bonnevie O. Controlled clinical trial of treatment with cimetidine for non-ulcer dyspepsia. Acta Med Scand 1985;217:281-7.
7. Coutant G, François I, De Nutte N, De Cock G, Borgers P, Rutgeerts L. Dose-response study of cisapride in the management of "non-ulcer dyspepsia". Prog Med 1987;43:91-6.
8. Kairaluoma MI, Hentilae R, Alavaikkro M, Kellosalo J, Stahlberg M, Jalovaara P, Olsen M, Jaervensivu P, Laitinen S. Sucralfate *versus* placebo in treatment of non-ulcer dyspepsia. Am J Med 1987;83:51-5.
9. Nesland AA, Berstad A. Effect of cimetidine in patients with non-ulcer dyspepsia and erosive prepyloric changes. Scand J Gastroenterol 1985;20:629-35.
10. Kleveland PM, Larsen S, Sandvik L, Kristensen P, Johannessen T, Hafstad PE, Sandbakken P, Loge I, Fjosne U, Petersen H. The effect of cimetidine in non-ulcer dyspepsia. Scand J Gastroenterol 1985;20:19-24.
11. Johannessen T, Fjosne U, Kleveland PM, Halvoisen T, Kristensen P, Loge I, Hafstad PE, Sandbakken P, Petersen H. Cimetidine responders in non-ulcer dyspepsia. Scand J Gastroenterol 1988;23:327-36.

12. Deruyttere M, Lepoutre L, Heylen H, Samain H, Pennvit H. Cisapride in the management of chronic functional dyspepsia: a multicentre double-blind, placebo-controlled study. Clinical Therap 1987;10:44-51.
13. Brooy S, Lovell D, Misiewicz J. The treatment of non-ulcer dyspepsia. Westminster Hospital Symposium Edinburgh Churchill, Livingstone 1978:131-7.
14. Naggler J, Mishovitz P. Clinical evaluation of domperidone in the treatment of chronic postprandial idiopathic upper gastrointestinal distress. Am J Gastroenterol 1981;76:495-9.
15. Rosch W. Cisapride in non-ulcer dyspepsia. Scand J Gastroenterol 1987;22:161-4.
16. Dal Monte PR, D'imperio N, Accardo P, Giuliani Piccari G, Mazzetti A. Pirenzepine in non-ulcer dyspepsia: a double-blind placebo-controlled trial. Advances in gastroenterology with the selective antimuscarinic compound-pirenzepine. Amsterdam, Excepta Medica 1982:163-9.
17. Hradsky M, Wikander M. Effect of pirenzepine in the treatment of non-ulcer dyspepsia: a double-blind study. Advances in gastroenterology with the selective antimuscarinic compound-pirenzepine. Amsterdam, Excepta Medica 1982:170-2.
18. Weberg R, Berstad A. Low-dose antacids and pirenzepine in the treatment of patients with non-ulcer dyspepsia and erosive prepyloric changes. Scand J Gastroenterol 1988;23:237-43.
19. Sarin SK, Sharma P, Chawla YK, Gopinath P, Nundy S. Clinical trial on the effect of domperidone on non-ulcer dyspepsia. Indian J Med Res 83 1986:623-8.
20. Nyrén O, Adami HO, Bates S, Bergstrom R, Gustavsson S, Loof L, Nyberg A. Absence of therapeutic benefit from antacids or cimetidine in non-ulcer dyspepsia. N Engl J Med 1986;314:339-43.
21. Talley NJ, Mc Neil D, Hayden A, Piper DW. Randomized double-blind placebo-controlled cross-over trial of cimetidine and pirenzepine in non-ulcer dyspepsia. Gastroenterology 1986;91:149-56.
22. Delattre M, Malesky M, Prinzic A. Symptomatic treatment of non-ulcer dyspepsia with cimetidine. Curr Ther Res 1985;37:980-91.
23. Mackinnon M, Willing RL, Whitehead R. Cimetidine in the management of symptomatic patients with duodenitis. Dig Dis Sci 1982;27:217-9.
24. De Nutte N, Van Ganse W, Witterhulghe M, Defrance P. Clin Therap, (in press).
25. Hannon R. Efficacy of cisapride in patients with non-ulcer dyspepsia. Curr Ther Res 1987;42:814-22.
26. Kang JY, Tay HH, Wee A, Guan R, Math HV, Yap I. Effect of colloidal bismuth subcitrate on symptoms and gastric histology in non-ulcer dyspepsia. A double-blind placebo-controlled study. Gut 1990;31:476-80.
27. Loffeld RJLF, Potters HVJP, Stobberingh E, Flendrig JA, Van Spreeuwel JP, Arends JW. *Campylobacter*-associated gastritis in patients with non-ulcer dyspepsia: a double-blind placebo-controlled trial with colloidal bismuth subcitrate. Gut 1989;30:1206-12.
28. Goethals G, Van de Mierop L. Cisapride in the treatment of chronic functional dyspepsia. Curr Ther Res 1987;42:261-7.
29. François I, De Nutte N. Non-ulcer dyspepsia: effect of the gastrointestinal prokinetic drug cisapride. Curr Ther Res 1987;41:891-8.
30. Gotthard R, Bodemar G, Brodin U, Jonsson KA. Treatment with cimetidine, antacid or placebo in patients with dyspepsia of unknown origin. Scand J Gastroenterol 1988;23:7-18.
31. Burette A, Glupczynski Y, Labbe M, Deprez C, Dereuck M, Deltenre M. *Campylobacter pylori*-associated gastritis: a double-blind placebo-controlled trial with amoxycillin. Acta Endoscopica 1987;17:251-7.
32. Corinaldesi R, Stanghellini V, Raiti C, Rea E, Salgemini R, Barbara L. Effect of chronic administration of cisapride on gastric emptying of a solid meal and on dyspeptic symptoms in patients with idiopathic gastroparesis. Gut 1987;28:300-5.

33. Mac Nulty CAM, Gearty JC, Crump B, Davis M, Donovan IA, Melikian V, Lister DM, Wise R. *Campylobacter pyloridis* and associated gastritis: investigator blind, placebo-controlled trial of bismuth salicylate and erythromycin ethylsuccinate. Br Med J 1986;293:645-9.
34. Rokkas T, Pursey C, Uzoechina E, Dorrington L, Simmons NA, Filipe MI, Sladen GE. Non-ulcer dyspepsia and short term De-Nol therapy: a placebo-controlled trial with particular reference to the role of *Campylobacter pylori*. Gut 1988;29:1386-91.
35. Skoubo-Kristensen E, Funch-Jensen P, Kruse A, Hanberg-Sorensen F, Amdrup E. Controlled clinical trial with sucralfate in the treatment of macroscopic gastritis. Scand J Gastroenterol 1989;24:716-20.
36. Olubuyide O, Ayoola EA, Okubanjo AO, Atoba HA. Non-ulcer dyspepsia in Nigerians. Clinical and therapeutic results. Scand J Gastroenterol 1986.21:83-7.
37. Lambert JR, Dunn K, Borromeo M, Korman HG, Hansky J. *Campylobacter pylori*. A role in non-ulcer dyspepsia? Scand J Gastroenterol 1989;24:7-13.
38. Gad A, Dobrilla G. *Campylobacter pylori* and non-ulcer dyspepsia: the final results of a double-blind multicentre trial for treatment with pirenzepine in Italy. Scand J Gastroenterol 1989;24:39-43.
39. Rauws EAJ, Langenberg W, Houthoff HJ, Zanen HC, Tytgat GNJ. *Campylobacter pyloridis*-associated chronic active antral gastritis. A prospective study of its prevalence and the effects of antibacterial and anti-ulcer treatment. Gastroenterology 1988;94:33-40.
40. Jian R, Ducrot F, Ruskoné A, Chaussade S, Rambaud JC, Modigliani R, Rain JD, Bernier JJ. Symptomatic, radionuclide and therapeutic assessment of chronic idiopathic dyspepsia. A double-blind placebo-controlled evaluation of cisapride. Dig Dis Sci 1989;34:657-64.
41. Van Ganse W, Reyntjens A. Clinical evaluation of cisapride in postprandial dyspepsia. Il Progresso Medico 1987;43(suppl1):77-81.
42. Deruyttere M, Milo R, Creytens G, Goethals C, Bourgeois E, Offner E. Therapy of chronic functional dyspepsia: multicentre cross-over study of cisapride and placebo. Il Progresso Medico 1987;43(suppl1):61-8.
43. Humphreys H, Bourke S, Dooley C, McKenna D, Power B, Keane CT, Sweeney EC, O'Morain C. Effect of treatment on *Campylobacter pylori* in peptic disease: a randomized prospective trial. Gut 1988;29:279-83.
44. Guslandi M. Comparison of sucralfate and ranitidine in the treatment of chronic non-erosive gastritis. A randomized, multicentre trial. Am J Med 1989;86:45-8.
45. Corinaldesi R, Raiti C, Stanghellini V, Monetti N, Rea E, Salgemini R, Paparo GF, Barbara L. Comparative effects of oral cisapride and metoclopramide on gastric emptying of solids and symptoms in patients with functional dyspepsia and gastroparesis. Curr Ther Res 1987;42:428-35.
46. Hendrix R, Van Lint J. Experience with cisapride in the treatment of chronic functional dyspepsia. Il Progresso Medico 1987;43(suppl.1):69-75.
47. Barbara L, Biasco G, Capurso L, Dobrilla G, Lalli A, Paganelli GH, Pallone F, Torsoli A. Effects of sucralfate and sulglycotide treatment on active gastritis and *Helicobacter pylori* colonization of the gastric mucosa in non-ulcer dyspepsia patients. Am J Gastroenterol 1990;85:1109-13.
48. Mwakyusa DH. Effects of domperidone in dyspepsia. East Afr Med J 1987;64:322-6.
49. Moriga M. A multicentre double-blind study of domperidone and metoclopramide in the symptomatic control of dyspepsia. Progress with domperidone, a gastrokinetic and anti-emetic agent. J R Soc Med 1980;36:77-9.
50. Saunders JHB, Oliver RJ, Higson DL. Dyspepsia: incidence of non-ulcer disease in a controlled trial of ranitidine in general practice. Br Med J 1986;292:655-68
51. Creytens G. Effect of the non-antidopaminergic drug cisapride on postprandial nausea. Curr Ther Res 1978;23:695-701.
52. Milo R. Non-cholinergic, non-antidopaminergic treatment of chronic digestive symptoms suggestive of a motility disorder: a two-step pilot evaluation of cisapride. Curr Ther Res 1984:36:1053-61.

53. Milo R. Use of the peripheral dopamine antagonist, domperidone in the management of gastrointestinal symptoms in patients with irritable bowel syndrome. Curr Med Res Opin 1980;6:577-84.
54. Bekhti A, Rutgeerts L. Domperidone in the treatment of functional dyspepsia in patients with delayed gastric emptying. Postgrad Med J 1979;55(suppl1):30-2.
55. Van de Mierop L, Rutgeerts L, Van den Langenbergh B, Staessen A. Oral domperidone in chronic postprandial dyspepsia. A double-blind placebo-controlled evaluation. Digestion 1979;19:244-250.
56. Van Ganse W, Coenegrachts J. Chronic dyspepsia: double-blind treatment with domperidone (R33812) or a placebo. A multicentre therapeutic evaluation. Curr Ther Res 1978; 23: 695-701.
57. De Loose F. Domperidone in chronic dyspepsia: a pilot open study and a multicentre general practice cross-over comparison with metoclopramide and placebo. Pharmatherapeutica 1979; 2:140-6.
58. Dobrilla G, Comberlato M, Steele A, Vallaperta P. Drug treatment of functional dypsepsia. A meta-analysis of randomized controlled clinical trials. J Clin Gastroenterol 1989; 11:169-77.

# 22

# Diagnostic strategy

G. VANTRAPPEN

*Universitaire Ziekenhuizen, Louvain, Belgique*

The most widely accepted definition of dyspepsia in English language publications is chronic or recurrent upper abdominal pain or distress, which may or may not be associated with nausea or vomiting, and is not necessarily related to food intake. On the European continent the term dyspepsia implies a syndrome of upper abdominal distress rather than pain. The distress is described in various ways: fullness, heaviness, early satiety, sensation of slow digestion, bloating, nausea, vomiting, etc. This definition is in better accordance with the etymological significance of dyspepsia: to digest badly.

The unqualified term "dyspepsia" is not really meaningful, because it is too vague. Other terms such as "non-ulcer dyspepsia" and "essential dyspepsia" have become popular in the medical literature. The term non-ulcer dyspepsia refers to a symptom complex suggestive of peptic ulcer disease in a patient shown not to have peptic ulcer at endoscopy. Although this term is already more precisely defined, it is still ambiguous and includes a number of identifiable diseases such as gastro-oesophageal reflux disease, irritable bowel syndrome and gallbladder or pancreatic disease. Essential dyspepsia is perhaps a better term as it refers to an upper abdominal pain or distress syndrome in which the above mentioned disorders, identifiable by standard investigations, have been excluded.

## Investigating patients with "dyspepsia": who?

The main aim of the gastroenterologist asked to investigate a patient with dyspepsia is to discard that diagnosis as soon as possible, by identifying and isolating specific disorders and retaining only those cases that can be labelled "essential" or "idiopathic" dyspepsia. The main problem is: how far should we go in our investigations to achieve that aim?

## History taking

The main disorders causing upper abdominal distress or pain labelled dyspepsia include peptic ulcer, gastro-oesophageal reflux disease, irritable bowel syndrome and gallbladder or pancreatic disease. The symptoms of essential dyspepsia may mimic those of peptic ulcer. In both conditions the pain is often located in the epigastrium, may have the same degree of severity, may be intermittent in nature and may occur before and/or 30 min to 3 hours after meals [1]. In contrast, night pain, relief of pain by food, and vomiting occur more frequently in peptic ulcer than in essential dyspepsia (75% *versus* 42%, 78% *versus* 50%, and 38% *versus* 14% respectively).

The symptoms of gastro-oesophageal reflux are often very typical. When a patient presents with acid regurgitation, or heartburn, i.e. an epigastric or low substernal burning sensation moving upward substernally, there is no need for sophisticated investigations to be sure that this patient has gastro-oesophageal reflux. Atypical symptoms include non-radiating pain in the epigastrium, substernal pain attacks and coughing spells or asthmatic dyspnoea on reclining at night.

Epigastric pain may be part of an irritable bowel syndrome. The term irritable bowel syndrome is as vague as that of essential dyspepsia. As there are neither pathological lesions nor pathophysiological markers, the disease can only be defined by its symptoms. The irritable bowel syndrome is characterized by disordered bowel habit, often with abdominal pain, but without organic lesions that may explain the symptoms. Disordered bowel habit is not part of essential dyspepsia. The most discriminating feature of the irritable bowel syndrome is a combination of three or more of the following six symptoms: relief of pain by defaecation, loose stools or more frequent stools with the onset of pain, abdominal distension, mucus per rectum, and a feeling of incomplete evacuation [2].

Essential dyspepsia may also mimic gallbladder disease. The location of the pain in the right upper quadrant, its radiation to the back and its occurrence in attacks are all in favour of gallbladder disease [3].

## Alarm symptoms

When taking a history of a patient with "dyspepsia", it is important to look for alarm symptoms, suggestive of organic, possibly serious disease. These symptoms include recent loss of weight without obvious reason, anaemia or blood loss per anum, dysphagia, fever, jaundice and an abdominal mass. The onset of symptoms after the age of 40 years has the same significance.

In contrast, when the symptoms have been present unchanged for a long period of time, when there is a positive family history of functional disease and when there are other "neurovegetative" symptoms, organic disease is much less likely. Therefore investigations are not needed from the onset in a young patient with recent non-alarming symptoms. When organic lesions have been excluded by previous investigations in a patient with a protracted but unchanged symptom pattern, investigation is also redundant.

*Diagnostic strategy*

## When to investigate?

Whenever careful history and clinical examination elicit alarm symtoms, such as recent weight loss, anaemia, blood loss, dysphagia, fever or an abdominal mass, investigations are needed regardless of the duration of the symptoms and the age of the patient. Organic or serious pathology must be excluded, in these cases.

When the patient presents with symptoms suggestive of a specific disease, the diagnostic or therapeutic decision will depend upon the nature of the suspected condition. In case of a functional disorder such as gastro-oesophageal reflux disease or irritable bowel syndrome, a six-week course of symptomatic therapy is warranted. Investigations should be carried out if, after this therapeutic trial, the symptoms have not completely resolved. When the symptoms suggest the presence of a specific organic disease such as peptic ulcer or gallbladder or pancreatic disease the appropriate investigations are indicated from the onset.

The most difficult problem is the patient who presents with atypical non-alarming symptoms. In a young patient, less than 40 years of age, symptomatic treatment may be started. Re-evaluation after six weeks is mandatory. If the symptoms have not completely resolved, investigations are indicated. Patients over the age of 40 years with chronic or recurrent dyspeptic symptoms should also be investigated from the onset. This is particularly true if a longstanding symptom pattern has recently changed in character.

The reason why investigations are ordered may be related to physician's fear of missing an important pathology, and thereby missing the opportunity to start possibly life-saving therapy at a time when it is still likely to be clinically useful. Such investigations often lead to a diagnosis through exclusion. The knowledge that serious pathology has been excluded is reassuring for most patients. Experience with chest pain of non-cardiac origin indicates that it is not always sufficient to tell the patient that the various invasive investigations that have been performed prove that nothing is wrong with his heart. If he continues to suffer chest pain attacks, he will soon believe that the doctor did not find what is wrong with his heart or that it is so serious that he does not wish to tell him. Therefore, whenever possible, it is advisable to try and come to a positive diagnosis.

## What investigations?

The investigation of patients with dyspepsia comprises two different steps. The first and most important aim is to arrive at a more specific diagnosis either by identifying a specific organic lesion or pathophysiological phenomenon, or by making a diagnosis of essential dyspepsia after having excluded all appropriate disease entities. The second step, which does not necessarily have to be taken, is the investigation into the nature of the pathophysiological disorder underlying the patient's symptoms.

Careful history is essential to construct a logical plan of investigations.

### "First-step" investigations

1. The nature of the alarm symptoms will determine the type of investigation that has to be carried out in order to exclude or identify suspected organic disease.

2. Similarly, when symptoms suggest a specific pathology, the investigation will depend upon the nature of the suspected disorder.

(a) Typical symptoms of gastro-oesophageal reflux only require investigation if they are accompanied by alarm symptoms or if a preceding six-week course of symptomatic treatment with $H_2$-antagonists, motility stimulating drugs or antacids proved to be ineffective. The first investigation to be done in this case is endoscopy. If endoscopy reveals the presence of reflux oesophagitis with erosions or ulceration, treatment is indicated. The type of treatment will depend on the severity of the lesions. Grade 1 and grade 2 oesophagitis may be treated by $H_2$-antagonists or motility stimulating drugs. More severe lesions may require high doses of $H_2$-antagonists, a combination of motility stimulating drugs and $H_2$-antagonists, or omeprazole.

If endoscopy does not show any objective lesions of reflux oesophagitis, further investigations such as 24-hour pH measurements and oesophageal manometry are indicated.

(b) When upper abdominal pain or distress is accompanied by a disordered stool pattern, a tentative diagnosis of irritable bowel syndrome is often made. In patients presenting with longstanding, unchanged symptoms, for which organic lesions have been satisfactorily excluded previously, investigations are not needed. As the diagnosis of irritable bowel syndrome is based in part on the absence of organic lesions that possibly may explain the symptoms, investigations should be carried out at the beginning to establish the diagnosis firmly; they should also be done whenever the presence of alarm symptoms or a change in symptom pattern casts doubt upon the initial diagnosis. In these cases we usually perform a total colonoscopy and ileoscopy, which will exclude the majority of ileocolonic diseases. Sometimes it will be necessary to proceed to a barium follow-through of the small intestine.

(c) The first examination to be carried out in patients with ulcer-like symptoms is upper gastrointestinal endoscopy. There is some evidence that erosive duodenitis should be considered as an acid-related disease and therefore should be treated in the same way as a duodenal ulcer.

(d) In patients with symptoms of gallbladder or pancreatic disease, ultrasonography of the upper abdomen will be the first step. If ultrasonography and oral cholecystography are negative, the risk of missing a biliary cause of pain is less than 1% [4]. Pancreatic disease is a rare cause of chronic epigastric pain or distress. Therefore CT-scan and endoscopic retrograde choledocopancreatography will only rarely be needed in the dyspeptic patient.

3. A difficult diagnostic problem is the investigation of the patient with aspecific symptoms, i.e. the patient who does not present with alarm symptoms and does not have symptoms suggestive of gastro-oesophageal reflux disease, irritable bowel syndrome, peptic ulcer or biliopancreatic disease. When investigations are indicated (i.e. in patients over the age of 40) the first aim will be to exclude organic pathology such as peptic ulcer or gastric carcinoma, reflux oesophagitis, and biliopancreatic disease. The appropriate investigations are upper gastrointestinal endoscopy and ultrasonography of the upper abdomen. This approach is different from the approach in patients with symptoms of gastro-oesophageal reflux. Heartburn and acid regurgitation are so specific that further investigations are not needed to be sure the patient has gastro-oesophageal reflux. Only if the symptoms do not respond satisfactorily to symptomatic treatment is endoscopy indicated. In contrast, non-specific epigastric pain or distress may be due to various organic and possibly very serious lesions and should therefore be investigated.

## Diagnostic strategy

When upper gastrointestinal endoscopy and ultrasonography are normal, and there is nothing to suggest that the colon is involved, the major organic lesions responsible for the non-specific symptoms are excluded, and a diagnosis of essential dyspepsia may be made.

This approach leaves the problem of *Helicobacter pylori* gastritis untouched. Although there is little doubt that *H. pylori* may cause acute and chronic active gastritis, there is insufficient evidence to indicate that gastritis due to this agent causes dyspeptic symptoms or that eradication of the organism results in longlasting symptomatic relief.

### Further investigations into the nature of essential dyspepsia

#### First-line treatment

Once the diagnosis of essential dyspepsia has been established, treatment should be started. The type of treatment to be given is not standardized. In all cases it should be stressed that, after the careful investigations that have been performed, organic or serious disease may confidently be excluded. This strong affirmation will reassure, at least temporarily, many patients.

In most patients reassurance is, of itself, not sufficient. Symptomatic treatment should be added. Although most acid-related conditions, for which $H_2$-receptor antagonists or antacids are indicated, have been excluded before a diagnosis of essential dyspepsia is made, $H_2$-blockers should be tried if part of the symptom pattern seems to be acid-related. For instance, in patients with irritable bowel syndrome and gastro-oesophageal reflux symptoms, $H_2$-blockers will be useful to combat heartburn and acid regurgitation.

It would seem logical to treat symptoms thought to be due to motility disorders by means of motility stimulating or inhibiting drugs. It is often difficult, however, to be sure about the presence or absence of motility disorders and even more so about the nature of the motility disorder without further investigations. When symptoms such as postprandial distress and early satiety, even after a light meal, suggest delayed gastric emptying, scintigraphic study of a radioisotope-labelled meal may clarify the gastric emptying pattern and justify the use of gastroprokinetic drugs [5].

Other symptoms such as nausea and vomiting, epigastric fullness or heaviness, and abdominal distension also suggest a motility disorder for which prokinetic drugs may be useful. Motility inhibiting drugs such as calcium channel blockers and anticholinergics will be given when the symptomatology is dominated by crampy pains.

When given in this clinical situation, treatment with motility modulating drugs is empirical and based on the assumption not only that a motility disorder is present but also that the disorder results either in defective propulsion or in painful "spasms".

If after a sufficiently long therapeutic trial with these drugs (combined with reassurance and psychotropic agents) the patient continues to have severe symptoms or insists upon a positive diagnosis, further investigations into the nature of the motility disorders are indicated.

#### Investigation into the nature of motility disorders

The two main techniques for investigating motility disorders are manometry and electromyography. The clinical application of gastrointestinal manometry is not so well standardized as that of oesophageal manometry. When studying gastric motility, care should be taken to have at least two recording points in the terminal antrum throughout the study period. The study of antroduodenal coordination requires multiple recording sites in antrum and duodenum. A Dent-sleeve in the pylorus allows pyloric activity to be monitored in relation to antroduodenal contractions. If one wants to study the presence or absence and the propagation characteristics of phase 3 of the migrating motor complex, at least three recording sites are required, spanning a length of at least 40 cm. If the characteristics of phase 2 or postprandial contractions and their organization into motility patterns are studied, the distance between the three (or more) recording sites should be no more than 3 to 4 cm.

Several motor abnormalities have been identified in manometric studies of dyspeptic patients. Decreased antral phasic pressure activity after a solid meal was observed in 72 of 104 dyspeptic patients [6]. In 40% it occurred as an isolated phenomenon; in the remaining 30% it was accompanied by intestinal motor abnormalities. Antroduodenal coordination, which may be important in gastric emptying, was not measured in this study. Frequently, a small intestinal manometric study is considered to be normal if a normal-looking phase 3 is present and if there are not gross abnormalities in the number or amplitude of the pressure waves. Abnormalities in phase 2 patterns are often overlooked, mainly because they are not well defined or because they are poorly recognized [7].

Electromyography of the stomach is still in an experimental phase. It is difficult to obtain technically satisfactory recordings of gastric slow waves and spikes by means of intraluminal electrodes. Only at the level of the distal antrum is the gastric lumen narrow enough to facilitate prolonged recordings without signal loss. Techniques are being developed to record the slow wave activity of the stomach with skin electrodes.

Several disorders of slow wave rhythm and slow wave conduction have been reported in association with dyspeptic symptoms, particularly with nausea and vomiting. These include brady- and tachygastria (normal rhythm is 3 per minute), tachyarrhythmia and ectopic pacemaker activity with oral propagation of slow waves. It has been shown that during a phase of tachyarrhythmia all mechanical activity is abolished, which may explain part of the symptoms [8].

Electromyography of the small intestine is more easy to perform. A technique has been described which allows continuous recording for long periods of time at eight or more different levels of the intestine simultaneously [9]. As this technique allows one to record not only the contractions but also the myogenic control mechanisms, it should give a better insight and a better definition of normal and abnormal motility patterns [8].

The relationship between manometric or electromyographic abnormalities of gastrointestinal motility and symptoms is often difficult to establish. To prove such a relationship, a constant association of symptoms with specific motility abnormalities has to be demonstrated. This requires prolonged (24 hours or more) recording, in order to increase the chances of recording the motility abnormalities at the time symptoms develop. An alternative possibility is to use provocation tests that mimic closely the familiar symptomatology and to record motility during the provocation test.

## References

1. Talley NJ, Piper DW. Comparison of the clinical features and illness behaviour of patients presenting with dyspepsia of unknown cause (essential dyspepsia) and organic disease. Aust NZ J Med 1986;16:352-9.
2. Manning AP, Thompson WG, Heaton KW, Morris AF. Towards positive diagnosis of the irritable bowel. Br Med J 1978;2:653-4.
3. Talley NJ, McNeil D, Piper DW. Discriminant value of dyspeptic symptoms: a study of the clinical presentation of 221 patients with dyspepsia of unknown cause, peptic ulceration, and cholelithiasis. Gut 1987;28:40-6.
4. De Lacey G, Gajjar B, Twomey B, Levi J, Cos AG. Should cholecystography or ultrasound be the primary investigation for gallbladder disease? Lancet 1984;1:205-7.
5. Jian R, Ducrot F, Piedeloup C, Mary JY, Najean Y, Bernier JJ. Measurement of gastric emptying in dyspeptic patients: effect of a new gastrokinetic agent (cisapride). Gut 1985;26:352-8.
6. Malagelada JR, Stanghellini V. Manometric evaluation of functional upper gut symptoms. Gastroenterology 1985; 88:1223-31.
7. Vantrappen G, Janssens J, Coremans G, Jian R. Gastrointestinal motility disorders. Dig Dis Sci 1986;31(9 suppl):5S-25S.
8. Vantrappen G, Schippers E, Janssens J, Vandeweerd M. What is the mechanical correlate of gastric dysrhythmia? Gastroenterology 1984;86:1288(abstr).
9. Coremans G, Janssens J, Vantrappen G, Chaussade S, Ceccatelli P. Migrating action potential complexes in a patient with secretory diarrhoea. Dig Dis Sci 1987;32:1201-6.

# 23

# Therapeutic strategy

J.-P. GALMICHE*, T. VALLOT**

*Clinique des maladies de l'appareil digestif, CHU Nord, 44035 Nantes Cedex, France
** Clinique des maladies de l'appareil digestif, CHU Bichat, 75018 Paris Cedex, France

**Introduction**

Non-ulcer dyspepsia (NUD) is a poorly defined clinical entity including a heterogeneous group of patients with various upper alimentary complaints [1]. Although it is a very common disorder [2], probably affecting 20 to 30% of the general population, its management remains difficult. In fact, NUD encompasses a wide variety of symptoms with various degrees of intensity and frequency; on the one hand many patients probably do not seek medical help and treat themselves with over-the-counter (OTC) medications (mainly antacids and now, in some countries, $H_2$-antagonists). On the other hand, there is a substantial group of patients who suffer chronically from a disabling disorder which may negatively influence their quality of life. Hence, repeated investigations, multiple drug prescriptions and absenteeism are frequently observed in these patients. Therefore, the social cost, although difficult to evaluate exactly, is probably very important in most of Western countries; for instance, in Sweden, NUD ranks fourth among all primary care diagnoses [3].

Due to the heterogeneity of this syndrome and the multifactorial nature of its pathogenesis [4], it is unlikely than one type of drug can benefit all patients [5]. It is therefore important to identify those patients who will respond positively to one type of treatment. In this connection, a group of gastroenterologists from different countries [1] tried to divide NUD in several categories, based largely on symptoms, which were thought to suggest different causative factors (i.e. the so-called "reflux-like dyspepsia", "dysmotility-like dyspepsia", "ulcer-like dyspepsia" and "essential dyspepsia"). Unfortunately symptoms correlate poorly with presumed pathophysiological factors; for instance only half of the patients with dysmotility-like dyspepsia have delayed gastric emptying when assessed with an objective method such as gastric scintigraphy [6]. Despite these difficulties, an attempt at defining a practical approach to the patient with NUD will be made in this chapter after a short review of the present knowledge on currently available drugs.

## An overview of clinical trials and drugs potentially useful in the treatment of NUD

### General considerations on controlled trials

Due to uncertainties in the underlying pathophysiological mechanisms many drugs have been actually tested or may be potentially useful in the treatment of NUD; these include mainly acid-lowering drugs, prokinetics, mucosal coating agents and therapies directed against *Helicobacter pylori*. The methodological difficulties encountered in therapeutic trials have already been analysed in a previous chapter (see Poynard *et al.*). However, taken together, these trials, although randomized and performed blindly, have led to conflicting results probably because of the heterogeneity of selection criteria, characteristics of patients enrolled and mode of recruitment, as well as assessment criteria. Finally, the proportion of drug responders is probably as important as the efficacy of the drug itself in interpreting the results, positive or negative, of many controlled trials. For instance, including a large number of patients with reflux-related symptoms in a trial of an antisecretory drug is likely to enhance the probability of a positive answer with a statistically significant benefit (see below). In this regard, some authors have emphasized the value of cross-over or even multi-cross-over designs compared to the traditional trials with parallel groups [5].

### Acid-lowering drugs

#### *Antacids and alginate/antacids*

Antacids are widely used by patients with NUD. Although antacids have been considered the mainstay of the treatment of gastro-oesophageal reflux disease (GORD) until the 80s, a critical review of placebo-controlled trials failed to demonstrate that they are better than placebo in relieving symptoms [7]. However, this negative conclusion should be qualified because patients with the mild forms of reflux-like dyspepsia are perhaps not enrolled in these trials. In this regard, a double-blind cross-over trial [8] showed that heavy consumers of antacids frequently described symptoms compatible with GORD and found antacids preferable to placebo in relieving heartburn.

In many pharmaceutical formulations, antacids and alginates are combined (e.g. Gaviscon®). These compounds usually have a low acid buffering capacity and are mainly directed against reflux itself with alginates floating as a raft on the surface of the gastric contents and preventing contact between the oesophageal mucosa and the acid material of the refluxate. There are now several placebo-controlled trials showing that alginate/antacid compounds are effective in relieving heartburn and reflux symptoms [9]. In France a large multicentre trial [10] performed in primary care patients with *reflux-like dyspepsia* showed that about 92% of patients were asymptomatic after a 2-week treatment with an alginate-antacid compound; moreover, even in those incompletely relieved by treatment, endoscopy showed no or mild lesions of oesophagitis in 60%.

## Therapeutic strategy

In patients with *ulcer-like dyspepsia,* defined as chronic or recurrent pain without concomitant symptoms of the irritable bowel syndrome, Nyrén et al. [3] showed that a 3-week administration of an antacid suspension (Novaluzid®), given at a dose as high as 10 ml one and three hours after meals and at bedtime (one 10 ml sachet corresponding to 85 mmol antacid capacity), was not superior to placebo. Nevertheless, after 3 weeks a 25% mean reduction in pain intensity score occurred irrespective of the treatment received, antacid or placebo. In another study [11] including patients with inflammation of the antral or duodenal mucosa, the proportion of patients with deterioration in antral gastritis at endoscopy was greater after a 6-week antacid treatment than after placebo or cimetidine. However, it is worth mentioning that in these two trials [3, 11] about 20 to 30% of patients were receiving NSAIDs. Finally, in patients with NUD and endoscopic signs of erosive prepyloric changes (EPC), Weberg and Berstad [12] also failed to demonstrate a significant benefit of a low dose 4-week antacid regimen on either symptoms or endoscopic lesions. Lastly, in patients with associated symptoms suggestive of flatulent *dysmotility-like dyspepsia* (i.e. nausea, bloating, meteorism), antacids were not found to be more effective than placebo by Gotthard et al. [13] nor by Weberg and Berstad [12].

In conclusion, there is no evidence of efficacy of antacids in NUD even when specially searching for a subgroup of responders among patients with ulcer-like symptoms (with or without inflammation of the antrum or duodenum at endoscopy and histology). Moreover, for the relief of symptoms in patients with reflux-like dyspepsia alginate/antacids should be preferred to pure antacids.

### $H_2$-receptor antagonists

$H_2$-receptor antagonists have now been tested in many randomized double-blind placebo-controlled trials (Table I); this treatment consisted of cimetidine (0.8 to 1.2 g daily) in all except one case in which ranitidine was used [21]. The compilation of all these studies [3, 13-23], as well as the result of a recent meta-analysis [24], clearly establish that $H_2$-antagonists are effective and useful drugs, at least in a subgroup of patients. Indeed, only one large well-conducted trial [3] led to negative conclusions; although no clear explanation can be proposed for this discrepancy, it is worth mentioning that this trial included patients receiving NSAIDs and that the assessment criteria depended on a quantitative symptomatic score and not on a qualitative "yes or no" response to treatment. In two other negative trials [15, 19], a high risk of type-II error (related to small numbers of patients), might explain the absence of a significant difference between the placebo group and those treated with the active drug.

Trials using a cross-over design [20] or a multi-cross-over model [16, 22] are interesting in identifying those patients who do respond to these drugs. This group of responders includes patients with prominent reflux symptoms [20, 22] and, perhaps, those with EPC or inflammation of the antro-duodenal area at endoscopic and/or histological assessments [17]. In contrast, patients with symptoms suggestive of the irritable bowel syndrome (IBS) are probably poor responders to $H_2$-antagonists.

The efficacy of cimetidine in patients with reflux-like dyspepsia has recently been confirmed in the US where cimetidine 200 mg caplets were given on demand (up to 4 caplets per day) to patients with moderate or severe heartburn or "sour stomach"; in this large scale double-blind trial low doses of cimetidine (the mean intake was

**Table I.** Placebo-controlled trials of $H_2$-receptor antagonists in non-ulcer dyspepsia. (From Dobrilla et al. [24] modified).

| Authors [reference] | Type of NUD | Study design | Treatment duration and dose | "Assessment criteria" | Statistical results (p value < or =) |
|---|---|---|---|---|---|
| Nyrén et al. [3] | Ulcer-like | R, DB, PG | C. 3 wk. 400 mgx2 | Pain intensity and duration | NS |
| Gotthard et al. [13] | All types | R, DB, PG | C. 6 wk. 400 mgx2 | Responders and symptom relief | 0.05 |
| Mackinnon et al. [14] | Ulcer-like duodenitis | R, DB, PG | C. 6 wk. 1g | Symptomatic and endoscopic improvement | 0.05 |
| Kelbaeck et al. [15] | Ulcer-like | R, DB | C. 3 wk. 1g | Reduction of symptoms | NS |
| Kleveland et al. [16] | Ulcer-like (previous ulcer) | MCO (6 periods) | C. 2-4 days. 0.8-1.2 g | Symptom relief | 0.02 |
| Nesland and Berstad [17] | Ulcer-like (EPC) | R, DB, PG | C. 4 wk. 400 mgx2 | Epigastric pain and EPC | 0.05 |
| Delattre et al. [18] | Ulcer-like | R, DB, PG | C. 2 wk. 200 mgx4 | Relief of dyspeptic symptoms | 0.05 |
| Lance et al. [19] | Ulcer-like | R, DB, PG | C. 4 wk. 1g | Symptom relief | NS |
| Talley et al. [20] | Essential and reflux like | R, DB, CO | C. 4 wk. 200 mgx4 | Abdominal pain episodes<br>Acid regurgitations | 0.0008<br>0.04 |
| Saunders et al. [21] | Ulcer-like | R, DB, PG | R. 6 wk. 150 mgx2 | Number of symptom free patients | 0.05 |
| Johannessen et al. [22] | Ulcer-like (6 periods) | R, DB, MCO | C. 2 days. 400 mgx3 | VAS Scores (responders had reflux symptoms) | 0.0001 |
| Singal et al. [23] | Ulcer-like and reflux like | R, DB, PG | C. 4 wk. 400 mgx2 | Patients with pain relief | 0.05 |

EPC: Erosive prepyloric changes — R: Randomized — DB: Double-blind — PG: Parallel groups — C: Cimetidine — R: Ranitidine — CO: Cross-over — MCO: Multi cross-over — VAS: Visual analog scale about 400 mg per day) proved significantly more efficacious than placebo or antacid relieving symptoms (Shriver et al., SKF unpublished data).

In conclusion, results with $H_2$-antagonists in NUD illustrate the risk of making a type-II error when including in the same trial patients with different symptom clusters. In our opinion, as in that of other workers [5, 16, 22], cross-over trials may represent the first step in the identification of responders whereas trials on parallel groups should ideally focus on selected populations.

## Pirenzepine

Pirenzepine is a selective anticholinergic compound acting on the $M_1$ muscarinic receptors. Several trials and a meta-analysis of these [24] concluded that is it effective in NUD with an overall therapeutic gain of 25%. However, these favourable studies have mainly been published in supplements of journals which are usually promoted by the manufacturers [24]. In contrast, the excellent double-blind randomized cross-over study performed by Talley et al. [20] failed to show any benefit with pirenzepine in patients with essential or reflux-like dyspepsia. Furthermore there was a trend for patients on pirenzepine to have an increased number of pain episodes compared with placebo; nausea was also exacerbated on pirenzepine as were regurgitations in patients with reflux-like dyspepsia. Lastly, 51% of patients receiving pirenzepine experienced dry mouth compared to 9% on placebo, which seems an unacceptable rate of unwanted side effects. Similar negative results and frequent adverse effects were also recently reported by Smith et al. [25]. Finally, this drug appears inferior to placebo as a first choice treatment of NUD and should never be used when there are symptoms suggestive of reflux or nausea.

## Prokinetic drugs

This class of drugs includes antidopaminergic compounds, metoclopramide and domperidone, and the newly developed prokinetic agent, cisapride, which is the most promising drug at the moment.

Among antidopaminergics, metoclopramide has been extensively evaluated in various conditions including gastroparesis secondary to diabetic dysautonomia or vagotomy; unfortunately few studies deal specifically with NUD [26, 27]. It is important to underline the fact that with the effective doses (40 mg per day) frequently required for treating symptomatic patients, adverse effects (drowsiness, bowel disturbance, dizziness and faintness) are frequent (the incidence being at least 10%) especially in children, young adults and women. However, severe cases of extrapyramidal effects are very rare.

Domperidone is a more recently developed dopamine antagonist related to butyrophenones which has nearly the same pharmacodynamic actions as metoclopramide on oesophageal and gastric motility [28]. However domperidone does not cross the blood-brain barrier and seldom causes extrapyramidal untoward effects; it may, however, produce symptoms related to hyperprolactinaemia (galactorrhoea, amenorrhoea). Several controlled trials and the meta-analysis of these studies performed by Dobrilla et al. [24] concluded that this well-tolerated prokinetic agent was effective in NUD (Fig. 1) with an overall therapeutic gain over placebo of 56% (95% confidence interval 46-74%).

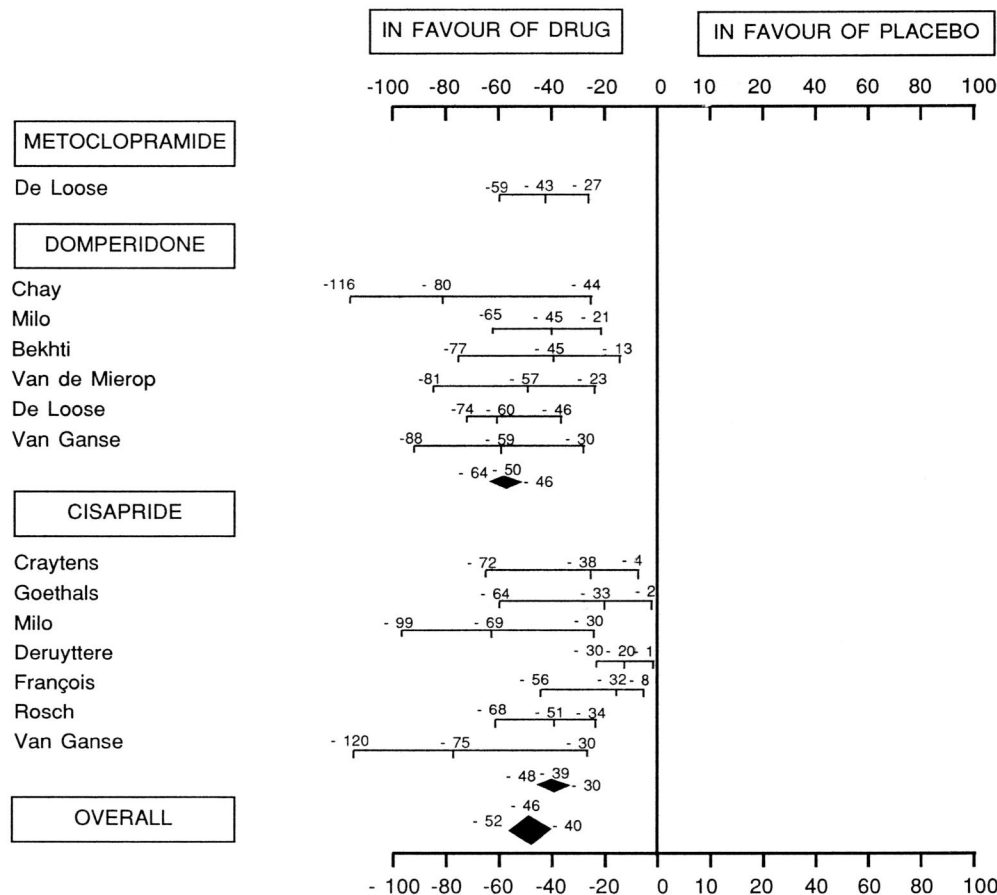

**Figure 1.** Differences in success rates between patients treated with placebo and antidopaminergic prokinetics (metoclopramide and domperidone) or cisapride in non-ulcer dyspepsia. (From Dobrilla et al. [24], with permission of the editor of the Journal of Clinical Gastroenterology). Number at end-points indicate 95% confidence limits.

Cisapride is a new prokinetic drug without antidopaminergic or direct cholinomimetic effects [for review, see 29, 30]. Its mechanism of action involves acetylcholine release but there is also some evidence that cisapride acts both as an agonist ($5HT_4$) and an antagonist ($5HT_3$) of serotonin. Cisapride strengthens the basal tone of the LOS and the amplitude of oesophageal body contractions. It accelerates gastric emptying but does not affect gastric acid secretion. A review [31] of 10 placebo-controlled trials of cisapride in the treatment of NUD showed that cisapride was superior to placebo in all of them. Cisapride (at a dose of 5 or 10 mg tid or qid for 2 to 8 weeks) seems effective on epigastric pain and concomitant symptoms

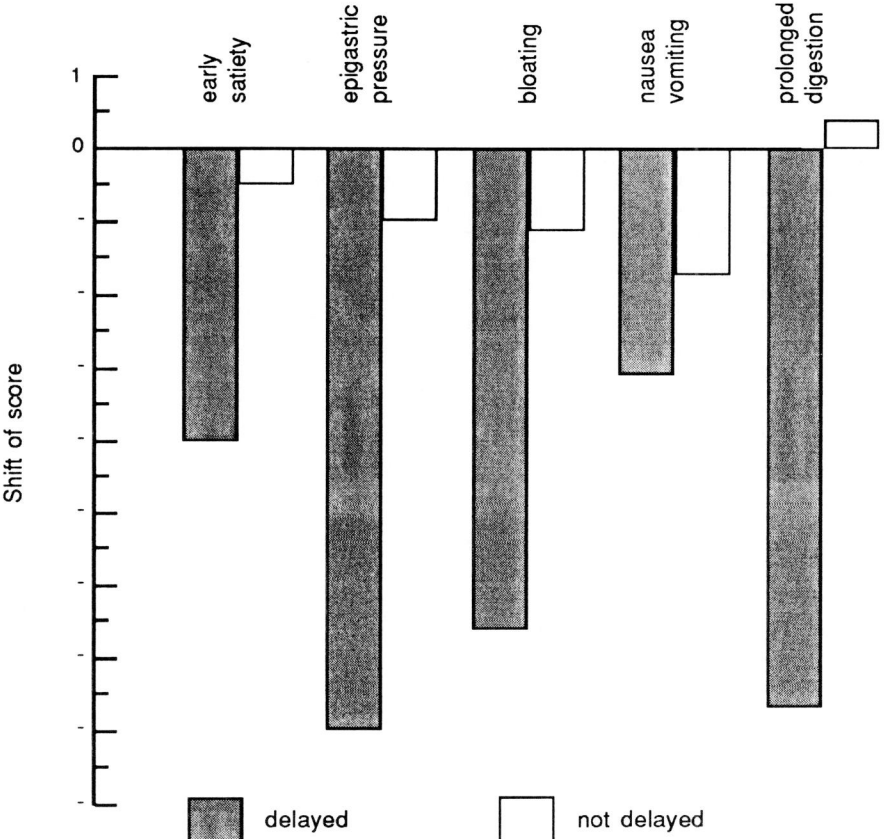

**Figure 2.** Shifts in specific symptom scores induced by cisapride at week 3 in subgroups of dyspeptic patients with gastric emptying delay (n=7) and without such a delay (n=8). Negative values indicate score reductions induced by cisapride. (Reproduced from Jian *et al.* [32], with permission of the editor of Digestive Diseases and Sciences).

including heartburn as well as postprandial discomfort (belching, bloating, early satiety, nausea). It is also well tolerated, with only few patients complaining of diarrhoea or increased bowel movements. Recently, an interesting study [32] identified a subgroup of patients with better alleviation of symptoms after 3 weeks of cisapride 40 mg daily; these responders had delayed gastric emptying (assessed by a dual isotopic method) at baseline (Fig. 2). Unfortunately this trial also illustrates the fact that symptoms are poorly correlated with the objective parameters of the gastric scintigraphic study since only the feeling of "slow digestion" was significantly associated with gastric stasis. These observations are in agreement with the results of trials including patients with both flatulent and ulcer-like or reflux-like dyspepsia where cisapride was always found to be better than placebo [31]. Finally, should long term clinical experience and further trials confirm the efficacy and safety of cisapride, it could represent a first choice drug in the treatment of NUD.

In conclusion, the role of prokinetic agents in the treatment of NUD patients will probably grow as far as our basic knowledge progresses in that field. In this regard, the development of new prokinetic agents is now in progress [see Scarpignato, page 213]. For example, several potent and structurally related 5-$HT_3$ selective receptor antagonists have been identified within the last few years [33]. Evaluation of these compounds in a large variety of animal models has indicated a wide potential use for gastrointestinal disorders including NUD since they can increase gastric emptying and reduce emesis. Similarly, recent studies showed that erythromycin, a macrolide antibiotic, acts on smooth muscle motilin receptors. The prokinetic effects of erythromycin on gastric emptying has been demonstrated in patients with severe diabetic gastroparesis [34]. Lastly, various CCK antagonists have also recently been described (lorglumide, loxiglumide, L364,718, etc.) with possible effects on postprandial motility and satiety [35]. The benefit of inhibiting CCK with loxiglumide in dyspeptic patients has recently been suggested in a pilot study [36]. Although it is difficult to define the role of these new prokinetics, in the future they could dramatically broaden our therapeutic armamentarium in NUD.

## Mucosal coating agents and therapeutics aimed at the eradication of *Helicobacter (Campylobacter) pylori*

### Sucralfate

Sucralfate, an aluminium salt of sulphated sucrose, is a non-systemic drug that forms an adherent complex with proteins of the normal and damaged mucosa of the stomach and duodenum. It acts as a protective barrier against various noxious agents, and adsorbs pepsin and bile salts. It stimulates bicarbonate and mucus secretion by prostaglandin $E_2$-dependent and prostaglandin-independent mechanisms and causes accumulation of epidermal growth factor in the mucosa. Sucralfate also protects the microcirculation and proliferative zone integrity and promotes epithelial restitution (37). Although the relative contribution of these different properties to the overall "cytoprotective" effect of sucralfate are not well-known, they have provided the rationale for trials with this drug in erosive and non-erosive gastritis associated to NUD. However, few studies have been published so far.

In their double-blind placebo-controlled trial performed in patients with chronic epigastric pain without concomitant symptoms of IBS and with no evidence of any organic disease other than macroscopic or microscopic gastritis/duodenitis, Kairaluoma *et al.* [38] found sucralfate (1 g three times daily half an hour before meals for 4 weeks) significantly better than placebo. Hence, 77% and 56% of patients had become symptom-free at the end of the trial in the sucralfate and the placebo groups, respectively. However the best response to treatment was achieved in patients with mild or moderate symptoms and no inflammation of their gastric or duodenal mucosa. Although the results were not reported in detail in this special group of patients, it is interesting to notice that about 40% of the subjects enrolled in this trial used NSAIDs. In another trial [39] sucralfate (1 g three times a day) was compared with ranitidine

(150 mg bid) in patients with chronic non-erosive gastritis defined as oedema, reddening, contact bleeding or petechial lesions. The severity of symptoms was assessed before and after 2, 4, 6 and 8 weeks of treatment. Sucralfate was significantly more effective than ranitidine in inducing healing or improvement of endoscopic and histological gastritis but ranitidine was significantly more efficacious at relieving pain during the first four weeks of the trial. At the end of the study, however, the same proportion (about 80%) of patients were symptom-free in both groups. This study illustrates once again the poor correlation between non-erosive gastritis and symptoms of NUD. Since many patients with these mild signs of gastritis are symptomless, these lesions should not justify medical therapy in the absence of dyspepsia. Finally the role of sucralfate in NUD is actually difficult to evaluate; in our opinion, more information is needed before it can be considered as one of the first choice drugs. Because of its pharmacological profile, trials with sucralfate should be encouraged in the treatment of patients with dyspeptic symptoms associated with NSAID use or as prophylaxis against NSAID intolerance [40].

## *Eradication of* **Helicobacter pylori**

There is considerable evidence of a high incidence of *Helicobacter pylori* infection in the gastric mucosa of patients with NUD. This spiral-shaped Gram negative bacterium has also been found in close association with peptic ulcer disease and "active" antral gastritis [41, 42] but its pathogenic role in these various disorders remains controversial. Although *H. pylori* is present in some 60 to 80% of dyspeptic patients, the possible mechanisms leading to dyspepsia are virtually unknown; in this connection it is important to note that the role of gastroparesis (whether as a causative factor or as a consequence of infection) has been ruled out by two studies [43, 44]. However, several preliminary uncontrolled studies using bismuth-containing preparations and/or antibiotics have suggested that a therapeutic approach directed against *H. pylori* could be effective on both symptoms [42] and gastritis [42, 45] associated with NUD. Recently, several trials [45-51] aimed at the treatment of *H. pylori* infection have been reported. Most controlled studies have tested the effects of colloidal bismuth subcitrate (DeNol®, Table II) and only one tested that of amoxicillin alone [51]. Taking together the relatively small number of patients with positive *H. pylori* status included in these trials and the fact that bismuth is not very effective on *H. pylori*, it is not surprising that these studies led to controversial results with respect to symptom relief. For instance, in the study of Loffeld *et al.* [49] the clearance of *H. pylori* at the end of treatment was lower (30%) than in other studies, in which it ranged from 59 to 89%. Finally CBS is better than placebo in clearing *H. pylori* from the gastric mucosa and in improving gastritis scores in patients with NUD. It is therefore probable that only those patients positive for *H. pylori* and with active antral gastritis will respond to this form of therapy. Future trials should be encouraged to include large numbers of such patients and to test more effective forms of antibacterial therapy, i.e. capable of achieving clearance and if possible eradication of the bacteria. In this connection, a recent meta-analysis of controlled trials of CBS and amoxicillin in NUD led to the conclusion that a treatment achieving at least a 75% clearance of *H. pylori* would be effective on symptoms of NUD [52]. However it seems wise to wait for the result of further studies before providing clear recommendations on the treatment of *H. pylori* infection in dyspeptic patients.

**Table II.** Placebo-controlled trials of bismuth salts in non-ulcer dyspepsia and effects of treatment on *Helicobacter pylori* (HP).

| Authors [reference] | Number | Bismuth salt | Study design | Duration of treatment (weeks) | Statistical results (p value < or =) | | | Clearance of HP (%)[a] |
|---|---|---|---|---|---|---|---|---|
| | | | | | Symptoms | Gastritis | Clearance | |
| McNulty et al. [46][b] | 50 | Salicylate | R, DB, PG | 3 | NS | 0.001 | 0.001 | (78) |
| Rokkas et al. [47] | 52 | CBS | R, DB, PG | 8 | 0.001 | 0.01 | 0.01 | (83) |
| Lambert et al. [48] | 78 | CBS | R, DB, PG | 4 | 0.05[c] | 0.01[c] | 0.05 | (59) |
| Loffeld et al. [49] | 50 | CBS | R, DB, PG | 4 | NS | 0.0007 | 0.00001 | (30) |
| Kang et al. [50] | 51 | CBS | R, DB, PG | 4 (+4 open treatment) | NS[d] | 0.025 | 0.001 | (89) |

Same abbreviations as in Table I. CBS: colloidal bismuth subcitrate.

— a - Percentage of patients cleared of HP in the bismuth group is indicated in parentheses.
— b - Three parallel groups (bismuth n=15; erythromycin n=17; placebo n=17). Twenty-two of these 50 patients had previous history of duodenal ulceration; 35 patients had symptoms of dyspepsia. No significant difference between placebo and erythromycin treated patients.
— c - In patients cleared of HP.
— d - Overall symptomatic response.

## Miscellaneous

Beside the previously discussed drugs many other therapeutic approaches have been proposed in NUD.

Sulglycotide, a cytoprotective agent isolated from pig duodenum, has been tested and compared to sucralfate in NUD patients with active gastritis and *H. pylori* infection [53]. Both agents induced marked regression of active gastritis whereas *H. pylori* colonization remained unchanged at the end of treatment. However the clinical relevance of these results is difficult to establish because the relationship between gastritis and symptoms is debated and because there was no placebo control group in this study.

The symptomatic effect of pancreatic enzymes was evaluated in a pilot study including dyspeptic patients recruited from general practice [54]. The evaluation was based on a comparison of the enzyme-associated and placebo-associated symptoms using a 24-day multi-cross-over model with treatment periods. No evidence of a short-term effect of pancreatic enzymes was found.

Lastly, while antidepressants or tranquillizers are frequently prescribed for dyspeptic patients, it is worth mentioning that no double-blind trial has really evaluated this practice. Therefore indications for using these drugs in NUD should be more restrictive, especially in some countries (e.g. France) where an abuse does exist.

## Strategy for the management of the dyspeptic patient

Because dyspeptic symptoms commonly occur in the general population [55, 56], it is important to realize that extensive and expensive investigations are not needed in most patients [4]. In fact only a minority of patients seek medical advice and self care seems an important factor in the management of dyspepsia [56, 57]. Advice may come to the patient from a variety of sources (e.g. family, friends, community pharmacists) and OTC medications (especially antacids) and dietary manipulations play an important role. Symptom severity and frequency as well as the effect of symptoms on physical function and daily living correlate poorly with consultation behaviour. In fact, fears that symptoms may be related to malignant and cardiac diseases or other serious illnesses seem very important [57]. In these patients, excluding an organic disease may help in reassuring the patient but it should not lead to over-investigation. Since the diagnostic strategy is discussed in the previous chapter [see Vantrappen] only those principles which are most important in the therapeutic approach will be recalled before we attempt to define some guidelines in the choice of drugs to be used in clinical practice.

### When to treat empirically and when to investigate?

The role of the general practitioner is very important in selecting which patients can be assigned to low-risk and high-risk groups [58].

Low-risk patients can be defined as young patients (under 45 years) without alarm symptoms and with no sign of organic disease on physical examination. In these patients, investigations can safely be deferred [1, 4], management can be at first symptomatic and a short trial of therapy (see below) can be prescribed. Although there is no good evidence in the literature of the efficacy of such recommendations, *dietary manipulations* (e.g. avoidance of coffee abuse and fatty foods) *and withdrawal of environmental factors* (smoking, alcohol and — if possible — analgesics or NSAIDs) are usually advised at this stage of treatment. Some specific foods are frequently incriminated by the patient himself but exclusion should be very cautious because the relation between foods and symptoms of dyspepsia is not established on a scientific basis in most cases of NUD. Similarly the role of psychosocial and lifestyle factors in NUD has frequently been underlined; for instance, these patients have been described as often unmarried or more anxious, neurotonic and depressed than the community controls [59]. They have also been found to have had unhappy childhoods or lower occupational status than their place of residence indicated [60]. However the clinical relevance of these differences and the role of major life event stress and social activities in the onset and course of NUD is controversial [61, 62]. Therefore, the psychological treatment of these patients should be limited to reassurance and careful explanation without any additional drug therapy in most cases. Finally many patients do respond to this conservative therapeutic approach and do not require further investigation. However, it must be re-emphasized that investigations, especially endoscopy (now usually completed by ultrasonography), are definitely indicated if there is no response or rapid recurrence of symptoms [63, 64].

Early investigations (without any previous empirical trial) should be performed in all patients above 45 years or in those with features suggestive of organic disease, especially in smokers or in those with a previous history of peptic ulcer [1]. Depending on symptoms and clinical presentation or progression, other diagnostic procedures [63] may be indicated (e.g. 24-h oesophageal pH monitoring, measurement of gastric emptying, biopsies and search for *H. pylori* infection).

**Which drugs to choose for empirical treatment?**

It is difficult to give practical guidelines because symptoms are poor predictors of therapeutic response and do not correlate with any specific pathophysiological disorder.

Until recently antacids have been considered the mainstay of symptomatic treatment in patients with NUD. Although they could serve as "a significant placebo" [4], in fact it seems more logical to consider alginate/antacids or prokinetic agents (especially cisapride) as the first choice drugs in patients with reflux-like dyspepsia.

The empirical use of $H_2$-receptor antagonists in NUD is controversial. Indeed, $H_2$-blockers may mask the symptoms and heal malignant gastric ulcers; they may also weaken the diagnostic value of a subsequent endoscopy, especially when there are superficial erosions of the antrum or duodenum. Empirical use of $H_2$-receptor antagonists may also lead to inappropriate long-term therapy and occasionally to untoward effects. However, all these arguments have been recently questioned and they are now considered not clinically relevant by many authors [65]. Hence, it is unlikely that the empirical use of $H_2$-receptor antagonists would mask the diagnosis of cancer because its prevalence is very low in young patients and because most patients with cancer have persistent symptoms suggestive of organic disease [66]. Moreover cimetidine and ranitidine are very well tolerated and probably among the safest drugs released, as shown by a considerable past clinical experience. In Denmark, cimetidine and ranitidine were transferred to the OTC status in 1989 and $H_2$-receptor antagonists have now replaced antacids as first choice drugs for mild dyspepsia without preceding diagnostic investigations. By the end of 1989 the total consumption had gone down and prices had been reduced by up to 35%. Cost-benefit analysis shows that the expected costs for treatment with $H_2$-receptor antagonist and antacids are similar because the greater effectiveness of the former compensates for their higher cost; comparing a strategy of empirical treatment with $H_2$-receptor antagonists with routine endoscopy shows the latter approximately doubles the costs for the treatment [67]. In our opinion the choice of $H_2$-receptor antagonists is probably reasonable when symptoms are suggestive of reflux or in patients with a history of ulcer-like dyspepsia without ulcer at previous endoscopies. Although many GPs already apply such a policy, it must be carefully monitored in a surveillance programme before the empirical use of $H_2$-receptor antagonists is confirmed and recommended on a larger scale.

## Can the results of investigations influence the choice of the drug?

When endoscopy shows *erosive prepyloric changes or duodenitis*, the overall results of therapeutic trials (Table I) strongly suggest that $H_2$-receptor antagonists are effective drugs. In fact in some patients the course of the disease seems very similar to that of peptic ulcer disease; in these cases long term maintenance therapy should be discussed when pain relief is effectively achieved with the drug and relapse shortly occurs at cessation of treatment. However in most cases it seems preferable to give the treatment on demand for relatively short periods of time (not exceeding 2 or 3 months).

At the moment biopsies should not be done routinely for the identification of *H. pylori* in NUD patients. However, in those patients who failed to respond to previous conventional therapies, such investigations are justified and, if positive, it is reasonable to try to eradicate the bacteria using one of the appropriate combinations of bismuth and antibiotics (mainly amoxicillin and metronidazole).

Oesophageal pH monitoring is now widely available for the diagnosis of GORD. In patients with rather atypical symptoms, the use of the event marker is crucial to document the role of reflux in the pathophysiology of symptoms of dyspepsia. Therefore, analysis should not only include a measure of oesophageal acid exposure but also the calculation of a symptom index [68]. In patients with well-documented reflux-related symptoms the role of long term treatment with prokinetics (especially cisapride) is certainly important because the pathophysiology of the disease is primarily that of a motility disorder.

In contrast to 24-h pHmetry, the isotopic measurement of gastric emptying is not easily accessible and should be restricted to patients with severe symptoms and a long history of dyspepsia which fail to respond to several attempts with various drugs. It is however an important assessment because a better symptomatic response to prokinetics may be expected in patients with delayed gastric emptying. In this connection, new drugs acting through a motilin agonism effect (e.g. erythromycin derivatives) or by blocking $5 HT_3$ receptors may prove useful in the future and they clearly deserve further investigation in this group of patients.

Lastly, there is a substantial group of patients with no objective abnormality despite several well-conducted investigations. After excluding organicity, a pragmatic individual approach including reassurance and a multi-cross-over trial [69] may be proposed in these difficult cases.

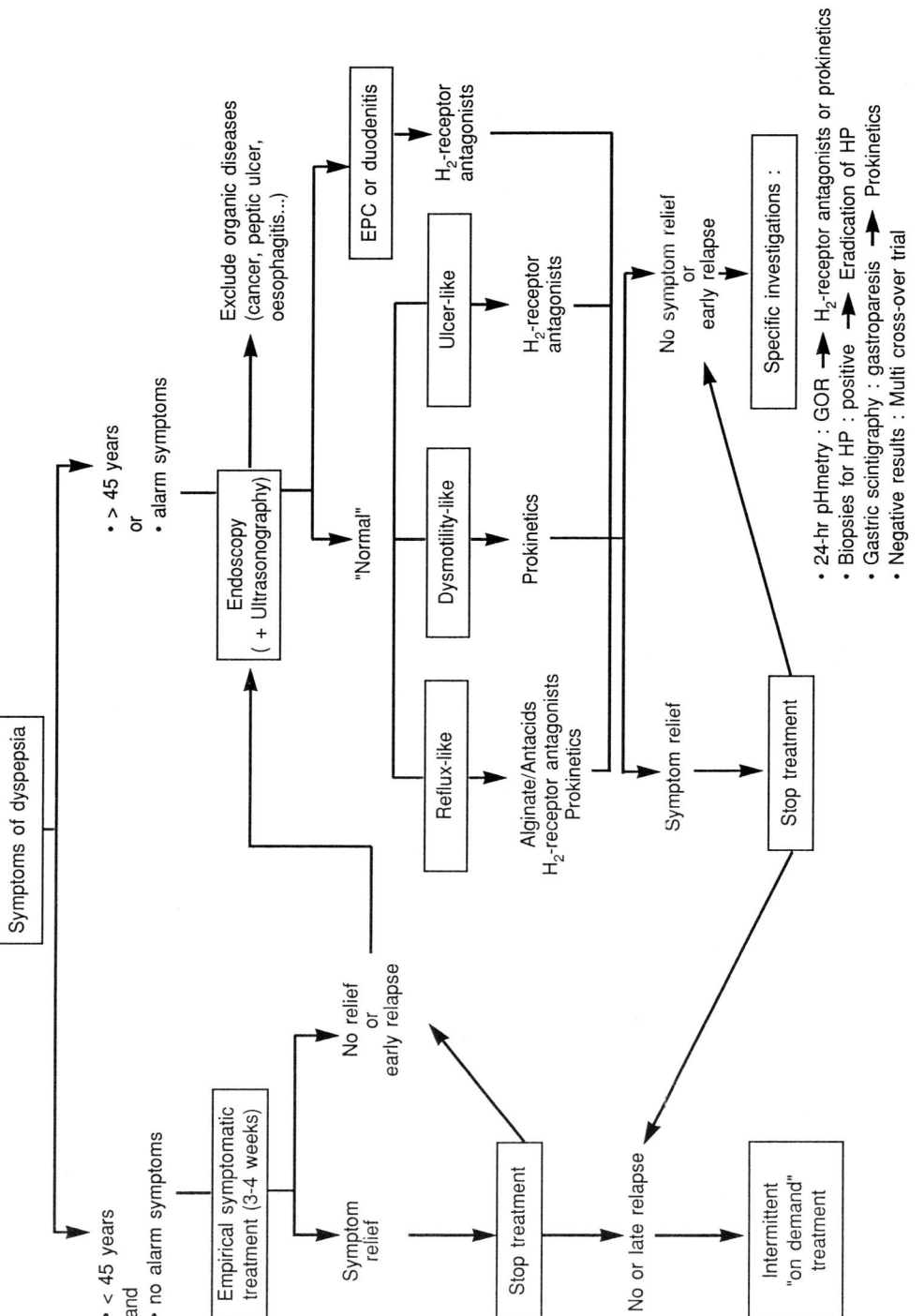

**Figure 3.** Flow chart for the management of the dyspeptic patients and guidelines for the choice of drugs according to the predominant symptoms and results of investigations. For the discussion of empirical (symptomatic) treatment, see the text.
EPC: erosive prepyloric changes at endoscopy [17]
HP: *Helicobacter pylori*

*Therapeutic strategy*

The prognosis of patients with NUD is not well-known. In one study [70] patients with unexplained (essential) NUD were followed up by telephone for a mean of 17 months per patient. Patients with more pain before diagnosis were significantly more likely to have pain over the follow-up. Similarly development of gastro-oesophageal reflux was also associated with more days of pain over the follow-up. In contrast demographic and environmental factors, the length of dyspepsia, and a past history of ulcer were of no significant prognostic value. Finally it seems quite difficult to predict accurately the prognosis of the patient with essential NUD and there is no definite evidence that symptoms may "burn out" with time [70].

In summary, practical guidelines for the management strategy in a dyspeptic patient are summarized in Figure 3. In fact, until we have more knowledge on the pathophysiological mechanisms involved in NUD and on its natural history, many patients will continue to raise difficult problems of management.

# References

1. Colin-Jones DG. Management of dyspepsia: report of a working party. Lancet 1988;12:576-9.
2. Jones R. Dyspeptic symptoms in the community. Gut 1989;30:893-8.
3. Nyrén O, Adami H, Bates S, Bergstrom R, Gustavsson S, Loof L, Nyberg A. Absence of therapeutic benefit from antacids or cimetidine in non-ulcer dyspepsia. N Engl J Med 1986;314:339-43.
4. Talley NJ, Phillips SF. Non-ulcer dyspepsia: potential causes and pathophysiology. Ann Intern Med 1988;108:865-79.
5. Petersen H, Loge I, Johannessen T, Fjosne U, Kleveland PM, Kristensen P, Sandbakken P, Hafstad PE, Halvorsen T. Dyspepsia: therapeutic response as a diagnostic tool. Scand J Gastroenterol 1987;128:108-13.
6. Jian R, Ducrot F, Piedeloup C, Mary JY, Najean Y, Bernier JJ. Measurement of gastric emptying in dyspeptic patients: effect of a new gastrokinetic agent (cisapride). Gut 1985;26:352-8.
7. Galmiche JP, Scarpignato C. Antacids in gastroesophageal reflux disease. In: Bianchi-Porro G, Richardson CT, eds. *Antacids in Peptic Ulcer Disease. State of the Art.* Verona, New York: Cortina International Raven Press, 1988;53-65
8. Graham DY, Smith JL. Why are some apparently healthy people heavy antacid users? Gastroenterology 1981;80:1161(abstr).
9. McHardy G. A multicentric, randomized clinical trial of Gaviscon in reflux oesophagitis. Southern Medical Journal 1978;71:16.
10. Bigard MA, Colin R, Galmiche JP, Rampal P, de Meynard C. Evolution des symptômes de reflux gastro-oesophagien (RGO) après 2 semaines de traitement par alginate-antiacide. Facteurs prédictifs et données endoscopiques chez les non-répondeurs. Gastroenterol Clin Biol 1990;14,A110(abstr).
11. Jonsson KA, Gotthard R, Bodemar G, Brodin U. The clinical relevance of endoscopic and histological inflammation of gastroduodenal mucosa in dyspepsia of unknown origin. Scand J Gastroenterol 1989;24:385-95.
12. Weberg R, Berstad A. Low-dose antacids and pirenzepine in the treatment of patients with non-ulcer dyspepsia and erosive prepyloric changes. A randomized, double-blind placebo-controlled trial. Scand J Gastroenterol 1988;23:237-43.
13. Gotthard R, Bodemar G, Brodin U, Jonsson KA. Treatment with cimetidine, antacid, or placebo in patients with dyspepsia of unknown origin. Scand J Gastroenterol 1988;23:7-18.

14. Mackinnon M, Willing RL, Whitehead R. Cimetidine in the management of symptomatic patients with duodenitis. A double-blind controlled trial. Dig Dis Sci 1982;27:217-9.
15. Kelbaek H, Linde J, Eriksen J, Munkgaard S, Moesgaard F, Bonnevie O. Controlled trial of treatment with cimetidine for non-ucler dyspepsia. Acta Medica Scand 1985;217:281-7.
16. Kleveland PM, Larsen S, Sandvik L, Kristensen P, Johannessen T, Hafstad PE, Sandbakken P, Loge I, Fjosne U, Petersen H. The effect of cimetidine in non-ulcer dyspepsia. Experience with a multi-cross-over model. Scand J Gastroenterol 1985;20:19-24
17. Nesland AA, Berstad A. Effect of cimetidine in patients with non-ulcer dyspepsia and erosive prepyloric changes. Scand J Gastroenterol 1985;20:629-35.
18. Delattre M, Malesky M, Prinzie A. Symptomatic treatment of non-ulcer dyspepsia with cimetidine. Curr Ther Res 1985;37:980-91
19. Lance P, Filipe MI, Wastell C. Non-ulcer dyspepsia, duodenitis and cimetidine. In: Wastell C, Lance P, eds. Cimetidine. *The Westminster Symposium, 6th.* Edinburgh: Churchill Livingstone, 1978;126-30.
20. Talley NJ, McNeil D, Hayden A, Piper DW. Randomized, double-blind, placebo-controlled cross-over trial of cimetidine and pirenzepine in non-ulcer dyspepsia. Gastroenterology 1986;91:149-56.
21. Saunders JHB, Oliver RJ, Higson DL. Dyspepsia: incidence of non-ulcer disease in a controlled trial of ranitidine in general practice. Br Med J 1986;292:665-8.
22. Johannessen T, Fjosne U, Kleveland PM, Halvorsen T, Kristensen P, Loge I, Hafstad PE, Sandbakken P, Petersen H. Cimetidine responders in non-ulcer dyspepsia. Scand J Gastroenterol 1988;23:327-36.
23. Singal AK, Kumar A, Broor SL. Cimetidine in the treatment of non-ulcer dyspepsia: results of a randomized double-blind, placebo-controlled study. Curr Med Res Opin 1989;11:390-7.
24. Dobrilla G, Comberlato M, Steeie A, Vallaperta P. Drug treatment of functional dyspepsia. A meta-analysis of randomized controlled clinical trials. J Clin Gastroenterol 1989;11:169-77.
25. Smith PM, Troughton AH, Gleeson F, Walters J, McCarthy CF. Pirenzepine in non-ulcer dyspepsia: a double-blind multicentre trial. J Int Med Res 1990;18:16-20.
26. Johnson AG. Controlled trial of metoclopramide in the treatment of flatulent dyspepsia. Br Med J 1971;2:25-6.
27. De Loose F. Domperidone in chronic dyspepsia: a pilot study and a multicentre general practice cross-over comparison with metoclopramide and placebo. Pharmatherapeutica 1979;2:140-6.
28. Brogden RN, Carmine AA, Heel RC, Spelght TH, Avery GS. Domperidone. A review of its pharmacological activity, pharmacokinetics, and therapeutic efficacy in the symptomatic treatment of chronic dyspepsia and as an antiemetic. Drugs 1982;24:360-400.
29. Fraitag B, Cloarec D, Galmiche JP. Le cisapride: pharmacologie, résultats thérapeutiques actuels et perspectives d'avenir. Gastroenterol Clin Biol 1989;13:265-76.
30. Mc Callum RW, Prakash C, Campoli-Richards DM, Goa KL. Cisapride. A preliminary review of its pharmacodynamic and pharmacokinetic properties, and therapeutic use as a prokinetic agent in gastrointestinal motility disorders. Drugs 1988;36:652-81.
31. Rosch W. Efficacy of cisapride in the treatment of epigastric pain and concomitant symptoms in non-ulcer dyspepsia. Scand J Gastroenterol 1989;24(suppl 165):54-8.
32. Jian R, Ducrot F, Ruskoné A, Chaussade S, Rambaud JC, Modigliani R, Rain D, Bernier JJ. Symptomatic, radionuclide and therapeutic assessment of chronic idiopathic dyspepsia. A double-blind placebo-controlled evaluation of cisapride. Dig Dis Sci 1989;34:657-64.
33. King FD, Sanger GJ. 5-$HT_3$ receptor antagonists. Drugs future 1989; 14(3):876-89.
34. Janssens J, Peeters TL, Vantrappen G, Tack J, Urbain JL, De Roo M, Muls E, Bouillon R. Improvement of gastric emptying in diabetic gastroparesis by erythromycin. N Engl J Med 1990;322:1028-31.
35. Bruley des Varannes S, Cloarec D, Dubois A, Galmiche JP. Cholécystokinine et ses antagonistes: effets sur la motricité digestive. Gastroentérol Clin Biol (in press).

36. Li Bassi, Rovati LC, Giacovelli G, Bolondi L, Barbara L. Effect of loxiglumide, a cholecystokinin antagonist, in non-ulcer dyspepsia. Gastroenterology 1990;98:A77(abstr).
37. Hollander D, Tarnawski A. The protective and therapeutic mechanisms of sucralfate. Scand J Gastroenterol 1990;25(suppl 173):1-5.
38. Kairaluoma MI, Hentilae R, Alavaikko M, Kellosalo J, Stahlberg M, Jalovaara P, Olsen M, Jaervensivu P, Laitinen S. Sucralfate *versus* placebo in treatment of non-ulcer dyspepsia. Am J Med 1987;83:51-5.
39. Guslandi M. Comparison of sucralfate and ranitidine in the treatment of chronic non-erosive gastritis. A randomized, multicentre trial. Am J Med 1989;86:45-8.
40. Larkai EN, Smith JL, Lidsky MD, Graham DY. Gastroduodenal mucosa and dyspeptic symptoms in arthritic patients during chronic non-steroidal anti-inflammatory drug use. Am J Gastroenterol 1987;82:1153-8.
41. Rokkas T, Pursey C, Uzoechina E, Dorrington L, Simmons NA, Filipe MI, Sladen GE. *Campylobacter pylori* and non-ulcer dyspepsia. Am J Gastroenterol 1987;82:1149-52.
42. Gad A, Hradsky M, Furugard K, Malmodin B, Nyberg O. *Campylobacter pylori* and non-ulcer dyspepsia. A prospective study in a Swedish population. Scand J Gastroenterol 1989;24(suppl 167):44-8.
43. Barnett JL, Behler EM, Appelman HD, Elta GH. *Campylobacter pylori* is not associated with gastroparesis. Dig Dis Sci 1989;34:1677-80.
44. Wegener M, Borsch G, Schaffstein J, Schulz-Flake C, Mai U, Leverkus F. Are dyspeptic symptoms in patients with *Campylobacter pylori*-associated type B gastritis linked to delayed gastric emptying. Am J Gastroenterol 1988;83:737-40.
45. Rauws EAJ, Langenberg W, Houthoff HJ, Zanen BC, Tytgat GNJ. *Campylobacter pyloridis*-associated chronic active antral gastritis. A prospective study of its prevalence and the effects of antibacterial and anti-ulcer treatment. Gastroenterology 1988;94:33-40.
46. Mac Nulty CAM, Gearty JC, Crump B, Davis M, Donovan IA, Melikian V, Lister DM, Wise R. *Campylobacter pyloridis* and associated gastritis: investigator blind, placebo-controlled trial of bismuth salicylate and erythromycin ethylsuccinate. Br Med J 1986;293:645-9.
47. Rokkas T, Pursey C, Uzoechina E, Dorrington L, Simmons NA, Filipe MI, Sladen GE. Non-ulcer dyspepsia and short term De-Nol therapy: a placebo-controlled trial with particular reference to the role of *Campylobacter pylori*. Gut 1988;29:1386-91.
48. Lambert JR, Dunn K, Borromeo M, Korman MG, Hansky J. *Campylobacter pylori*. A role in non-ulcer dyspepsia? Scand J Gastroenterol 1989;24(suppl 160):7-13.
49. Loffeld RJLF, Potters HVJP, Stobberingh E, Flendrig JA, Van Spreeuwel JP, Arends JW. *Campylobacter*-associated gastritis in patients with non-ulcer dyspepsia: a double-blind placebo-controlled trial with colloidal bismuth subcitrate. Gut 1989;30:1206-12.
50. Kang JY, Tay HH, Wee A, Guan R, Math MV, Yap I. Effect of colloidal bismuth subcitrate on symptoms and gastric histology in non-ulcer dyspepsia. A double-blind placebo-controlled study. Gut 1990;31:476-80.
51. Barberis C, Lamouliatte H, De Mascarel A, Megraud F, Bernard P, Quinton A. Controlled study of amoxicillin in *Campylobacter pylori*-associated gastritis. In: Megraud F, Lamouliatte H, eds. *Gastroduodenal Pathology and Campylobacter pylori*. Elsevier, Excerpta Medica, Amsterdam: 1989;581-5.
52. Lamouliatte H, Cayla R, Bernard PH, Quinton A, Boulard A. Méta-analyse des essais randomisés dans les dyspepsies non ulcéreuses associées à *Helicobacter pylori*. Gastroenterol Clin Biol 1991;15:A119(abstr).
53. Barbara L, Biasco G, Capurso L, Dobrilla G, Lalli A, Paganelli GM, Pallone F, Torsoli A. Effects of sucralfate and sulglycotide treatment on active gastritis and *Helicobacter pylori* colonization of the gastric mucosa in non-ulcer dyspepsia patients. Am J Gastroenterol 1990;85:1109-13.
54. Kleveland PM, Johannessen T, Kristensen P, Loge I, Sandbakken P, Dybdahl J, Petersen H. Effect of pancreatic enzymes in non-ulcer dyspepsia. A pilot study. Scand J Gastroenterol 1990;25:298-301.

55. Bruley des Varannes S, Galmiche JP, Bernades P, Bader JP. Douleurs épigastriques et régurgitations: épidémiologie descriptive dans un échantillon représentatif de la population française. Gastroenterol Clin Biol 1988;12:721-8.
56. Jones R, Lydeard S. Prevalence of symptoms of dyspepsia in the community. Br Med J 1989;298:30-2.
57. Jones R. Epidemiology of dyspeptic symptoms in primary care. In: Practical guidelines for the management of dyspepsia. Proceedings of a Smith Kline and French Symposium held in Geneva, 16-17 March 1990;9-13.
58. Heatley RV, Rathborne BJ. Dyspepsia: a dilemma for doctors? Lancet 1987;2:779-82.
59. Talley NJ, Fung LH, Gilligan IJ, McNeil D, Piper DW. Association of anxiety, neuroticism, and depression with dyspepsia of unknown cause. A case-control study. Gastroenterology 1986;90:886-92.
60. Talley NJ, Jones M, Piper DW. Psychosocial and childhood factors in essential dyspepsia. A case control study. Scand J Gastroenterol 1988;23:341-6.
61. Talley NJ, Piper DW. A prospective study of social factors and major life event stress in patients with dyspepsia of unknown cause. Scand J Gastroenterol 1987;22:268-72.
62. Talley NJ, Ellard K, Jones M, Tennant C, Piper DW. Suppression of emotions in essential dyspepsia and chronic duodenal ulcer. A case-control study. Scand J Gastroenterol 1988;23:337-40.
63. Barbara L, Camilleri M, Corinaldesi R, Crean GP, Heading RC, Johnson AG, Malagelada JR, Stanghellini V, Wienbeck M. Definition and investigation of dyspepsia. Consensus of an international *ad hoc* working party. Dig Dis Sci 1989;34:1272-6
64. Kagevi I, Lofstedt S, Persson LG. Endoscopic findings and diagnoses in unselected dyspeptic patients at a primary health care centre. Scand J Gastroenterol 1989;24:145-50.
65. Krag E. Implications of $H_2$-receptor antagonist use in dyspepsia: a case study. Proceedings of a Smith Kline and French Symposium held in Geneva 16-17 March 1990;34-9.
66. Williams B, Luckas M, Ellingham JHM, Dain A, Wicks ACB. Do young patients with dyspepsia need investigation? Lancet 1988;2:1349-51.
67. Jonsson B. Management of dyspepsia: the value of cost-benefit analysis. Proceedings of a Smith Kline and French Symposium held in Geneva 16-17 March 1990;40-5.
68. Barré P, Bruley des Varannes S, Masliah C, Cloarec D, Le Bodic L, Galmiche JP. Le marqueur d'événements: un progrès dans l'interprétation de la pH-métrie œsophagienne. Gastroenterol Clin Biol 1989;13:3-7.
69. Johannessen T, Fosstvedt D, Petersen H. Experience with a multi cross-over model in dyspepsia. Scand J Gastroenterol 1988;(suppl 147):33-7.
70. Talley NJ, McNeil, Hayden A, Colreavy C, Piper DW. Prognosis of chronic unexplained dyspepsia. A prospective study of potential predictor variables in patients with endoscopically diagnosed non-ulcer dyspepsia. Gastroenterology 1987;92:1060-6.

# 24

# Prospects and priorities for research in non-ulcer dyspepsia

R.C. HEADING

*Department of Medicine, Royal Infirmary, Edinburgh, Scotland, UK*

Non-ulcer dyspepsia is now attracting much research interest as new observations reported in the recent literature, and reviewed in the preceding chapters of this volume, suggest explanations of its basis. New directions for possible further research can immediately be seen. It is inevitable, however, that when important new observations on many unrelated aspects of a subject are reported in rapid succession, there is difficulty in understanding their relative contribution and formulating a coherent strategy for further research. For example, should *Helicobacter* infection now be a major focus of research in non-ulcer dyspepsia? Is dysmotility a cause or a consequence of dyspeptic symptoms? Is non-ulcer dyspepsia fundamentally a disorder of sensation, rather than a consequence of a variety of unrelated gastrointestinal tract disorders? All three of these concepts, and others besides, have been supported by recent experimental evidence, so that many gastroenterologists are even more confused than they were previously about the pathogenic mechanisms which may underlie non-ulcer dyspepsia and the principles which should govern rational management of these patients in clinical practice.

How can we identify the directions of future research which have the best prospect of integrating the disparate strands of present thinking and make real scientific and practical progress? One simple principle which has proved a sound foundation for determining research strategy is that as much care should be given to identifying the right questions as will be given to seeking the answers. It is therefore appropriate in this paper to consider three fundamental questions which must be asked before any specific research can be undertaken. These are: (1) What is non-ulcer dyspepsia? (2) Which patients should be studied? (3) What are the principal research objectives?

## What is non-ulcer dyspepsia?

Lack of agreement on definition of the word dyspepsia, and derived terms such as non-ulcer dyspepsia, has been emphasized in many published papers, with the implication that better agreement on definitions is important to future research progress [1-7]. It is self-evident that substantial variation in the definition of dyspepsia limits the comparability of published studies and most investigators would regard standardization of the terminology as helpful. It is also apparent that critical review of the terminology in current use focuses attention not only on the words used by physicians, but also on the concepts associated with them.

In essence, dyspepsia (from the Greek δυσ = bad, and πεπτειν = to digest) is widely understood by physicians to denote a variable combination of recurrent or persistent symptoms which appear to be referable to the upper gastrointestinal tract. Provided some sort of upper abdominal pain or discomfort is included, almost any combination of the symptoms listed in Table I may be described as dyspepsia and thus the word itself does not carry any implication of precision as a description of symptoms.

Non-ulcer dyspepsia is an ungainly term now usually considered to denote dyspepsia for which clinical assessment, upper gastrointestinal endoscopy and, where appropriate, other investigations have failed to reveal a cause [4, 6, 7]. The terms non-organic dyspepsia and functional dyspepsia are synonymous. There is some strength to the argument that "functional dyspepsia" should be preferred, so that unexplained dyspepsia can be perceived in the context of the whole spectrum of functional gastrointestinal disorders, within which oesophageal, biliary, bowel and anorectal functional disorders are also recognized [8].

Attention is now being directed to detailed analysis of symptom patterns, with the suggestion that many dyspeptic patients may be categorized as having ulcer-like dyspepsia, reflux-like dyspepsia or dysmotility-like dyspepsia [6]. The identification of different types of dyspepsia would seem to be of value, especially if different symptom patterns were found to be associated with different underlying disorders. However, it is important to recognize that neither the practical value nor the biological significance of this type of categorization has yet been established. The extent to which different investigators would agree in allocating patients to the ulcer-like dyspepsia, reflux-like dyspepsia or dysmotility-like dyspepsia categories has not been determined and of course there is no certainty that greater precision in the analysis of symptoms

**Table I.** Dyspeptic symptoms.

Abdominal pain or discomfort
Postprandial fullness
Abdominal bloating
Belching
Early satiety
Anorexia
Nausea
Vomiting
Heartburn
Regurgitation

will lead to the identification of specific disorders responsible for non-ulcer dyspepsia. Indeed, recent experience of peptic ulcer disease and of gastro-oesophageal reflux disease suggests the contrary, in that symptom patterns are so frequently non-specific that diagnosis from the clinical history is often not possible [9, 10]. There is no well-founded reason for believing that relationships between symptoms and their cause is any closer in non-ulcer dyspepsia.

Despite these reservations, greater precision and consistency in the identification of individual dyspeptic symptoms are clearly desirable, and may permit the identification of genuine symptom patterns which have diagnostic value.

## Which patients should be studied?

Many investigations, especially those involving physiological studies of gastrointestinal function, will wish to focus on patients referred to gastroenterology centres. Useful information may be gained from such studies, particularly if specific symptom patterns can be correlated with particular abnormalities of gastrointestinal function. However, it is essential to recognize that a very large number of individuals who suffer from dyspepsia do not seek any medical attention at all. Questionnaire studies as well as information on over-the-counter antacid purchase indicate that many patients treat upper gastrointestinal symptoms on their own initiative and are apparently content with the outcome [11, 12]. Consequently, patients seen by primary care physicians are unlikely to be representative of all those affected, and patients seen by gastroenterologists are even more highly selected. There is an obvious risk that misleading conclusions will be drawn if hospital-based studies are not matched by comparable studies in the community.

## What are the principal research objectives?

Identification of strategic objectives is fundamental to any research programme so that individual research projects may be appraised in the context of their likely contribution to the overall goals. For non-ulcer dyspepsia, it is possible to suggest a broad distinction between scientific objectives and therapeutic objectives. Presumably the former are (1) identification of causes and mechanisms of non-ulcer dyspepsia and (2) identification of means of modifying those causes and mechanisms. The principal therapeutic objectives may be identified as (1) the alleviation of symptoms and (2) the prevention of recurrence.

Many of the specific topics of current research interest have been fully reviewed in preceding chapters and it is not appropriate to duplicate such review here. Nevertheless, it is useful to consider some aspects of current research in the context of these objectives.

### Gastro-oesophageal reflux

It is well recognized that gastro-oesophageal reflux may be responsible for troublesome heartburn and acid regurgitation in patients who show no evidence of oesophagitis at endoscopy [13]. It is also well established that many patients with reflux disease demonstrable by prolonged oesophageal pH monitoring present to gastroenterologists with symptoms which are not sufficiently specific to point to the correct diagnosis [10, 14]. It is therefore surprising that there has hitherto been little direct appraisal of the frequency with which gastro-oesophageal reflux is demonstrable by pH-metry in patients categorized as having non-ulcer dyspepsia. In one recent study, however, gastro-oesophageal reflux was demonstrable in 17% of such patients [15], and in another study was identified in 21% [Klauser AG, Müller-Lissner SA, personal communication]. If these figures can be confirmed, it would seem that unrecognized gastro-oesophageal reflux is responsible for about one in five instances of non-ulcer dyspepsia, and that appropriate use of existing diagnostic methodology, particularly oesophageal pH monitoring, may be sufficient to identify the source of symptoms.

**Delayed gastric emptying**

Impaired antral motility and delayed gastric emptying have been identified in up to 50% of patients with non-ulcer dyspepsia and considerable interest has focused on gastric stasis as a possible "cause" of the symptoms [16, 18]. It is becoming clear, however, that this concept does not stand up to scrutiny. Direct observations have found poor correlations between symptoms and objectively demonstrable gastric emptying delay, and no consistent improvement in symptoms has been identified when gastric emptying delay is corrected [19-20]. In addition, it is difficult to understand why gastric emptying delay of the magnitude observed in non-ulcer dyspepsia should itself be a cause of symptoms. Although it may be abnormal for, say, 70% of a given test meal to be present in the stomach one hour after ingestion, this percentage may normally be present at 30 minutes after meal ingestion. There is no reason why the former should be considered a direct cause of symptoms when the latter clearly is not.

Delayed gastric emptying may nevertheless be a marker of abnormal motor function which produces symptoms. The relationships between symptoms and upper gastrointestinal motor function certainly require further study, but of a much more sophisticated nature than straightforward gastric emptying measurements. In particular, the relationships between motor function and sensory mechanisms in the stomach and duodenum would seem to merit attention.

Further reason to study the basis of sensation is suggested by the results of recent clinical trials of cisapride in non-ulcer dyspepsia. Therapy with this drug appears not only to improve the global symptom status of patients with non-ulcer dyspepsia when compared with placebo therapy, but there seems to be improvement in most of the individual symptoms (heartburn, epigastric pain, bloating, etc.) which have been recorded [18, 21, 22]. If these observations are correct, it is necessary to ask how a drug which is a stimulant of gastrointestinal contractile activity can produce parallel improvement in such diverse symptoms. The possibility must be entertained that gastrointestinal motor activity somehow modulates visceral sensation, and alters what is consciously perceived. While this is no more than speculation, the observations made with cisapride at least reinforce the case for more direct study of visceral sensory mechanisms.

## Non-ulcer dyspepsia and the irritable bowel syndrome

There is preliminary evidence suggesting that as in the irritable bowel syndrome and the irritable oesophagus, patients with non-ulcer dyspepsia have a lowered threshold for visceral sensation in comparison with healthy subjects [23]. There are obviously many other parallels, as well as areas of overlap between non-ulcer dyspepsia and the irritable bowel syndrome — probably one quarter of patients with dyspepsia also have symptoms which fulfil the criteria of the irritable bowel syndrome [24]. If this is more than chance association, it would seem worthwhile to investigate the mechanisms that produce dyspeptic symptoms in some IBS patients but not in others.

## Psychological and social factors

Many physicians believe that psychological and social factors make a major contribution to non-ulcer dyspepsia and that in clinical practice it is important to recognize their existence so as to avoid unnecessary investigation and concern directed at the patient's gastrointestinal tract. While there is no doubt that many aspects of gastrointestinal function are influenced by psychological state, formal study has suggested that psychopathology is not a major cause of non-ulcer dyspepsia. For example, it appears that although anxiety, depression and neuroticism are more common in non-ulcer dyspepsia patients than in the general population, they are not significantly more frequent than may be found in patients with organic gastrointestinal disease (Fig. 1) [24, 25]. Similarly, formal study has not established adverse life events

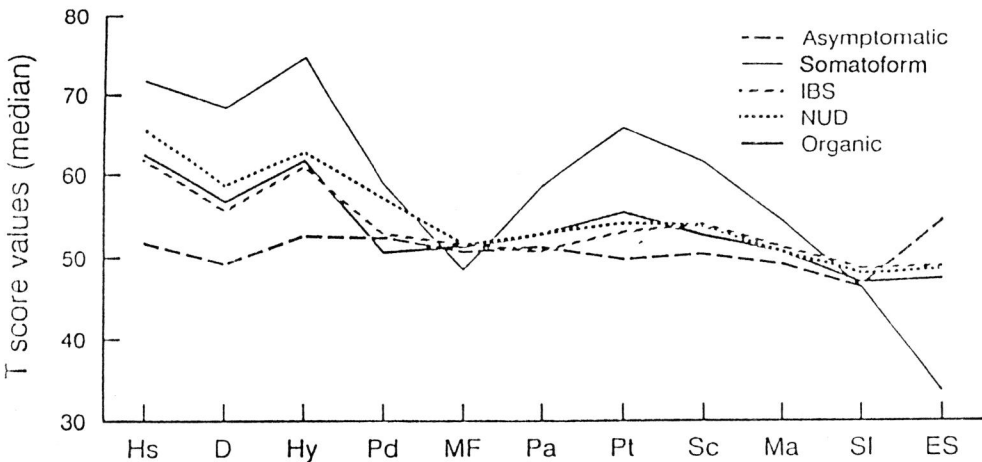

**Figure 1.** Median scores of the MMPI clinical scales (and one research scale) by diagnostic group. Hypochondriasis (Hs), depression (D), hysteria (Hy), psychopathic deviate (Pd), masculinity-femininity (MF), paranoia (Pa), psychasthenia (Pt), schizophrenia (Sc), hypomania (Ma), social introversion (SI), and ego strength (ES). The figure shows that patients with the IBS, NUD, and organic gastrointestinal disease (organic) have similar MMPI scores. Patients with somatoform disorder (somatoform) and healthy controls differ from the other groups on a number of the scales. (From Talley et al. [25]).

as a major association of non-ulcer dyspepsia, nor do social factors appear to be critical in determining the non-ulcer dyspepsia patient's lifestyle or decision to seek medical advice about symptoms [26-28].

The extent to which personality or life events may determine a patient's decision to seek health care is an important issue for future research in non-ulcer dyspepsia. If it is health-care-seeking, rather than the condition itself, which is associated with particular personality characteristics, physicians are at risk of gaining a false impression that personality traits contribute directly to the disorder. Of course, neuroticism and social isolation are likely to influence any patient's ability to accept and cope with chronic symptoms, and non-ulcer dyspepsia patients are no exception. To date, no additional relevance of psychological and social factors has been established in respect of non-ulcer dyspepsia but the issue is of considerable importance and deserves continuing attention.

## Clinical trials of therapy

The therapeutic research objectives proposed above draw attention to some particular issues relevant to clinical trials of therapy. If the alleviation of symptoms is a major goal of therapy, it is necessary to accept the subjective nature of symptoms and to recognize the variability of their significance for individual patients. In comparison with some other medical disciplines, gastroenterologists have been slow to introduce quality of life assessments to evaluation of the effects of therapy, and when this weakness is recognized in addition to the crudeness of symptom severity evaluation in recent clinical trials, it seems clear that the whole basis of evaluating chronic gastrointestinal symptoms is in need of modernization. Of course, it must be recognized that the quality of life appraisal protocols which are relevant to the assessment of physical disability may be less satisfactory in assessing gastroenterological conditions such as non-ulcer dyspepsia. Nevertheless, the same principles should easily enable our symptom analyses to be refined so that clinically relevant indices of therapeutic outcome are obtained. In particular, this requires systematic evaluation of the distress caused by the symptoms, the extent to which they interfere with the patient's normal lifestyle and, of course, whether the therapy produces improvement in well-being to a level the patient finds acceptable.

The development of appropriate systems of symptom evaluation, including quality of life assessment, must be one of the major priorities in the sphere of therapeutic research in gastroenterology. In the context of upper gastrointestinal disorders, the Graci score developed for the assessment of gastro-oesophageal reflux symptoms is a useful innovation along these lines [29].

Finally, the natural history of non-ulcer dyspepsia is still poorly characterized, and this presents a considerable problem for the interpretation of many clinical trials. It is obviously desirable to establish whether the high placebo response rates observed in such trials are merely an indication of a high frequency of spontaneous remission, or whether a genuine treatment effect is obtained from the close medical attention and reassurance which participants in clinical trials inevitably receive.

**Table II.** Proposed priorities for research in non-ulcer dyspepsia.

1. Refine symptom definitions and ensure investigators can use them consistently.
2. Study community and primary care based dyspepsia in parallel with hospital patients.
3. Confirm gastro-oesophageal reflux disease as a common cause of NUD.
4. Develop modern systems of symptom evaluation, including quality of life appraisal, for all clinical trials.
5. Initiate further basic science and clinical investigation into mechanisms and modulation of visceral sensation.

## Conclusions

Because the cause of symptoms in patients with non-ulcer dyspepsia is by definition unexplained, the initial reaction of many scientifically-inclined physicians will be to advocate research which seeks new mechanisms and abnormalities which might be responsible for the problem. However, consideration of the research objectives suggests that such an approach is inappropiate. Although further study of the importance of specific abnormalities such as gastroduodenal dysmotility, *Helicobacter* infection, and psychological and social factors is unquestionably desirable, substantial progress will not be possible without improved specification of the nature of dyspeptic symptoms and an understanding of the frequency and natural history of non-ulcer dyspepsia in the community. It is not certain, however, that better analysis of symptom patterns will necessarily permit accurate clinical diagnosis in individual patients, nor that it will lead directly to identification of pathogenic mechanisms responsible for those symptoms.

Table II lists topics which appear to have a good claim for the immediate attention of research teams interested in non-ulcer dyspepsia and it is suggested that both clinical investigators and basic scientists should give special attention to the mechanisms which are responsible for visceral sensation. It is clearly a subject which presents a number of difficulties for investigators but dyspepsia is defined by the presence of symptoms, and these are frequently similar in patients with and without demonstrable upper gastrointestinal disease. Whether disorders of visceral sensation are or are not important as an underlying cause of non-ulcer dyspepsia remains to be established, but there is now enough evidence to indicate that gastrointestinal sensation is a subject which justifies substantial research effort.

## References

1. Rhind JA, Watson L. Gallstone dyspepsia. Br Med J 1968;1:32.
2. Crean GP, Card WI, Beattie AD, Holden RJ, James WB, Knill-Jones RP, Lucas RW, Spiegelhalter D. "Ulcer like dyspepsia". Scand J Gastroenterol 1982;17(suppl 79):9-15.
3. Thompson WG. Non-ulcer dyspepsia. Can Med Assoc J 1984;130:565-9.
4. Talley NJ, Piper DW. The association between non-ulcer dyspepsia and other gastrointestinal disorders. Scand J Gastroenterol 1985;20:896-900.
5. Nyrén O, Adami HO, Gustavsson S, Lindgren PG, Loof L, Nyberg A. The "epigastric distress syndrome". A possible disease entity identified by history and endoscopy in patients with non-ulcer dyspepsia. J Clin Gastroenterol 1987;9:303-9.

6. Colin-Jones DG, Bloom B, Bodemar G, Crean G, Freston J, Gugler R, Malagelada J, Nyrén O, Petersen H, Piper D. Management of dyspepsia: report of a working party. Lancet 1988;1:576-9.
7. Barbara L, Camilleri M, Corinaldesi R, Crean GP, Heading RC, Johnson AG, Malagelada JR, Stanghellini V, Wienbeck M. Definition and investigation of dyspepsia. Consensus of an international *ad hoc* working party. Dig Dis Sci 1989;34:1272-6.
8. Drossman DA, Thomson WG, Talley NJ, Funch-Jensen P, Janssens J, Whitehead WE. Identification of subgroups of functional gastrointestinal disorders. Gastroenterol Int 1990;3:159-72.
9. Talley NJ, McNeil D, Piper DW. Discriminant value of dyspeptic symptoms: a study of the clinical presentation of 221 patients with dyspepsia of unknown cause, peptic ulceration and cholelithiasis. Gut 1987;28:40-6.
10. Klauser AG, Schindlbeck NE, Müller-Lissner SA. Symptoms in gastro-oesophageal reflux disease. Lancet 1990;335:205-8.
11. Jones R, Lydeard S. Prevalence of symptoms of dyspepsia in the community. Br Med J 1989;298:30-2.
12. Graham DY, Smith JL, Patterson DJ. Why do apparently healthy people use antacid tablets? Am J Gastroenterol 1983;78:257-60.
13. Schindlbeck NE, Heinrich C, Konig A, Dendorfer A, Pace F, Müller-Lissner SA. Optimal thresholds, sensitivity, and specificity of long-term pH-metry for the detection of gastro-esophageal reflux disease. Gastroenterology 1987;93:85-90.
14. Wienbeck M, Berges W. Esophageal disorders in the etiology and pathophysiology of dyspepsia. Scand J Gastroenterol 1985;20(suppl 109):133-43.
15. Waldron B, Cullen PT, Kumar R, Smith D, Jankowski J, Hopwood D, Sutton D, Kennedy N, Campbell FC. Evidence for hypomotility in non-ulcer dyspepsia: a prospective multifactorial study. Gut 1991;32:246-51.
16. Camilleri M, Malagelada JR, Kao PC, Zinsmeister AR. Gastric and autonomic responses to stress in functional dyspepsia. Dig Dis Sci 1986;31:1169-77.
17. Kerlin P. Postprandial antral hypomotility in patients with idiopathic nausea and vomiting. Gut 1989;30:54-9.
18. Jian R, Ducrot F, Piedeloup C, Mary JY, Najean Y, Bernier JJ. Measurement of gastric emptying in dyspeptic patients: effect of a new gastrokinetic agent (cisapride). Gut 1985;26:352-8.
19. Jian R, Ducrot F, Ruskoné A, Chaussade S, Rambaud JC, Modigliani R, Rain JD, Bernier JJ. Symptomatic, radionuclide and therapeutic assessment of chronic idiopathic dyspepsia. A double-blind placebo-controlled evaluation of cisapride. Dig Dis Sci 1989;34:657-64.
20. Corinaldesi R, Stanghellini V, Raiti C, Rea E, Salgeminini R, Barbara L. Effect of chronic administration of cisapride on gastric emptying of a solid meal and on dyspeptic symptoms in patients with idiopathic gastroparesis. Gut 1987;28:300-5.
21. Deruyttere M, Milo R, Creytens G, Goethals C, Bourgeois E, Offner E. Therapy of chronic functional dyspepsia: multicentre cross-over trial of cisapride and placebo. Progr Med 1987;43(suppl 1):61-8.
22. Rosch W. Cisapride in non-ulcer dyspepsia. Results of a placebo-controlled trial. Scand J Gastroenterol 1987;22:161-4.
23. Mearin F, Cucala M, Azpiroz F, Malagelada JR. Origin of gastric symptoms in functional dyspepsia. Gastroenterology 1989;96:A337(abstr).
24. Talley NJ, Fung LH, Gilligan IJ, McNeil D, Piper DW. Association of anxiety, neuroticism, and depression with dyspepsia of unknown cause. A case-control study. Gastroenterology 1986;90:886-92.
25. Talley NJ, Phillips SF, Bruce B, Twomey CK, Zinsmeister AR, Melton LJ. Relation among personality and symptoms in non-ulcer dyspepsia and the irritable bowel syndrome. Gastroenterology 1990;99:327-33.

26. Stockton M, Weinmann J, McColl I. An investigation of psychosocial factors in patients with upper abdominal pain: a comparison with other groups of surgical outpatients. J Psychosom Res 1985;29:191-8.
27. Talley NJ, Jones M, Piper DW. Psychosocial and childhood factor in essential dyspepsia. A case-control study. Scand J Gastroenterol 1988;23:341-6.
28. Talley NJ, Piper DW. Major life event stress and dyspepsia of unknown cause: a case-control study. Gut 1986;27:127-34.
29. Spechler SJ, Williford WO, Krol WF. Development and validation of a gastroesophageal reflux disease activity index graci. Gastroenterology 1990;98:A130(abstr).

LOUIS-JEAN
avenue d'Embrun, 05003 GAP cedex
Tél. : 92.53.17.00
Dépôt légal : 667 — Septembre 1991
Imprimé en France